Tuberculosis Control in Migrating Population

Wei-ye Yu • Pu-Xuan Lu • Wei-guo Tan
Editors

Tuberculosis Control in Migrating Population

PMPH PEOPLE'S MEDICAL PUBLISHING HOUSE

Springer

Editors
Wei-ye Yu
Department of Tuberculosis
The Shenzhen Center for Chronic Disease Control
Shenzhen
Guangdong
China

Pu-Xuan Lu
Department of Radiology
The Shenzhen Center for Chronic Disease Control
Shenzhen
Guangdong
China

Wei-guo Tan
Department of Tuberculosis
The Shenzhen Center for Chronic Disease Control
Shenzhen
Guangdong
China

ISBN 978-981-32-9762-3 ISBN 978-981-32-9763-0 (eBook)
https://doi.org/10.1007/978-981-32-9763-0

This Springer imprint is published by the registered company Springer Nature Singapore Pte Ltd.
The registered company address is: 152 Beach Road, #21-01/04 Gateway East, Singapore 189721, Singapore

Preface

With the rapid development of economy, international communication, tourism, migration, and labor, as well as world population mobility increase significantly. Such migration and mobility pose a serious challenge to the prevention and control of tuberculosis. Shenzhen, a new and open city in southern China near Hong Kong, has more than 10 million immigrants from all over China. Only a few cities in China and even in the world have such large population of immigrants. Large-scale population mobility makes tuberculosis epidemic control much more difficult. It can seriously endanger human health. We have carried out a systematic research on this important issue in human health for many years, constructed and implemented tuberculosis control strategy, initiated tuberculosis management and control model, and set up a tuberculosis control strategy for migrating population. Such strategy of monitoring system for tuberculosis control of migrating population in China has greatly reduced the epidemics of tuberculosis in the migrating population in Shenzhen; therefore, the incidence of tuberculosis has been effectively controlled. Such successful results have been well recognized by the WHO and the China Tuberculosis Control Organization.

In order to achieve the important WHO goal of "Eradicating Tuberculosis" by 2035, we need to make a marked progress in the discovery, registration, referrals, reception, and management of tuberculosis patients in migrating population. Additionally, it is of great importance to promote the strategy and measures for the advanced management and control of tuberculosis in the migrating population. Hence, we have organized data from more than 40 senior scholars who are actively in tuberculosis prevention and control and clinical research, including experts in prevention and control, infectious diseases, pulmonary, imaging, pathology, and experimental research. We also compiled the latest research results in tuberculosis prevention and control from China and abroad and composed a book entitled "*Tuberculosis Control in migrating population.*" The book is divided into ten chapters covering the epidemic of tuberculosis in migrating population, the strategies and technologies for control of tuberculosis, the diagnosis and treatment of tuberculosis, the management of tuberculosis in migrating population, and the prevention and control of tuberculosis in schools. We also present a new technology of emergency treatment during public health emergency, prevention and control of drug-resistant tuberculosis, double infection of TB/HIV, and so on. During the course of writing this book, we tried to keep track of the latest developments in the TB control in migrating population, prevention and treatment of drug-resistant tuberculosis, and HIV-associated tuberculosis.

This book is the first one in China and abroad focusing on prevention and control of tuberculosis among migrating population. This book provides comprehensive introduction and elaboration of prevention and control strategies, as well as integrates various research results. We compiled this book in such a way that it contains abundant content, several outstanding points, the lush pictures, strong practicability, and unique characteristic. It is a valuable book for medical workers and medical students in tuberculosis prevention and control, respiratory and infectious disease control, imaging department, laboratory, pathology department, and other medical workers. At the same time, it is intended to provide a useful reference for the relevant medical workers in the world, especially in the "*the Belt and Road*" countries and regions.

Shenzhen, China Wei-ye Yu
Shenzhen, China Pu-Xuan Lu
Shenzhen, China Wei-guo Tan
May 12, 2019

Contents

About the Editors

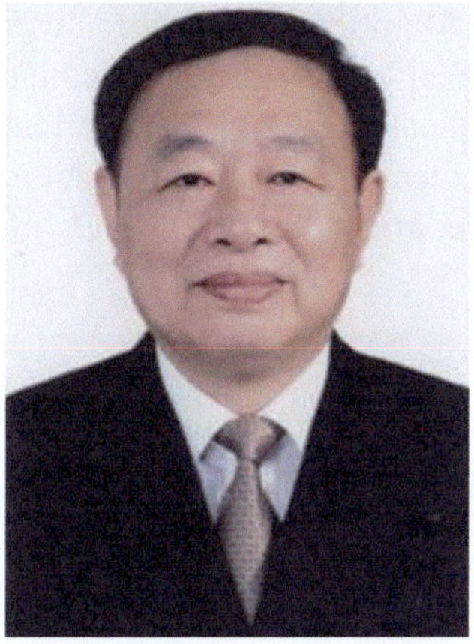

Wei-ye Yu, MD, PhD Appointments and Positions:

- Director of Shenzhen Center for Chronic Disease Control. Chief Physician, Professor
- Master Student Supervisor of Guangdong Medical University

Research Directions:

- Prevention, clinical treatment, and scientific research of tuberculosis (including extrapulmonary tuberculosis such as tuberculous meningitis, bone tuberculosis, and genitourinary tuberculosis)

Research Productions:

- Professor Yu has published more than 50 papers which are related to tuberculosis prevention, diagnosis, or treatment. As a co-editor-in-chief, he has published six medical monographs, among which the monograph entitled *Diagnostic Imaging of Emerging Infectious Diseases* was published by Springer. He has completed or is hosting lots of research projects, including the National Major Scientific and Technological Special Project during the Eleventh and Twelfth Five-Year Plan Period and the National Key Research and Development Plan Project. Furthermore, he has won seven awards, including the second prize of the Scientific and Technological Progress Award of the Chinese Anti-Tuberculosis Association in 2017, the second prize of the Scientific and Technological Progress of Shenzhen Municipality in 2014, the third prize of the Scientific and Technological Progress of Guangdong Province in 2013, the third Prize of the Scientific and Technological Progress Award of the Chinese Preventive Medicine Association in 2007, the third prize of the Scientific and Technological Progress Award of Guangdong Province in 2007, the third-class merit from the People's Government of Guangdong Province, and the third-class merit from the People's Government of Shenzhen Municipality.

Social Positions:

- Chairman of the Internet Technology Branch of the Chinese Anti-Tuberculosis Association, Executive Vice Chairman of the Grassroots Tuberculosis Infection Control Committee of the Chinese Anti-Tuberculosis Association Vice President of the Beijing Innovation Alliance on Tuberculosis Diagnosis and Treatment, Vice Chairman of the Guangdong Provincial Antituberculosis Association, Vice Chairman of the Guangdong Provincial Leprosy Prevention and Treatment Association, Chairman of the Tuberculosis Branch of the Shenzhen Medical Association Member of the Tuberculosis Branch of the Chinese Medical Association, Executive Director of Shenzhen Medical Doctor Association, Executive Director of Shenzhen Medical Association, Deputy editor-in-chief of the Electronic Journal of Emerging Infectious Disease.

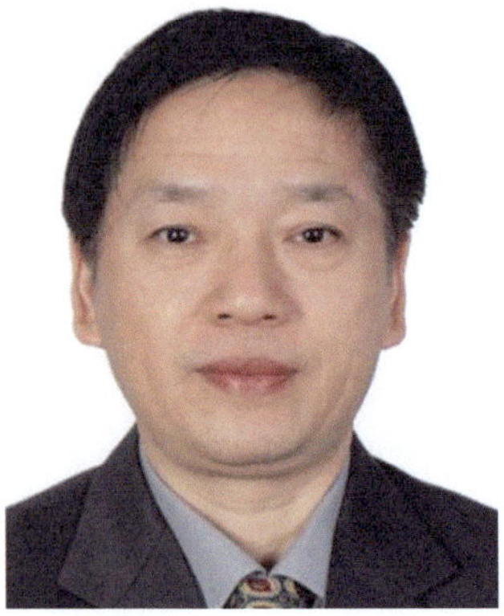

Pu-Xuan Lu is a professor and graduate supervisor of Guangdong Medical University and director of Department of Radiology, Shenzhen Center for Chronic Disease Control.

His academic titles include:

- Chief editor of Electronic Journal of Emerging Infectious Disease.
- Deputy chair, Radiology of Infectious Disease group at radiology branch of Chinese Medical Society.
- Deputy chair, Radiology of Infectious Disease group at Chinese Radiology Society.
- Deputy chair, Radiology branch of Chinese Sexually Transmitted Disease and HIV/AIDS Society.
- Deputy chair, Beijing Diagnostic Imaging Technology Innovation Alliance.
- Deputy chair, Radiology branch of Provincial Health Management Society of Guangdong, China.
- Editorial Committee Member, Journal of Radiology of Infectious Disease.

His research fields include:

- Diagnostic imaging and differential diagnosis of emerging infectious diseases, such as SARS, MERS, AIDS, human-infected avian influenza, tuberculosis, hepatitis, and other infectious diseases as well as clinical and basic sciences of emerging infectious diseases.
- Professor Lu has edited or co-edited more than ten academic treaties. *Diagnostic Imaging of Emerging Infectious Diseases* has been published by Springer in Nov 2015, which obtained national key award for book output in May 2017 by the General Administration of News and Publishing, China. In the recent 5 years, Professor Lu has directed and finished 5 national and provincial as well as international

collaborative research projects. He has published more than 150 research papers, including SCI indexed 43 research papers. And he received 12 awards from Chinese Medical Society, Chinese Preventive Medicine Society, Guangdong provincial government, and Shenzhen city government.

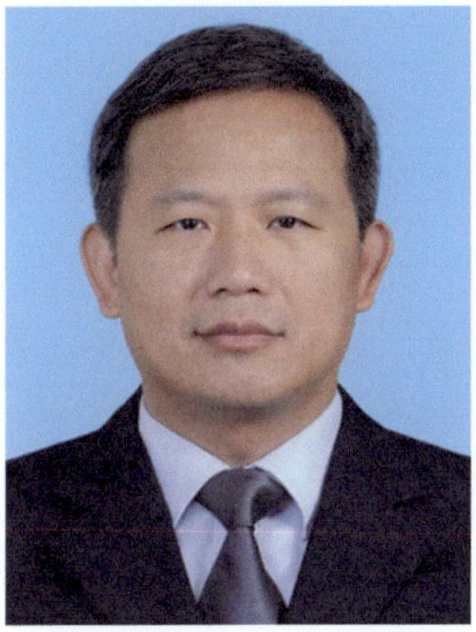

Wei-guo Tan, MD is a chief physician graduated from Sun Yat-sen University of Medical Science and Beijing Tuberculosis and Pulmonary Tumor Research Center. Presently, he is the Vice president of Pulmonary Disease Control Institute in Shenzhen Center for Chronic Disease Control and Secretary general of frontline tuberculosis control committee of Anti-Tuberculosis Association of China. He has more than 20 years of experiences in tuberculosis diagnosis, treatment, and prevention; he is in charge of more than 10 scientific research projects and has published plenty of high rank scientific papers.

Contributors

Bu-dong Chen Department of Radiology, Beijing Ditan Hospital, Capital Medical University, Beijing, China

Tao Chen The Third People's Hospital of Shenzhen, Shenzhen, Guangdong, China

Xiao-ling Che Shenzhen Center for Chronic Disease Control, Shenzhen, Guangdong, China

Guo-fang Deng The Third People's Hospital of Shenzhen, Shenzhen, Guangdong, China

Yu-zheng Fan Shenzhen Nanshan Center for Chronic Disease Control, Shenzhen, Guangdong, China

Hong-yun Guan Shenzhen Nanshan Center for Chronic Disease Control, Shenzhen, Guangdong, China

Lin Guo Shenzhen Smart Imaging Healthcare Co. Ltd., Shenzhen, Guangdong, China

Xu-jun Guo Shenzhen Nanshan Center for Chronic Disease Control, Shenzhen, Guangdong, China

Juan He Shenzhen Nanshan Center for Chronic Disease Control, Shenzhen, Guangdong, China

Fang-xiang Hu Baoan Chronic Diseases Prevent and Cure Hospital, Shenzhen, Guangdong, China

Le-cai Ji Shenzhen Center for Chronic Disease Control, Shenzhen, Guangdong, China

Hong-Jun Li Department of Radiology, Beijing You'an Hospital, Capital Medical University, Beijing, China

Mu-Lan Li Shenzhen Smart Imaging Healthcare Co. Ltd., Shenzhen, Guangdong, China

Sheng-yuan Liu Shenzhen Nanshan Center for Chronic Disease Control, Shenzhen, Guangdong, China

Shou-jiang Liu Shenzhen Nanshan Center for Chronic Disease Control, Shenzhen, Guangdong, China

Chun-rong Lu Shenzhen Center for Chronic Disease Control, Shenzhen, Guangdong, China

Yi-ting Luo Shenzhen Center for Chronic Disease Control, Shenzhen, Guangdong, China

Pu-Xuan Lu Department of Radiology, The Shenzhen Center for Chronic Disease Control, Shenzhen, Guangdong, China

Fleming Lure College of Engineering, University of Texas, El Paso, TX, USA

Jin-zhou Mei Baoan Chronic Diseases Prevent and Cure Hospital, Shenzhen, Guangdong, China

Li-ai Peng Baoan Chronic Diseases Prevent and Cure Hospital, Shenzhen, Guangdong, China

Yu-xin Shi Shanghai Public Health Clinical Center, Fudan University, Shanghai, China

Chun-fa Song Shenzhen Nanshan Center for Chronic Disease Control, Shenzhen, Guangdong, China

Wei-guo Tan Department of Tuberculosis, The Shenzhen Center for Chronic Disease Control, Shenzhen, Guangdong, China

Hui Wang The Third People's Hospital of Shenzhen, Shenzhen, Guangdong, China

Yun-xia Wang Baoan Chronic Diseases Prevent and Cure Hospital, Shenzhen, Guangdong, China

Wei Wei Shenzhen Nanshan Center for Chronic Disease Control, Shenzhen, Guangdong, China

Li-juan Wu Shenzhen Nanshan Center for Chronic Disease Control, Shenzhen, Guangdong, China

Qing-fang Wu Shenzhen Center for Chronic Disease Control, Shenzhen, Guangdong, China

Li Xie Shenzhen Center for Chronic Disease Control, Shenzhen, Guangdong, China

Ru-Ming Xie Beijing Ditan Hospital, Capital Medical University, Beijing, China

Ya-rui Yang Shenzhen Nanshan Center for Chronic Disease Control, Shenzhen, Guangdong, China

Zheng Yang Shenzhen Center for Chronic Disease Control, Shenzhen, Guangdong, China

Wei-ye Yu Department of Tuberculosis, The Shenzhen Center for Chronic Disease Control, Shenzhen, Guangdong, China

Fan Zhang Shenzhen Nanshan Center for Chronic Disease Control, Shenzhen, Guangdong, China

Juan-juan Zhang Baoan Chronic Diseases Prevent and Cure Hospital, Shenzhen, Guangdong, China

Mei-juan Zhang Baoan Chronic Diseases Prevent and Cure Hospital, Shenzhen, Guangdong, China

Qiu-ting Zheng Shenzhen Center for Chronic Disease Control, Shenzhen, Guangdong, China

Qiu Zhong Chinese Antituberculosis Association, Guangzhou, Guangdong, China

Yang Zhou The Third People's Hospital of Shenzhen, Shenzhen, Guangdong, China

Zhi-peng Zhuo Shenzhen Center for Chronic Disease Control, Shenzhen, Guangdong, China

Overview of Tuberculosis

1

Wei-ye Yu, Yun-xia Wang, Jin-zhou Mei, Fang-xiang Hu, and Le-cai Ji

1 Prevalence of Tuberculosis

1.1 Concept of Tuberculosis and Its Evolution

Tuberculosis (TB) is a chronic infectious disease caused by the infection of *Mycobacterium tuberculosis* (Mtb) which spreads via respiratory tract. Lungs are the most commonly infected human organ whose infection accounts for above 80% of tuberculosis. Therefore, TB is also known as pulmonary TB [1]. There had been a long history of TB before its pathogenesis, spreading routes, treatment, and prevention of TB have been elucidated.

According to literature records, the human being has fought against tuberculosis, a classic infectious disease, for more than 4000 years. Early in the seventh century BC, TB-like symptoms were recorded in Assyria. Due to insufficient knowledge about its etiology and mechanism of transmission, pandemics of TB occurred till the twentieth century [2].

During the Hippocratic period in the ancient Greek in the fifth century BC, TB (lately known as phthisis) was the most widely spread disease and it was always fatal. At that time, many scholars in medicine, including Hippocrates, believed that TB is a hereditary disease. However, Aristotle disagreed and he believed that TB is an infectious disease. But because no evidence demonstrated his opinions, Aristotle was referred to as an outcast for a long period of time.

In the following centuries, two distinct schools emerged in Europe with a geographic boundary concerning the etiology of TB. In the northern Europe, TB was believed as a hereditary disease, while in the southern Europe, it was believed as an infectious disease. The distinction was partially due to geographic distribution of TB. At that time, it was believed that the wide spread of TB was caused by nomadic activities of Indo-European herdsmen. It was then confirmed that its pathogen, Mtb, is derived from M. bovis and the speculation of hereditary disease was abolished.

In the year 1720, Benjamin Marten, a doctor from Britain, firstly proposed that TB is an infectious disease but it was not confirmed. At the beginning of the nineteenth century, pandemic of TB occurred due to well-matched population density and natural conditions. In 1816, Rene Theophile Hyacinthe Laennec, the inventor of stethoscope, firstly elucidated the pathogenesis of TB and many terms he proposed concerning clinical intrapulmonary and extrapulmonary lesions of TB have been currently applied in clinical practice. In 1839, Johann Lukas Schönlein, a German doctor, firstly nominated the disease as tuberculosis. In 1865, Jean-Antoine villemin confirmed that TB is communicable from infected cadaveric tissue. In 1882, Robert Koch demonstrated his discovery of Mtb. And he won the Nobel Prize for medicine in 1905 in recognition of his contribution to pathogenesis of TB. In the nineteenth and twentieth centuries, due to the improved hygienic condition and quarantine of the infected population, the incidence of TB gradually decreased year by year.

Although the pathogen of tuberculosis, Mtb, has been isolated in the end of the nineteenth century, it costs nearly 50 years to develop a feasible treatment regimen. From the year 1914–1944, Selman A. Waksman dedicated himself to a hypoxic chemical drug that is applicable to human and he finally discovered streptomycin. However, Mtb is a microorganism that is strongly adaptable to the environment. If only one medication is applied to treat TB, Mtb tends to produce resistance to it. That is why the modern standard anti-tuberculosis regimen is a quadruple medication whose application is intended to prevent drug resistance.

W.-y. Yu (✉)
Department of Tuberculosis, The Shenzhen Center for Chronic Disease Control, Shenzhen, Guangdong, China

Y.-x. Wang · J.-z. Mei · F.-x. Hu
Baoan Chronic Diseases Prevent and Cure Hospital, Shenzhen, Guangdong, China

L.-c. Ji
Shenzhen Center for Chronic Disease Control, Shenzhen, Guangdong, China

W.-y. Yu et al. (eds.), *Tuberculosis Control in Migrating Population*, https://doi.org/10.1007/978-981-32-9763-0_1

In 1921, Bacille Calmette-Guerin (BCG) vaccine was first applied to human, which then gained widespread application in Europe. Along with the application of effective anti-tuberculosis medications, such as sodium aminosalicylate, isoniazid, and pyrazinamide, a new era of combined medications for tuberculosis began. In 1959, a trial conducted in a medical center in India demonstrated that the effects of medication for tuberculosis have no difference between outpatients and inpatients. And it was proposed in the study that directly observed treatment should be applied to assure regular medication treatment in outpatients with tuberculosis.

In 1982, in a campaign celebrating the 100th anniversary of Mtb discovery by Robert Koch, an anti-tuberculosis institution in Republic of Mali, Africa proposed to establish the world anti-tuberculosis day. The proposal was soon adopted by the council of the International Anti-tuberculosis Association. But the memorial activities were launched in local areas. Till the end of 1995, March 24th was established as the world anti-tuberculosis day by the World Health Organization (WHO). In 1996, an official document was issued in China by the former Ministry of Health to initiate activities on March 24th, the world anti-tuberculosis day, each year in response to the WHO.

1.2 WHO and Evolution of Strategies for Tuberculosis Control

After the World War II, to keep peace and promote cooperation in economic, social, and human rights development, multiple sovereign governments including France, China, Soviet Union, Britain, and the USA initiated the establishment of the United Nations in 1945. At the establishment of the United Nations, the presidents of multiple countries proposed the establishment of a global health organization. And the World Health Organization (WHO) was finally established on April 7th, 1948. Since then, WHO has made joint efforts worldwide in fight for the infectious diseases such as influenza and HIV/AIDS as well as non-infectious diseases such as cancer and heart diseases.

In the 1960s and 1970s of the twentieth century, the short-term treatment for tuberculosis achieved success due to successive discoveries of effective anti-tuberculosis drugs. Since then, the treatment evolved into the directly observed treatment, short-course (DOTS) and has been gradually standardized. The standard DOTS has then been successfully applied in some countries of Africa, Asia, and Europe. At the 44th World Health Assembly in 1991, the WHO was informed that many countries lost their control to epidemics of tuberculosis due to neglects of the threats of tuberculosis to human health. Therefore, in April 1993, the WHO declared red alert of tuberculosis worldwide and re-assessed the post-strategies for tuberculosis control. In 1994, a new framework for tuberculosis control was proposed [3]. In 1995, the WHO officially proposed the modern anti-tuberculosis strategy (DOTS strategy) including the framework for tuberculosis control and DOTS, which was then promoted worldwide.

Since 1997, the WHO has been issuing the World Tuberculosis Report each year. The report provides important reference for scholars and clinicians in their understandings about epidemics of tuberculosis worldwide as well as newly developed diagnostic techniques, treatment regimens, and management strategies [4].

Due to limitations by the coverage and accessibility of the DOTS strategy, infection of HIV/AIDS, smoking, insufficient health care resources, and non-standard treatment regimen, the effects of DOTS strategy on tuberculosis control have been gradually weakened. Targeting the limitations in implementing the DOTS strategy, the WHO initiated a new strategy for tuberculosis control worldwide in March 2006, the Stop TB strategy. Meanwhile, the WHO established the goals to greatly reduce the global TB burden, to realize the Millennium Development Goals (MDGs) of the United Nations, and to reduce the morbidity and mortality of TB by 50% in the year 2015 based on the data of 1990, and to eradicate TB in the year 2050 (with an incidence of TB being less than 10 per million). TB is hopefully no longer a threat to the public health in the year 2050, according to the WHO.

In the World Tuberculosis Report of 2014, the WHO proposed the global strategy for tuberculosis after the year 2015, namely the End TB strategy. The general goal of the End TB strategy is to terminate the epidemics of tuberculosis worldwide. The WHO also proposed that the mortality rate of tuberculosis reduces by 75% and 95% in 2025 and 2035, respectively; and the morbidity rate of tuberculosis reduces by 50% and 90% in 2025 and 2035, respectively, compared to the data of 2015. In the year 2035, hopefully, no family has catastrophic expense on TB, according to the report [5].

1.3 Prevalence of TB Worldwide

According to data released in the 2018 World Tuberculosis Report by the WHO [6], TB is one of the top 10 deadly diseases worldwide and is the main cause of death from infection of singular pathogen. Its mortality rate is higher than that of HIV/AIDS. It has been estimated that the new cases of TB were 10 million worldwide in the year 2017 and the incidence rate was 133 per 0.1 million. The patients included 5.8 million male patients, 3.2 million female patients, and 1 million children. The adult patients aged above 15 years accounted for 90%, and the cases of TB complicated by HIV/AIDS accounted for 9% with 72% in Africa. In the 10 million new cases of TB worldwide, two-thirds were from India, China, Indonesia, Philippines, Pakistan, and the other three countries. The total number of cases in 30 countries with high TB burden accounted for 87% of all the cases worldwide. The incidence rate of TB showed great variance in different countries. The incidence rate of TB in most high-income countries is lower than 10 per 0.1 million, while the incidence rate of TB in the 30 countries with high TB burden ranged from 150 to 400 per 0.1 million. But the incidence rate of TB in some countries including Mozambique, Philippines, and South Africa was higher than 500 per 0.1 million. A longitudinal study for etiology of tuberculosis demonstrated that in 10.4 million patients with pulmonary TB in the year 2016, 1.9 million can be attributed to malnutrition, 1 million to compromised immunity induced by HIV/AIDS, and 0.8 million to smoking and diabetes [7]. In the year 2016, the cure rate of TB was 82% worldwide, which was lower than 83% in 2015 and 86% in 2013 [6].

According to a study in patients with TB receiving no intervention, within 10 years after definitive diagnosis of TB by sputum smear positive, death occurred in about 70% patients. During the same period of time, 20% patients of TB with sputum smear negative but sputum culture positive died [8]. It has been reported that [6] in the year 2017, about 1.3 million patients with TB but HIV negative died from TB worldwide, showing a decrease of 29% and 5% compared to the years of 2000 and 2015, respectively. And about 0.3 million patients with TB and HIV positive died from TB in the year 2017, showing a decrease of 44% and 20% compared to the years of 2000 and 2015, respectively. According to the report, the mortality rate (every 0.1 million population) of TB decreased by 42% from the year 2000 to 2017. During the 5 years from 2013 to 2017, the mortality rate of TB showed a sharpest decrease in Europe and South-east Asia by 11% and 4% yearly, respectively. The mortality rate of TB worldwide was about 17%, with a yearly decrease of 3%, while the yearly decrease of its incidence rate was only 2%. To achieve the goal of stop TB in the year 2020, the yearly decrease of its incidence rate should be 4–5% and the mortality rate should reach 10% in the year 2020.

According to the report, drug-resistant TB is still a threat to the human health. In the year 2017, the new cases of multidrug-resistant TB and rifampicin-resistant TB were 0.1607 million, being slightly higher than 0.1531 million in the year 2016, and about 47% cases of drug-resistant TB were from India (24%), China (13%), and Russia (10%). Meanwhile, about 0.23 million patients with multidrug-resistant TB or rifampicin-resistant TB died [6]. In the year 2017, about 3.5% initially treated patients with TB and 18% re-treated patients with TB were diagnosed with extensive drug-resistant TB worldwide. In terms of treatment, in the year 2017, about 0.1391 million patients with drug-resistant TB worldwide received treatment, showing an increase compared to 0.1297 in 2016. However, those receiving treatment only accounted for 25% of the estimated number of patients with drug-resistant TB [6]. Concerning the outcome of treatment, the cure rate of drug-resistant TB was only about 55% worldwide, which still remained a low level.

According to the report, most deaths of patients with TB can be avoided by early diagnosis and timely standard treatment. In the years from 2000 to 2016, the early diagnosis and standard treatment have saved about 53 million lives of patients with TB [9]. Although many patients with TB can be accurately diagnosed and cured, gaps exist in the diagnosis and treatment of TB. In most countries with high TB burden, poverty, HIV/AIDS, malnutrition, and tobacco play more extensive and profound role in the prevention and control of TB [7]. A report about 119 countries with middle and low income indicated that the investment for prevention and control of TB amounted to 6.9 billion US dollars in the year 2018, showing an increase of 0.6 billion and 3.6 billion US dollars compared to the years of 2016 and 2006, respectively. And the domestic financial outcome accounted for above 86% [6]. Although the investment for prevention and control of TB has successively increased for more than 10 years, there is still an about 2.3 billion US dollars shortfall in funding worldwide [6, 7]. To make up the shortfall, domestic financial funding should be increased for prevention and control of TB in the countries with middle income, international financial help for countries with low income is also necessary.

Currently, 7 countries including Ghana, Kenya, Burma, Philippines, Moldova, Timor-Leste, and Vietnam have completed survey for disease burden in families [7]. The surveys in Burma and Vietnam indicated that the patients with TB and their families are facing heavy economic burden, which is consistent with the data that the expenses on disease by patients themselves account more than 30% of all the health care cost. The data from the Global TB Drug Facility (GDF) indicated that each patient with common TB spends about 40 US dollars for 6-month medication treatment and each patient with drug-resistant TB spends far more than that for treatment [7].

According to the report, the diagnostic technology for TB showed barely any new development. Currently, 20 anti-tuberculosis drugs are in Stage I, II, or III clinical trials, including 11 newly combined drugs. According to the results of the Stage IIb clinical trial, Bedaquiline and Delamanid acquired approval or conditional approval by the supervision agency. In addition, multiple regimens of new combinations are still in Stage II or III clinical trials. In 2018, 12 candidate vaccines are in clinical trials, including 4 vaccines in the Stage I clinical trials, 6 in the Stage II clinical trials, and 2 in the Stage III clinical trials.

1.4 Prevalence of TB in China

China as the country with the second largest population is also the second largest country of patients with TB and one of the high TB burden countries. In China, the number of new cases ranks as one of the highest in statutory class A and B infectious diseases. To timely understand the prevalence of TB all over the country, five epidemiological sampling surveys for TB were conducted in 1979, 1984–1985, 1990,

2000, and 2010, which provide basic epidemiological data for infection status, morbidity and mortality, and geographic distribution of TB [10–14].

According to literature report, at the early stage after foundation of P. R. China, the epidemics of TB were serious due to low economic level, insufficient health-care resources, and poor environmental conditions. In the year 1949, the morbidity and mortality rates of TB were 1750 per 0.1 million and 200 per 0.1 million and TB constituted a serious threat to human health in China [15]. Along with the economic development and improvement of living conditions, the morbidity and mortality rates of TB decreased by 70% (523 per 0.1 million) and 90% (21 per 0.1 million) compared to the data of 1949, respectively. However, from the global perspective, TB is highly prevalent in China, with high morbidity rate, high mortality rate, high drug-resistance rate (initial drug-resistance rate of 28.1%), and a decrease of annual decline rate (2.8%) [15]. To control the epidemic of TB in China, the Ministry of Health adopted a series of measures to improve the national regulations for prevention and treatment of TB, to establish and improve the national network for prevention and treatment of TB, to increase the funding for prevention and treatment of TB after the year 1991, such as to initiate TB Control Program in the World Bank Loan and to reinforce TB control program. By the year 2000, the national morbidity rate, mortality rate, and initial drug-resistance rate of TB in China had decreased to 346 per 0.1 million, 9.8 per 0.1 million, and 18.6%, respectively. Compared to the data of 1990, the morbidity rate, mortality rate, and initial drug-resistance rate decreased by 33.8%, 53.1%, and 33.8%, respectively, with annual decline rates of 4.0%, 8.3%, and 4.0%, respectively [11, 16]. Although the national prevalence of TB in China sharply decreased, there was still low detection rate of TB non-standard treatment and management of TB [11]. According to the 5th national epidemiological sampling survey for TB in 2010, the mortality rate of TB was 3.7 per 0.1 million, showing a decrease of 62.2% and annual decline rate of 9.3% compared to the data of 2000. The morbidity rate of TB was 459 per 0.1 million and drug-resistance rate to detected 11 drugs was 42.1% [10]. Due to variance in statistic methods and detected drugs, the morbidity rate and drug-resistance rate of TB in 2010 cannot be directly compared to the data of 2000. The results of survey indicated that the prevalence of TB in China was characterized by decreasing morbidity rate, increasing new cases, aggravating drug resistance, great regional variance in prevalence of TB, and increased percentage of asymptomatic TB cases [10].

China is also one of the high burden countries with drug-resistant TB. According to the data from the national baseline survey for drug-resistant TB in 2007–2008, the drug-resistance rate in initially treated patients with TB was 5.8% (175/3037) and the multidrug-resistance rate of re-treated patients with TB reached 25.3% (226/892). Compared to the data from the national epidemiological survey for TB in 2000, the epidemic of drug-resistant TB was aggravating [17, 18]. According to the data of the 2018 World Tuberculosis Report, the reported cases of drug-resistant TB in China were estimated to be 58,000, with the new cases of drug-resistant TB accounting for 7.1%. Currently, the cases of rifampicin-resistant TB were 108,000, with the new cases accounting for 12% and the re-treated cases accounting for 69% [6]. Compared to the data in 2017, the number of reported cases of drug-resistant TB remained the same and the number of reported cases of rifampicin-resistant TB decreased by 10,000. The epidemic of drug-resistant TB in China is severe. For Chinese governments, it is necessary to reinforce works in control of TB epidemics, including detection of drug-resistant and multidrug-resistant TB, construction of service system for prevention and treatment of TB, management of treatment and financial investment [19, 20].

2 Current TB Control

Pulmonary TB is one of the major infectious diseases, which is an old and serious threat to human health. During the 12th Five-Year plan in China, the prevalence of TB generally tends to decrease, with obviously decreased morbidity and mortality. The goal of the 12th Five-Year plan was ultimately achieved. A total of 4.27 million cases of active pulmonary TB were detected and managed and the cure rate remained above 85% [21].

However, China remained a country with high TB burden. There are still challenges in the prevention and control of TB, including gradually aggravating prevalence of drug-resistant TB, gradually enlarging population with HIV/TB, incomplete mechanism and system for prevention and treatment of TB, severe prevalence of TB in the middle-west and rural areas, difficult detection and management of TB in the migrating population. These situations should be improved by reasonable strategies for prevention and control of TB during the 13th Five-Year plan in China.

2.1 Commitment of the Chinese Government Concerning the Eradication of TB

Currently, the general goal in the prevention and control of TB is to stop prevalence of TB in the world in the year 2035. Specifically, the number of deaths from TB and the number of new cases should be decreased by 95% and 90%, respectively, in the year 2035, compared to the data of 2015. And the specific goals in 2020, 2025, and 2030 have also been established. These goals can be achieved based on the comprehensive patient-centered prevention and treatment of TB, strong policies as the supporting system, and reinforced research and innovation [22].

Stop TB strategy by the WHO is intended to achieve its first goal in the year 2020, namely the numbers of deaths from TB and the new cases should be decreased by 35% and 20%, respectively, in the year 2020, compared to the data of 2015. And the patients with TB and their families should no longer pay for the catastrophic expenses on the treatment of TB [23].

On November 16–17, 2017, the 1st global ministerial conference of the WHO was held in Moscow. The theme of the conference was to eradicate TB in the era of sustainable development: multi-sector joint response. And the conference was intended to accelerate the implementation of Stop TB strategy proposed by the WHO and to eliminate the discrepancies in health-care accessibility and MDR-TB crisis. The conference advocated domestic and international commitments, achievements, and responsibilities to achieve the goals of Stop TB proposed by the WHO and Sustainable Development proposed by the United Nations [24]. In the conference, the ministers signed the declaration in accelerating movements to stop TB.

To accelerate movements to stop TB, presidents of many countries participated in the first high-level meeting of the United Nations Assembly on tuberculosis in New York of the USA on September 26, 2018. Multisectors were called politically for promotion of movements to stop TB.

2.2 Completion of a New Service System for Prevention and Treatment of TB

It has been definitively required in the 12th Five-Year plan for tuberculosis control and the Management for Prevention and Treatment of Tuberculosis issued in 2013 that a three-level network for prevention and treatment of TB should be constructed, and a new service system with designated hospitals, basic health-care institutions, and disease control institutions should be constructed. The new service system for prevention and treatment of TB emphasizes distinct responsibilities of different institutions. In addition, the responsibility of diagnosis and treatment of TB is transferred from the disease control institutions to the designated hospitals. The new service system has adapted to the needs of current prevention and treatment of TB and is in accordance with its future sustainable development. Since the implementation of the 12th Five-Year plan for prevention and treatment of TB, the new service system has been continually enriched and reinforced. The survey of designated hospital for diagnosis and treatment of TB in China in 2015 indicated that there have been 1,600 designated hospitals for diagnosis and treatment of TB [25] and coordination between different institutions has been explored.

The new service system for prevention and treatment of TB is gradually establishing. However, excessive diagnostic examinations and anti-tuberculosis drug abuse in treatment may exist in the designated hospitals. In some remote areas, the designated hospitals for diagnosis and treatment of TB are poorly equipped and the new technologies for detection and diagnosis of TB cannot be applied. There are discrepancies concerning the service quality of diagnosis and treatment in different designated hospitals. And the clinicians earn low income in the designated hospitals for diagnosis and treatment of TB and are not highly motivated for clinical practice. Some working staffs in prevention and treatment of TB have low incomes but high risks of occupational exposure. In addition to unstable allowance, the professional team remains unstable, which increases the difficulty in preventing and treating TB.

2.3 Advancement of Modern Strategy for Control of TB

The modern strategy for control of TB is centered on the control of infection source. In more than one decade with 100% coverage of DOTS. There have been free charge policy and incentive policy. In the free charge policy, the patients are provided with free charge X-ray for once and sputum smear for three times, and the patients with active pulmonary TB are provided with free charge anti-tuberculosis drugs according to the national uniform treatment regimen. And in the incentive policy, the basic level health-care staffs are provided with sickness subsidy and management grants. Based on these policies, some detections are added for free of charge and subsidies for health-care staffs are increased by the local government of China. Based on these policies and measures, the compliance of the patients is improved and the community-based health-care staffs are highly motivated for their clinical practice. Therefore, TB control is improved.

In China, patients finding is performed via multiple routes. Surveillance and screening of TB are performed in the high-risk populations, including the migrating population, students and teachers in schools, patients with type II diabetes, the senior citizens, patients with HIV/AIDS, custodial population, welfare population, and patients with drug-resistant TB. Gao et al. summarized the screening and control of TB in the high-risk populations [26]. They believed that the control of TB in the high-risk populations would be further emphasized along with increased government attention, increased financial funding, active social participation, and reform of health care institutions.

Combined with the technology of internet plus, DOTS can be reinforced and its effects can be improved by medication video, electronic medication kit, and other new technologies. Home isolation treatment can also be performed. Along with the application of new technologies, information technologies, and mass data in diagnosis and treatment of TB, we can achieve the planning goals under the strong leadership of government and efforts of anti-tuberculosis professionals.

3 Development in the Diagnosis of Pulmonary Tuberculosis

Pulmonary tuberculosis, as an infectious disease, poses serious threat to human health. In the middle of the nineteenth century, Pasteur, a French scientist, established the theory of communicable pathogenic microbiology. Thereafter, the European scholars in medicine began to recognize that tuberculosis is communicable. In 1865, Villemin discovered that the clinical specimens from patients with TB can infect rabbits and other animals. And then the discoveries of leprosy bacillus and other pathogenic bacteria as well as developments in staining technology and coagulated serum medium promoted the development of pathogenic bacteriology. On March 24, 1882, Robert Koch, a German scientist, published a historic report, which revealed that the pathogen of tuberculosis is *Mycobacterium tuberculosis*. The discovery about pathogen of TB marked the birth of bacteriology of tuberculosis. Koch contributed to identification of Mtb as the pathogen of TB, microscopy of glass slide for Mtb and plate culture, which constituted the basis for the bacteriological diagnosis and identification of TB. Based on the bacteriological diagnosis and identification of TB, immunology and modern clinical therapeutics of TB were developed. Till today, the well-known three principles in identifying pathogenic bacteria developed by Koch have been observed in identification of pathogenic bacteria. The discovery by Koch provoked people's expectation to avoid sufferings of TB. And scholarly studies soon focused on the Mtb itself, diagnosis and treatment of TB, and Mtb vaccines, with emergence of a research climax on TB. Koch and his contemporaries developed many concepts and technologies, which are now valuable legacies of medicine. And many basic bacteriological methods and bacteriological diagnosis have been applied till today.

TB is caused by infection of Mtb. Currently, there has been no effective vaccine to control the infection of Mtb. Treatment of patients with TB is the key point in the strategy of TB control. It has been generally believed that detection of Mtb is the basis for the definitive diagnosis of TB [27]. Therefore, the bacteriological diagnosis of TB is the beginning of TB control and the responsibility of the laboratory of tuberculosis bacteriology is to detect Mtb in the specimens of the patients. Routine smear microscopy and culture in TB bacteriology are the classical techniques when our ancestors discovered Mtb in the end of the nineteenth century, which have been effective nowadays. However, the techniques have their own defects, which render that bacteriology of tuberculosis remains to be the most important research field for clinical practice of tuberculosis. It has been expected that the clinical bacteriological diagnosis of TB should be rapid, specific, sensitive, accurate, and simple with low cost that adapts to clinical laboratories. However, research for almost 100 years has not achieved breakthrough developments. And the recent development in molecular diagnosis brings a ray of hope for an ideal technology in bacteriological diagnosis of TB [28].

3.1 Bacteriological Examination

Smear Detection

Acid-fastness is a physical property of certain bacteria, specifically their resistance to decolorization by acids during laboratory staining procedures. Once stained as part of a sample, these organisms can resist the acid and/or ethanol-based decolorization procedures common in many staining protocols. The acid-fastness of genus Mycobacteria is due to the high mycolic acid content of their cell walls, which is responsible for the staining pattern of poor absorption followed by high retention [29]. In addition, Corynebacteria and Nocardia may also be partially acid-fast due to their content of mycolic acid. Based on the knowledge, we know that acid-fastness is not specifically Mycobacteria but a possible preliminary implication. Therefore, when rod shaped bacteria with acid-fastness is detected in a clinical specimen, acid-fast bacillus positive rather than Mtb positive should be reported. In clinical practice, acid-fast bacillus is considered to be equal to Mtb as indicators in the diagnosis of TB [30–32].

Culture Detection

Mtb is facultative bacteria which is aerobic and has no complex requirement for nourishment. It can grow in test tubes at appropriate temperature. Compared to smear for microscopy, culture detection is more sensitive and shows positive for sputum specimen with a concentration of 100 bacteria/ml. After isolation culture, the *Mycobacterium tuberculosis* complex (MTBC) and *Mycobacterium tuberculosis* strain can be identified and drug sensitivity can be tested. Culture detection can provide bacteriological basis for Mtb infection [33].

Nucleic Acid Amplification

Since the polymerase chain reaction (PCR) was developed in the year 1983, the new technology of gene diagnosis with advantages of rapidity, high sensitivity, and high specificity has been expected to open up a new era for the diagnosis of TB [34]. PCR is an in vitro enzyme driven amplification of specific sequence segment in the nucleic acid of Mtb medicated by a pair of specific oligonucleotide primers. The target sequence specific to Mtb is denatured, renatured, and elongated in a series of 20–30 repeated thermal cycles and the sequence is exponentially amplified for detection. High standards of technology and reagents are required in performing PCR. Clinical observations have demonstrated that PCR has a high false positive rate in clinical diagnosis. And many scholars attempted to improve the technique for its clinical application, such as nested PCR and PCR plus nucleic acid probe [35]. Growth independence is the advantage of nucleic acid amplification but the source of detected target sequence cannot be determined from living or dead bacteria. Therefore, its application in the diagnosis of TB is limited.

Bacteriological examination plays an important role in the diagnosis of TB and the definitive diagnosis of TB mainly depends on culture positive, which is also the golden standard for other laboratory diagnostic methods. Currently, routine bacteriological diagnosis for TB is not satisfying. Smear for microscopy is simple with low cost, but it shows low sensitivity and no strain specificity. And its specificity is decreasing along with increasing cases of non-Mtb infection. Although culture for detection is highly sensitive, the report is sometimes delayed and it always fails to detect the growth-heterotypic Mtb.

The technique of molecular diagnosis is highly sensitive, but with a high false positive rate. However, it provides the most rapid and accurate preliminary diagnosis of TB and we should take the full advantage of it. Recently, the drug-resistant gene of Mtb can be rapidly detected by using techniques of molecular biology such as PCR-SSCP and sequence analysis, including rpoB gene mutation of Mtb strain that is resistant to rifampicin, kaG, inhA, and aphC genes mutation that is resistant to isoniazid, kasA gene mutation, pncA gene mutation that is resistant to pyrazinamide, mps and ms genes mutation that is resistant to streptomycin, rs gene mutation that is resistant to amikacin/kanamycin, embCAB gene mutation that is resistant to ethambutol, and gyrA and gyrB genes mutation that is resistant to quinolones as well as IrA gene mutation that inhibits coding of transcription proteins. In addition, it has been reported that resistance to clarithromycin by Mtb is possibly related to rs gene mutation; resistance to ethionamide, inhA gene mutation; and resistance to seromycin, urA/dadB genes mutation. These discoveries marked the advancements in the molecular biology of TB [36].

3.2 Imaging Diagnosis of Pulmonary TB

Chest High Voltage Photography

Chest high voltage photography is chest photography with an electric voltage of no less than 120 kV. It is characterized by short wave length of X-ray with strong penetrating power, low dosage of X-ray absorption by tissues, decreased density discrepancies of different tissues, decreased covering effect on the films, increased data, and enhanced image readability. The increase of electric voltage correspondingly decreases the electric current, which greatly reduces damages to human body and enhances the clarity of images. The advantages of chest high voltage photography include (1) increased data on films with decreased density of soft tissues and ribs and decreased covering effect; (2) clear demonstration of lesions adjacent to mediastinum and posterior to the cardiac shadow; (3) demonstration of internal structures of the lesions, such as calcification and cavity.

Computed Tomography (CT)

Computed tomography is abbreviated as CT. With the development of technology, CT has developed into current spiral CT and ultrahigh speed (electron beam) CT. And its scanning mode has developed from translation plus rotation and rotation plus rotation into static plus rotation, namely slip ring and spiral scan. The number of detector in CT scanner has been increasing and their arrangement has developed from continuous dense type into multilayer type, namely multilayer spiral CT scanner. The scanning time has been shortened from 3–5 min to 0.2–1 s. CT scan is characterized by clear demonstration of transverse sections of human body, high resolution power, clear demonstration of TB lesions at different stages, and accurate demonstration of hilar and mediastinal lymphadenectasis. In addition, modern computers are empowered with powerful image post-processing technology, such as multilayer reconstruction and virtual endoscopic reconstruction. In addition to harvest of clear images of transverse sections by thin layer scanning, virtual 3-dimentional images can be synthesized. CT has been an important imaging technique in the diagnosis of pulmonary TB and it has outweighed chest X-ray photography.

Magnetic Resonance Imaging (MRI)

Magnetic resonance imaging (MRI) was firstly developed by scholars from the USA, Bloch and Purcell. In 1978, Damadian firstly applied the technology in clinical practice and named it as MRI. The underlying mechanism is proton resonance of hydrogen atom. Hydrogen atom is the substance in human body with the largest number, containing only one proton that is the most unstable. Under the effect of external magnetic field, resonance of proton can be produced. That is to say, the protons in hydrogen atoms in human body are arranged disorderly with different directions of magnetic moments. When these self-spinning and disorderly protons are placed in a powerful and homogeneous external magnetic field, they are re-arranged along with the magnetic lines of force of the external magnetic field. At this time, when triggered by radio-frequency pulse from a specific second magnetic field, the hydrogen nuclei absorb the energy to produce resonance. Because hydrogen atoms are widely distributed in human body, the hydrogen protons are used as probes and transmitter-receivers to collect MRI signals and their distribution within human body. In MRI, human body is placed in a powerful and homogeneous magnetic field and the protons in hydrogen atoms are magnetized for directional arrangement. A specific radio-frequency is in processional motion around the magnetic field. The radio-frequency pulse with the same frequency as the proton processional motion is applied to trigger and deflect the magnetic moment of proton. And the self-spinning protons leave the planes of magnetic field to produce resonance at a certain frequency. When the electromagnetic wave is cut off, the self-spinning of protons in resonance gradually recovers to the original low energy thermal equilibrium, namely relaxation. At this time, the hydrogen nuclei radiate electromagnetic wave with the same frequency, which is known as resonant electromagnetic wave. The resonant electromagnetic wave is received for spatial coding in a computer to determine the spatial distribution of detected nuclei. A converter is then applied to reconstruct image for its display on a monitor, which is known as the image of MRI. By MRI, the substance with short T1 long T2 signal produces strong self-spinning echo wave of MRI signal, while the substance with long T1 short T2 signal produces weak signal due to low signal of flowing void effect. MRI is non-invasive and is capable of harvesting 3-dimensional image of any plane in human body. In addition, it can demonstrate cardiac chambers and vascular lumen with no application of reagent and facilitate differentiation of benign and malignant neoplasms based on T1 and T2 signals. Due to these advantages, it has gained wider application in clinical diagnosis.

3.3 B-mode Ultrasonography

B-mode ultrasonography is an important part of modern diagnostic imaging in clinical practice. Based on different penetration and reflection of ultrasound on different tissues and lesions, the images are constructed to accurately display the outlines, ranges, and properties of organs and lesions. The image by B-mode ultrasonography provides direct view of tissues and organs. It is non-invasive and provides dynamic observation with no radiation effects. Nowadays, it has been widely applied in the diagnosis of thoracic and abdominal diseases. Due to strong reflection of ultrasound to the gas containing lungs and interference of bone tissues in the thoracic wall, ultrasonography can hardly demonstrate micro-structures in deep lungs. Therefore, it is commonly believed that ultrasonography is not appropriate for the examination of thoracic cavity. However, many thoracic diseases can be demonstrated by ultrasonography such as fluid containing lesions, parenchymal lesions in lungs and atelectasis. In such cases, the lesions contact to the thoracic wall to form acoustic window, which increases the penetration of acoustic beam and clear ultrasound image can be harvested.

Thoracic TB

B-mode ultrasonography demonstrates early thoracic TB as abscess of the thoracic wall that is no-echo or weak-echo dark area. The lesion is fusiform along the intercostal space that is internally and externally dumbbell shaped. In its advanced stage, when the abscess invades the bone, the bone lamella is irregularly thin with interrupted or absent echo from the bone cortex. The abscess cavity is demonstrated with irregular flakes or spots like strong echo and accompanying acoustic shadow. Prolonged ultrasonography demonstrates internal surface of thoracic wall with purulent dark area, which protrudes towards the lung field with irregular boundary. There is also irregular weak sinus echo.

Tuberculous Pleurisy

In the cases of pleural effusion, the parietal and visceral pleura are separated and the space is demonstrated as fluid no-echo dark area. Encapsulated effusion is demonstrated as limited dark area with no echo or extremely weak echo. And the dark area is characterized by oblate in shape, medially protrusion towards the lung, and the two ends in sharp angle. The emergence of homogeneous light spot in the fluid dark area commonly indicates bloody effusion, while irregular and different sized light spots with uneven distribution indicate purulent effusion. In sitting position, liquid level dark area under strong gas echo or spots of gas strong echo in the liquid dark area are considered to be hydropneumothorax. B-mode ultrasonography has important clinical value in the diagnosis of pleural effusion, with a diagnostic accordance rate of above 98%. In the diagnosis of pleural effusion, it has the advantages in (1) detecting the location and quantity of pleural effusion; (2) qualifying thoracic shadow; (3) definitively diagnosing pleural effusion in the cases with a small quantity of effusion that is hardly demonstrated by chest X-ray; and (4) accurately and safely guiding puncture and drainage.

3.4 Fibrobronchoscopy

Principles of Fibrobronchoscopy

In a fibrobronchoscope, tens of thousands fiberglass with favorable light conductivity are orderly arranged whose both ends are fixed with ethoxyline resin to form light transmitting bundle and image guide bundle. The diameter of single fiber for light transmission is 15–30 m, while the diameter of single fiber for image guide is 5–20 m. The key point for light transmission and image guide is complete optical isolation of each fiberglass. That is to say, each fiberglass is coated with transparent substance with lower reflective index than the fiberglass to transmit light bundle along the fiberglass with no leakage. Therefore, the image from fibrobronchoscope is actually consisted of countless light spots. The fiberglass is subject to aging and rupture. When one fiberglass is broken, there is a black spot in the image guide bundle and thus the brightness of transmitted light is affected.

The Common Demonstrations of Bronchial TB by Fibrobronchoscopy

The mucosa of affected bronchus is demonstrated with congestion and edema. The interbronchial crest is widened and the cartilage rings are poorly defined. There is also bronchial lumen stenosis of different degrees.

On the mucosal surface of affected bronchus, there is erosion or singular/multiple ulcers, which may be covered by caseous substance or thick moss like secretions. The mucosal and submucosal congestion and edema are demonstrated around the ulcers.

The affected bronchus is demonstrated with mucosal and submucosal granuloma and accompanying luminal stenosis or obstruction. The lesions may be misdiagnosed as bronchogenic carcinoma.

Broncholymphatic fistula may be demonstrated and there are congestion and edema around the fistular orifice. When the patient coughs, caseous substances may be discharged from the fistular orifice. The old fistular orifice is demonstrated as small brownish depression.

The affected trachea and bronchus are demonstrated to be funnel shaped or even with occlusion due to obvious cicatricial stenosis. Meanwhile, the lesion may be complicated by irreversible atelectasis, which is commonly sequela of untreated or inappropriately treated serious tracheal or bronchial TB.

3.5 Serological Diagnosis

After years of studies on the serological diagnosis of TB, attempts have been made in the methodology, purified specific antigen, monoclonal antibody of the corresponding antigen, and recombinant antigen [37]. Serological diagnosis of TB is expected to provide valuable information on the diagnosis of Mtb negative TB, extrapulmonary TB, and pediatric TB. But the results are hardly satisfying. Multiple antigens have been defined in the serological diagnosis of TB, but the recombinant antigens have achieved unsatisfying results in the diagnosis of smear positive and smear negative TB [38–40]. And their clinical application is unpromising. Therefore, the serological diagnosis plays assistant role in the diagnosis of TB.

3.6 Detection of Cellular Immune Response

Anti-tuberculosis immunity is a T cell centered immune response participated by multiple immune cells. The activated T cells and macrophages play their roles in mediating immune responses via production of cytokines. The cytokines are a series of immune active factors with variant properties, sources, and effects, which form a highly efficient network. Based on the mechanism, the observation of cellular immune response and detection of cytokines, such as IFN-γ, TNF-a, Il-2, Il-4, I-12, and IL-10, in patients with suspected diagnosis of TB can provide significant data for the further diagnosis. And as the Th2T characteristic cytokine, IFN-γ has gained the most intensive scholarly attention in related scientific research [41, 42].

Generally speaking, bacteriological examination is the most reliable laboratory test for the diagnosis of TB. However, being the same as the other diagnostic techniques, bacteriological examination has its advantages and limitations. The clinicians should know well about the weight of each technique. Currently, the diagnosis of TB is still a comprehensive diagnosis based on the clinical face-to-face assessments. No laboratory test or diagnostic imaging can substitute the clinicians in diagnosing TB. Therefore, clinical experience plays important role in the diagnosis and treatment of TB.

References

1. Wang, C. Screening for biological markers specific to pulmonary tuberculosis and identification of genes responsible for its susceptibility. Zhejiang University, 2016.
2. Niemi R. A brief history of Mycobacterium tuberculosis' Etiology. [2018-11-9]. http://www.intellectualventureslab.com/invent/brief-mtb-history.
3. He GX, Wang LX. Evolution of strategies for tuberculosis control. Forum Prev Med. 2008;14(6):481–4.
4. World Health Organization. Global tuberculosis control: surveillance, planning, financing: WHO report 2006. Geneva: World Health Organization; 2006.
5. World Health Organization. Drug-resistant TB: surveillance & response: supplement to the global tuberculosis report 2014. Geneva: World Health Organization; 2014.
6. World Health Organization. Global tuberculosis report 2018. Geneva: World Health Organization; 2018.
7. World Health Organization. Global tuberculosis report 2017. Geneva: World Health Organization; 2017.
8. Tiemersma EW, Van Der Werf MJ, Borgdorff MW, et al. Natural history of tuberculosis: duration and fatality of untreated pulmonary tuberculosis in HIV negative patients: a systematic review. PLoS One. 2011;6(4):e17601.
9. World Health Organization. Tuberculosis: fact sheet. [2018-11-9]. http://www.who.int/mediacentre/factsheets/fs104/en/.
10. Wang LX, Cheng SM, Chen MT, et al. Report of the 5th national epidemiological sampling survey for tuberculosis in 2010. Chin J Anti-tuberc. 2012;8:485–508.
11. Technique Guidance Team of the National Epidemiological Sampling Survey for Tuberculosis. Report of the 4th national epidemiological sampling survey for tuberculosis. Chin J Tuberc Respir. 2002;1:6–10.

12. Duanmu HJ, Liu YX, Shi HS, et al. Data analysis of the 3rd national epidemiological sampling survey for tuberculosis. Dis Surv. 1995;7:215–7.
13. Leaders Team of the National Epidemiological Sampling Survey for Tuberculosis. Comprehensive brief of the national epidemiological sampling survey for tuberculosis in 1979. Chin J Anti-tuberc Commun. 1982;2:3–6.
14. Kan GQ, Zhang LX. Implications of the 2nd national epidemiological sampling survey for tuberculosis. Chin J Anti-tuberc Commun. 1989;3:97–101.
15. Song WH. Global emergency of tuberculosis and the control of TB in China. Chin J Epidemiol. 1997;18(2):109–11.
16. Liu YH, Jiang GL, Zhao LP, et al. The 4th national epidemiological sampling survey: analysis of drug resistance by Mycobacterium tuberculosis. Chin J Tuberc Respir. 2002;4:32–5.
17. Wang SF, Zhao B, Song YY, et al. The risk factors of drug resistant tuberculosis in China: data analysis of the national baseline survey for drug resistant tuberculosis in 2007. Chin J Anti-tuberc. 2013;4:221–6.
18. The Technique Guidance Team of the National Epidemiological Sampling Survey for Tuberculosis. Report of the national epidemiological sampling survey in 2000. Chin J Anti-tuberc. 2002;2:3–46.
19. Shen X, Song SC, Lei SG. Prevalence and control strategy for drug resistant tuberculosis. Occup Health. 2017;4:566–8.
20. Cheng SM. Current control of multidrug resistant tuberculosis and recommendations. Chin J Trop Med. 2017;3:213–5.
21. General Office of State Council, P. R. China. The national 13th five-year plan for prevention and treatment of tuberculosis. http://www.nhfpc.gov.cn/bgt/gwywj2/201702/7b2a362da2da4841a362f8eb36575b67.shtml.
22. Interpretation of the 2015 world tuberculosis report: evolution of control strategies for tuberculosis. http://www.chinatb.org/kxyj/gjkydt/201602/t20160223_125564.htm.
23. Implementing the End TB strategy: the essentials. http://www.who.int/tb/publications/2015/end_tb_essential.pdf?ua=1.
24. TheFirstGlobalMinisterialConferenceofWorldHealthOrganization. http://www.who.int/tb/endtb-sdg-ministerial-conference/zh/.
25. Li L, Liu YH, Ma Y, et al. Evolution of the service system for prevention and treatment of tuberculosis in China and its implications. Chin J Anti-tuberc. 2016;38(11):904–7.
26. Gao JH, Cen ZY, Tan YQ. Development in screening and control of tuberculosis in high-risk populations in China. J Youjiang Med. 2016;44(1):105–8.
27. National Anti-tuberculosis Association of China. Standard procedures in the bacteriological diagnosis of tuberculosis. Chin J Anti-tuberc. 1996;18:28–31.
28. Pan YX, Wu W. Molecular markers for bacteriological surveillance during treatment of tuberculosis. Chin J Tuberc Respir. 2001;24:393–5.
29. Chen XY. Research progress of tuberculosis diagnosis. Chin J Clin. 2013;41(3):11–4.
30. Zhang TM. Sub-clinical tuberculous sepsis. Chin J Tuberc Respir. 2001;24:622–4.
31. Mithison DA. The action of antituberculosis drug in short-course chemotherapy. Tubercle. 1985;66:219–25.
32. Van Grietnuysen AJ, JaMorgan MA, Horstmeier CD, et al. Comparison of a radiometric method (bactec) and conventional culture media for recovery of mycobacteria from smear-negative specimens. J Clin Microb. 1983;18:384–8.
33. Nsz AR, Buiting AGM. Comparison of fluorescent Bactec 9000MB system, Septi Check AFB system and LowersteinJensen medium for detection of mycobacteria. J Clin Microb. 1996;34:2391–4.
34. Chen XY, Wang HP, Jin YS, et al. Detection of Mycobacterium tuberculosis DNA by Taqman PCR and its clinical application. Chin J Tuberc Respir. 2000;23(5):284–8.
35. Han XQ, Ma Y, Gao WW, et al. Detection of drug resistant Mycobacterium tuberculosis by bacteriophage biological amplification, DNA sequence analysis and single-strand conformation polymorphism analysis. Chin J Tuberc Respir. 2004;27:815–9.
36. Hu ZY, Ni LD, Jin AJ, et al. Methodological study on rapid detection of Mycobacterium tuberculosis by bacteriophage biological amplification. Chin J Tuberc Respir. 2004;27:801–5.
37. Xie LMY, Gao WW, et al. Significance of interferon-γ release from mononuclear cells of peripheral blood after antigen stimulation in the diagnosis of Mycobacterium tuberculosis infection. Chin J Tuberc Respir. 2005;28:545–9.
38. Aubert-Pivert EM, Chedeverge FM, Lopez-Ramirez GM, et al. Cytokine transcripts in pediatric tuberculosis: a study with bronchoalveolar cells. Tuber Lung Dis. 2000;80:249–58.
39. Campos-Neto A, Rodrigues-Junior V, Pedral-Samparo DB, et al. Evaluation of DPPD, a single recombinant Mycobacterium tuberculosis protein as an alternative antigen for the Mantoux test. Tuberculosis. 2001;81(5-6):353–8.
40. David ST, Mukunkan U, Brahmadath KW, et al. Detecting mycobacterium for diagnosing tuberculosis. Indian J Med Res. 2004;119:259–66.
41. Ewer K, Deeks J, Alvarez L, et al. Comparison of T-cell-based assay with tuberculin skin test for diagnosis of Mycobacterium tuberculosis infection in a school tuberculosis outbreak. Lancet. 2003;361:1168–73.
42. Houghton RL, Lodes M, Dillon DC, et al. Use of multiepitope polyproteins in serodiagnosis of active tuberculosis. Clin Diagn Lab Immunol. 2000;9:883–91.

Epidemiology of Tuberculosis in Migrating Population

2

Yun-xia Wang, Mei-juan Zhang, Juan-juan Zhang, Qing-fang Wu, and Li-ai Peng

1 Status Quo of the Migrating Population

1.1 Overview of the Migrating Population

So far, there has been no consistent scholarly definition for the migrating population. *Report of Population Migration in China across the Century and the migrating Population* issued by Population Institute, Renmin University of China defined the migrating population as population living in the county or subdistrict for more than 6 months with registered permanent residence at the same place or living in the county or subdistrict for no more than 6 months but not at the place with registered permanent residence for more than 6 months subtracting those the population with the registered permanent residence at the other county or subdistrict in the city [1]. The definition of migrating population emphasizes the registered permanent residence, period of time, and living place. The migrating population refers to the specific migrating population with changed living place but no corresponding change of the registered permanent residence. Therefore, the migrating population is technically the population with changed living place with no corresponding change of the registered permanent residence, namely population with separated living place and registered permanent residence with exceptions of those migrating populations for schooling, travelling, visiting relatives and friends, and participating in the military army. The migrating population is closely related to the policies of registered permanent residence. In a broad sense, the migrating population refers to those leaving the place of registered permanent residence and living in another place. And in a narrow sense, the migrating population refers to those migrating people spontaneously participating in socioeconomic activities to make a living with exceptions of those with a short-term stay at a place rather than their living place [2]. The occupations that the migrating population commonly engages in include manufacturing (such as architecture, factories, and mining industry), transporting, agriculture, forest industry, commercial, and service industry.

The policy of registered permanent residence in China renders co-existence of the migrating population and the population with changed registered permanent residence. And in most other countries, such distinction does not exist. Therefore, in the international scholarly society, some pairs of concepts are applied in the studies of population migration in China, such as permanent migration and temporary migration, migration with registered permanent residence, and migration with no registered permanent residence, official migration, and non-official migration. The latter terms of these three pairs of concepts are the migrating population. Population migration and non-permanent migration are not characteristic of China. Internationally, studies on circulation of population in developing countries are active. The studies revealed that circulation of population is a common phenomenon in developing countries that is commonly covered by routine data [3]. And the policy of registered permanent residence and its related policies are not the only reason for temporary living of the migrating population at a place with no registered permanent residence [4]. In the countries with no policy of registered permanent residence, the abilities of migrating population and their families as well as configuration strategy of family resource and interests between the places of influx and their original living place are factors limiting the circulation and migration of populations. In addition, innate fluctuation of labor market at the influx place due to the change of market needs, separation of the labor market between the capital intensive primary sectors and labor intensive secondary sectors, and the corresponding employment strategy of the enterprises are all factors influencing the migration and circulation of migrating population.

Y.-x. Wang (✉) · M.-j. Zhang · J.-j. Zhang · L.-a. Peng
Baoan Chronic Diseases Prevent and Cure Hospital, Shenzhen, Guangdong, China

Q.-f. Wu
Shenzhen Center for Chronic Disease Control, Shenzhen, Guangdong, China

W.-y. Yu et al. (eds.), *Tuberculosis Control in Migrating Population*, https://doi.org/10.1007/978-981-32-9763-0_2

1.2 Migration of Population in the Developed Countries

In the period of mid-nineteenth century to mid-twentieth century, the main developed countries experienced the process of rapid urbanization. There have been large-scale migrations of populations during the rapid industrialization and urbanization in these developed countries. And the direction of population migration was in consistent to the direction of industrial development and industrial agglomeration. In the 1980s of the twentieth century, about 2.5–3 million people worldwide migrated into another country and the tendency has been no signs of attenuation [4, 5].

In the migrating migrant workers of the USA, 74% visited clinics once or twice during the past 3 years, 22% never visited clinics, and 61% were deprived of health-care service by laws. However, the federal government has paid enough attention to the prevention and treatment of TB in the migrating migrant workers [6, 7]. A survey in the USA revealed that 20% of the 313 patients with active TB are illegal immigrant and 6% of the patients are afraid of troubles from the immigration office and dares not to see a doctor [7].

The migration population living in urban and rural areas of Australia has been increasing, which is partially because immigration plan was introduced and expanded in some states and regions by the Australian government. The immigration plan was in response to the comment on the living environments and societies of immigrants in rural and urban areas in Australia. The approximate data about size of immigration populations in urban and rural areas of Australia, labor force participation rate and unemployment rate of Australian born population, median of weekly income per person, and percentage of highly skilled occupation were released. The difference of education level in immigrants was the most significant, with the education level in urban immigrants far higher than that in other populations, especially university education. The gender difference in the immigrants was much higher than that in Australian born population. In recent years, the education level, occupational skills, and incomes of Australian immigrants showed significant increase.

1.3 Migration Populations in the Developing Countries of Africa and Latin America

Along with the reform of social and political policies in Africa, the imbalance of regional economic development has been aggravating and the allocation of productive force has been changed. The population has been migrating at an unprecedented speed in Africa, which, to a large extent, changed the spatial distribution of population in Africa. The migration of population in Africa is characterized by migration towards the economic zones, coastal areas as well as industrial and mining centers. The developments of industry, agriculture, and transportation in coastal areas give rise to more employment opportunities to the migrating population, which intensely attract the flow of inland population into the coastal areas. The flow of population is especially obvious in the western Africa. And the population rapidly flows into the copper mine areas, such as Zaire and Zambia, gold and diamond mine area of southern Africa, and oil patches in northern Africa and Nigeria. In addition, large rural population in Africa migrates into urban areas, which accelerates urbanization in Africa. With migration of large rural population into cities, many countries in Africa have been facing some serious socioeconomic and public health issues, such as shortage of housing, unemployment, traffic jams, environmental deterioration, insecurity, and insufficient health-care resources.

Based on insufficient industrialization in Latin America, migration of rural population into cities and the excessive concentration of population cause the phenomenon of over urbanization. An overview to Latin American indicated that the urban population increased by 45.2% in the 1950s of the twentieth century, 45% in 1960–1970, 43.6% in 1970–1980, and 40.3% in 1980–1990. The urban population has expanded to more than 0.3 billion in 1990 from 30 million in 1930 [8]. In the USA, the percentage of urban population increased from 30% to 70% within almost 100 years, while it reached the same percentage in Brazil within 40 years [9]. Over urbanization is also characterized by more rapid urbanization than industrialization. Although the urbanization in Latin America is driven by industrialization, the development of industrialization is far slower than the urbanization. The economic development lags far behind the migration of population and labors. Till mid of 1970s in the twentieth century, the urban population in Latin America accounted for 60% of the total population, while the industrial population accounted for less than 20–30% [10]. The lagging of industrialization behind the urbanization causes serious social problems, such as insufficient employment opportunities for rapid inflow of population and labors within a short period of time. Therefore, the population migrating into cities commonly lives in poverty due to unemployment or semi-employment. They cannot obtain stable income and social security. In addition to poverty and unemployment, over urbanization also causes urban environmental pollution, traffic jams, insecurity, and insufficient supplies of electricity and water. The incidence rates of poverty, drug abuse, robbery, and raping are comparatively high in slum areas. And the increasingly serious social problems, to some extent, negatively affect the development of urban and even national economy.

In south-east Asia, many people in Indonesia work at one place, while consume and invest at another place. These people keep double identities for a long period of time. On the Djawa island of Indonesia, at least one person works in cities for a certain period of time in 25% farmer families. And the total number amounts to 3.75 million. Another survey in 37 villages on the Djawa island in 1992–1993 revealed that in most families, there is at least one person working in cities and they work in cities via non-permanent migration. Actually, from the 1970s to 1990s of the twentieth century, the scale and importance of circulating population have been increasing [11].

1.4 Status Quo of Migrating Population in China

Compared to developed countries and many developing countries, the studies on migrating population started late. Before the implementation of reform and open up policy, population migration had been strictly controlled in China. Non-permanent migration of population after implementation of reform and open up policy in China has emerged in many developing countries [12].

China is a country with vast land, with great variance in provincial economic development. Therefore, the migrating population in each province shows different features. The east coastal cities are the place of population influx, while the under-developed middle-west area is the original resident place of the migrating population. Along with the development of socialist market economy, the migrating population has been increasingly large. They leave their places of registered permanent residence for better lives [13]. A survey by the National Bureau of Statistics of P. R. China indicated that the interprovincial migrating population is nearly 40 million, with predominantly young and middle-aged adults. The migrating population aged between 15 and 35 years accounts for above 80% of the total migrating population, with an average age of 27.9 years. In the migrating population, 86.7% has registered permanent residence in rural areas. And they are engaged in low-salary or high-risk occupations, such as manufacturing, wholesale and retail, architecture, mining, and service industry. A sampling survey of the migrating population in six cities of China conducted in 2004 indicated that the migrating population with a monthly income of under ¥1000 accounts for above 90% of the total migrating population, and about 45% of the migrating population has a monthly income of under ¥500. The survey revealed that the majority of the migrating population in the influx cities is low-income population, compared to income of local labor. Meanwhile, the housing of the migrating population is mainly dormitory, self-rent, and shared rent, with extremely percentage of self-purchase apartment.

Shenzhen is the pioneering city in the reform and open up of China, which is closely adjacent to Hong Kong and Macao. Labor intensive industries, such as processing trade, electronics, clothing, and toys, are densely distributed in Shenzhen, which have attracted a large migrating population. Therefore, Shenzhen has become the city with the largest migrating population in China. According to the recent statistics on population in Shenzhen, the population with registered permanent residence in Shenzhen is only 3.67 million, the population with registered permanent residence plus the migrating population is 10.77 million. But the managed population reaches 20 million. The high mobility of population in Shenzhen increases the incidence of TB.

The migrating population is one of the vulnerable groups. They work at high-risk workplace with low socioeconomic status. Their accessibility to health-care service is poor and the majority of migrating population has insufficient knowledge about health and incorrect knowledge about infectious diseases. And their health care seeking behaviors are not good enough to protect them from diseases. Therefore, the migrating population commonly encounters delayed diagnosis and thus unfavorable therapeutic effects, which further develop into serious outcomes. So far, the public health issues emerging along with influx of large migrating population are highly emphasized by national and local governments. Along with socioeconomic development, the attention to the migrating population has been increasing and the related policies have been implementing. The strategies for prevention and control of TB in accordance with epidemiological data of TB in each country have been formulated, improved, and implemented.

2 Prevalence of TB in Migrating Population

2.1 Prevalence of TB in Migrating Population

Migrating population is a global issue. According to a report by the United Nations, the migrating population has reached 244 million in 2015 worldwide [14]. TB in migrating population has been a major challenge in control and stop TB strategy in countries with high TB burden and even in countries with low incidence of TB. In the 30 countries with low incidence of TB, including Canada, Cuba, Israel, Jamaica, Jordan, and New Zealand [15], the incidence of TB has been decreasing in local residents but increasing in the migrating population. And the increase of TB incidence is positively related to the enlargement of migrating population. A molecular epidemiological study in European Union revealed that the cross infection of TB between migrating population and local residents are bidirectional. Studies have demonstrated that the infection rate of TB from migrating population to local residents is 18.3% and 5.8%, respectively, while the infection rate of TB from local residents to migrating population is 16% and 7.9%, respectively. In rarely countries, the infection of TB from migrating population to local residents is zero or extremely limited.

In the USA, a country with a large migration population, the incidence rate of TB remains low. In 2017, the incidence rate of TB in the USA is only 2.8 per 0.1 million. But the USA is also facing the challenge of TB in migrating population [16]. According to statistics, 69.8% of patients with TB in 2017 are in the migrating population and the incidence rate of TB in the migrating population is 15 times as high as that in local residents. In Canada, the situation is almost the same. The incidence rate of TB in the migrating population is 23 times as high as that in the local residents. Patients with TB in the migrating population account for 90% of all the patients with TB.

The TB burden in the European Union should also be paid close attention, with an obviously higher incidence rate of TB in the migrating population than that of local residents [17]. In France, the incidence rate of TB is 9 times as high as that in the local residents, being 35.1 per 0.1 million and 4.3 per 0.1 million, respectively. In Britain, the incidence rate of TB in the migrating population increased from 75.5 per 0.1 million in 2000 to 81.6 per 0.1 million in 2010. But the incidence rate of TB in the local residents of Britain remained 4 per 0.1 million during the same period of time. Generally speaking, the epidemics of TB in the European Union have been decreasing. But since 2001, the percentage of patients with TB in the migrating population has been increasing. Till 2010, 25.1% patients with TB are from the migrating population in the total number of reported cases, which are rarely distributed in the north and east Europe. The percentages of patients with TB in migrating population show national variance, ranging from 0.2% in Romania to 85.8% in Sweden. The percentages of patients with TB in the migrating population in Cyprus, Ice Island, Malta, Holland, Norway, and Sweden are 82.0%, 72.7%, 78.1%, 73.5%, 85.3%, and 85.8%, respectively. The total number of patients with TB in the migrating population in the six countries accounts for above 70% in the total number of patients with TB in the European Union. The percentages of patients with TB in the migrating population in Belgium (54.6%), Denmark (60.2%), Estonia (6.6%), Germany (45.7%), Luxembourg (58.6%), and Silvigna (23.8%) have been decreasing in recent decades.

The 36 countries in the Western Pacific Region are the countries with heavy TB burden, with the patients of TB account for 23% of the global TB burden. And 97.6% of the patients with TB are new cases or relapse cases. In the Western Pacific Region, the patients with TB in China account for 62%, followed by Philippines and Vietnam, being 18% and 7.4%, respectively, with great regional variance of the TB report rate.

In China, a country with heavy TB burden, TB in the migrating population is a challenge to the prevention and control of TB. Along with the implementation of reform and open up policy, a large number of peasant workers have flowed into the coastal cities from the villages in the middle west part of China. Due to poor housing and economic conditions as well as high intensity of labor, the migrating population of peasant workers constitutes the high-risk population of TB in the densely populated cities. And the incidence rate of TB in the migrating population of peasant workers remains higher than that in the local residents of the cities [18, 19]. Due to their high mobility, low socioeconomic status, and insufficient knowledge about prevention and treatment of TB, the drug resistance rate of TB remains high in the migrating population. In addition to the low cure rate and high risk of spreading TB, TB in the migrating population is a challenge to the prevention and control of TB in China. According to statistics, the registered number of TB patients in the migrating population of China is around 70,000/year, accounting for around 8% of the total registered number of TB patients in China. In the economically developed cities, such as Beijing and Shanghai, the percentage of registered TB patients in the migrating population reaches as high as above 43% [20]. The new cases of smear-positive TB in the migrating population account for 7% of the total new cases of smear-positive TB in China [21] and the percentage has been increasing by 9.4% each year [22]. In Zhejiang province of China, the new cases of TB in the population of registered permanent residence have been decreasing, while the percentage of new cases in the migrating population has been increasing each year, from 20.26% in 2005 to 36.45% in 2011. Based on the data, it has been demonstrated that the main reason for slowly decreasing incidence of TB in China is the increasing incidence of TB in the migrating population. In addition, the new registry rate of TB patients and the new registry rate of smear-positive TB patients in the migrating population are commonly higher than those in local residents. And the 2-month negative conversion rate in smear-positive TB patients and cure rate of TB are lower than those in local residents. In 2001 and 2002, the new registry rates of smear-positive TB in the migrating population of Zhejiang, China were 311.6 per million and 312.7 per million, respectively, which were 2.03 times and 1.62 times as high as those in the local residents, respectively [23]. In Panyu district of Guangzhou, the 2-month negative conversion rate of smear-positive TB in the migrating population is 83.3% and the cure rate is 84.97%, which were lower than those in the local residents, being 89.0% and 91.0%, respectively.

2.2 Prevalence of TB in Migrating Population

Temporal Distribution

Temporal distribution of a disease provides important reference for general prevention and control of diseases. In addition, the temporal distribution of a disease facilitates the allocation of limited resources at different stages of a disease to avoid outbreak of a certain disease. TB is a chronic infectious disease, with report of cases all year round. Due to regional variance in climate and geographic environment, the number of reported cases of TB shows seasonal variance. Most studies have demonstrated a seasonal peak of TB, which is mainly in springs and summers. And in most countries and regions, the incidence of TB is the type of single peak, with rare occurrence of double peaks. In Hong Kong of China, the peak incidence of TB is in summer. But in Spain, the peak incidence of TB is in summers and autumns and in Japan, in springs and summers. In the north India, the incidence peak of TB is in April to June and the incidence valley of TB is in November and December, with obvious seasonal fluctuation. But in the south India, the incidence of TB shows no seasonal fluctuation. The seasonal variance of its incidence in one region does not represent the national incidence. And the seasonal variance in different regions may be different. Rare studies have been reported on the seasonal distribution of TB in the migrating population.

In China, the incidence of TB remains stable all year round. But due to the traditional custom of family union at the Spring Festival, a large population flow from large cities into their hometown in the end of each year and go back to large cities at the beginning of the new year. Such flow of population constitutes the characteristically Chinese migration of population once a year. Because of the Chinese migration of population, the reported cases of TB at the beginning and end of a year comparatively decrease, with a temporal distribution of low incidence at the beginning and end of a year but high incidence during the other months of a year [24]. Du et al. [21] reported the monthly registry change of smear-positive TB patients in the migrating population in China. The study revealed that the number of monthly registry reaches the highest during April to June, with monthly registry being up to above 10% of the yearly registry, and the number of registry is the lowest in February.

Regional Distribution

The geographic distribution of TB cases can also reflect the geographic and spatial changes of human migration. In Britain, 57% of the patients with TB in the migrating population is from south Asia, while another 27% from sub-Saharan Africa. In Holland, the patients of pulmonary TB in the migrating population are mainly from Somalia, Morocco and Turkey. In Italy, 36.6% of the patients with TB in the migrating population is from middle east Asia and another 21.7% from Africa [17]. But in the USA, the original countries of the patients with TB in the migrating population include Mexico (19.0%), Philippines (12.3%), India (9.4%), Vietnam (8.3%), and China (6.3%) [16].

China is a country with vast land and regional variance of TB is obvious. Especially due to the dual structure of urban and rural areas and socioeconomic discrepancies between the east and the west, a large population flows from under-developed west to well-developed east and from villages to cities. And the problem of TB in the migrating population is significant. Jia et al. [20] reported that most TB patients with no registered permanent residence at their living place agglomerate in the eastern coastal area and thus the east coastal area is the key area for prevention and control of TB in the migrating population in China. Beijing, Tianjin, and Shanghai are the most seriously affected areas of TB in the migrating population [21]. Among new cases of smear-positive TB in the migrating population in China, 68% is from the east area. In the areas of Beijing, Tianjin, and Shanghai, the new cases of smear-positive TB in the migrating population account for 39.1% of all the new cases of smear-positive TB in the three areas. The obviously increasing incidence of TB in the migrating population gradually aggravates the epidemics of TB in Beijing. Liu et al. [25] studied the provincial distribution of patients with TB in the migrating population. The study revealed that the patients with TB in the migrating population mainly inflow into Guangdong, Zhejiang, Jiangsu, Shanghai, Fujian, and Beijing, accounting for 84.7% of the total number of patients with TB in the migrating population. The patients with TB in the migrating population mainly outflow from Sichuan, Guizhou, Hunan, Hubei, Anhui, Jiangxi, Chongqing, and Jiangsu, accounting for 71.5% of the total number of patients with TB in the migrating population. Therefore, the middle-west area is the main original place of patients with TB in the migrating population and the east coastal area is the main influx place of patients with TB in the migrating population. Meanwhile, 40% of patients with TB in the migrating population migrate within provinces, including Guangdong, Shandong, Henan, Jiangsu, Sichuan, Fujian, Zhejiang, and Guangxi Zhuang Autonomous Region. What cannot be ignored is that the reported cases of TB in the west area of China have been increasing during recent 2 years. Along with the implementation of action plans on Western Development and the China-proposed Belt and Road Initiative, more and more migrating workers are employed in the west area of China and the population tends to migrate into large cities in the west area of China. The tendency of migration indicated that we should pay close attention to the prevention and control of TB in the migrating population in large cities of the west area of China. Spread of TB should be prevented in the population.

Populations Distribution

Due to special features of the migrating population, the distribution of TB in the migrating population shows populations variance from TB in the local residents.

Age Distribution

Knowledge about age distribution of a disease facilitates protection of a specific age population and discovery of high-risk population. In addition, knowledge about age distribution of a disease provides a basis for prevention and control of a disease. Due to different immunity and exposure of different age groups, the incidence of TB shows variance in different age groups. In the European Union, patients with TB in the migrating population are mainly young adults, with more than 50% being aged 25–44 years, while more than 50% of patients with TB in local residents are aged above 45 years. The average age of patients with TB in the local residents is 46.3 years, while in the migrating population, 37.5 years. The patients with TB in the migrating population are almost 9 years younger than the patients with TB in local residents.

In the patients with TB in the migrating population of China, the age group of 15–55 years accounts for the largest percentage, being 88.9% [21], with a mean of 30.8 ± 16.9 years [26]. And in patients with TB in the migrating population of China, the age group of 20–39 years accounts for 75.8% [23]. This is probably because the age group is the main body of the migrating population. But in patients with TB in the local residents, middle-aged and elderly patients show a higher percentage. Meanwhile, the patients with TB in the migrating population are the main labors of families and their outflow is for higher income and better life of their families. During recent years, along with aggravating aging of population, the percentage of the age group of 55–74 years is increasing in patients with TB [27].

There have been rare studies on age distribution of TB in the migrating population in the western Pacific area. But the study on the whole population revealed that the reported cases of TB have been increasing along with increase of age, with exception of Mongolia. The reported cases of TB are the least in age group of 0–14 years, especially in Vietnam the unweighed mean of reported cases in both males and females is 0.68 per 0.1 million per year. In the populations with age of above 15 years in the western Pacific area, the variance of TB reporting rate is the least in Mongolia, with the highest TB reporting rate (in the age group of 55–64 years) being 1.1 times as high as the lowest TB reporting rate (in the age group of ≥65 years) in male patients. In Laos, the TB reporting rate shows the greatest variance, with the highest TB reporting rate (in the age group of ≥65 years) being 17 times as high as the lowest TB reporting rate (in the age group of 15–24 years) in male patients.

In the countries with high TB burden in the western Pacific area, the TB reporting rate of new bacteriologically defined cases has decreased in all the age groups (0–14 years, 15–24 years, 25–34 years, 35–44 years, 45–54 years, 55–64 years, and ≥65 years) from 2000 to 2013. But the TB reporting rate of new bacteriologically defined cases remained stable in the 3 younger age groups (0–14 years, 15–24 years, and 25–34 years) of female patients in Vietnam, while it decreased in the other 4 elder age groups (35–44 years, 45–54 years, 55–64 years, and ≥65 years). In Philippines, the report rates of bacteriologically defined new cases in younger groups (0–14 years, 15–24 years, and 25–34 years) have been increasing along with age, while those in elder groups (35–44 years, 45–54 years, 55–64 years, and ≥65 years) have been decreasing along with age. However, the report rate in the age group of ≥65 years is close to that in the age group of 45–54 years. In China, the report rate of bacteriologically defined new cases shows significant gender difference. The report rate in males has been increasing along with age. But in females, the report rate in age group of 15–24 years has been close to that in the age group of 55–64 years. In Mongolia and Papua New Guinea, the report rate does not show a tendency to increase or decrease along with age.

Gender Difference

Due to gender differences in socioeconomic behaviors, social backgrounds, and expected roles, males and females are at different disease risks. More and more studies indicated that gender is an important factor influencing epidemic of diseases as well as their prevention and treatment. The gender difference in distribution of TB exists extensively in different countries and regions, which may be attributed to its collaborative effects with biological and sociological factors.

Men take more responsibilities in personal, family, and social lives and they participate in more intense physical labor than women. In addition, they are more susceptible to unfavorable personal habits such as smoking and alcoholism. All of these may cause compromised immunity to fight against diseases. Therefore, the incidence rate of TB is higher in males than in females. The data of the West Pacific Region and countries of high TB burden in the region in 2013 indicated that the bacteriologically defined new cases of TB in males are more than those in females, with a gender ratio of 2.2:1. The ratio of bacteriologically defined new cases of TB in males to females is the highest in Vietnam, being 2.9:1, while the lowest in Cambodia, being 1.2:1. In migrating population, the reported incidence of TB is also higher in males than in females. The data from European Union or European Economic Area in 2010 indicated that the reported incidence of TB shows a gender ratio of 2:1 and the ratio is 1.5:1 in the migrating population [17].

In China, the trend is similar. The percentage of male patients with TB in migrating population is significantly higher than that of female patients, with a gender ratio of about 2:1 [23, 26]. The gender ratio is the highest in Zhejiang province of China, being 2.12:1. Along with economic development, especially the development of service industry, the percentage of female patients with TB in migrating population is higher than that of female patients in local residents.

Race Difference

The patients with TB in migrating population also show race difference. Take the USA as an example [16], in the migration populations in the USA, the incidence rate of TB is the highest in Asian Americans (27 per 0.1 million), followed by non-Latino black Americans (22 per 0.1 million). In the local residents of the USA, black Americans account for the highest percentage in patients with TB (37.1%), followed by Latino white Americans (29.5%).

Occupation Distribution

In China, as an important part of city populations, the migrating population commonly participate in temporary jobs at the building sites and factories. Therefore, the patients with TB in the migrating population are mostly workers (including peasant workers), accounting for 47.8%; and more patients with TB in the migrating population work in industries of domestic service and are unemployed. A study also demonstrated that unemployed migrating population accounts for the highest percentage of patients with TB in the migrating population, followed by peasants and peasant workers [27]. Another study in Chongqing of China indicated that the percentage of peasant workers has been decreasing in patients with TB in migrating population, while the percentages of students, peasants, waiters, and waitresses, and those unemployed in domestic service have been increasing. In patients with TB in the migrating population, the labor workers account for 48.9% [26], with 89.6% working in industries of architecture, crop farming, and other temporary jobs [23].

Percentage of New Smear-Positive TB Patients in the Migrating Population

Due to the spread of TB along with droplets from respiratory tract, the smear-positive TB patients are the main source of infection of TB. The high percentage of smear-positive TB patients, to some extent, aggravates the spreading of TB. A study in Shenzhen of China indicated that the new smear-positive TB patients account for 44.8% [28]. Meanwhile, due to the high mobility of the migrating population, the new smear-positive TB patients constitute the mobile source of infection, which aggravates the spreading of Mtb in different populations.

Patients with TB in the Migrating Population are Mainly Initially Treated Patients

In China, patients with TB in the migrating population are mainly initially treated patients. In Shenzhen, one of the most densely distributed place for migrating population in China [28], the initially treated patients with TB account for as high as 90.61% in patients with TB in migrating population. That is probably because they are mostly healthy when they leave the place of their registered permanent residence. Another reason for the high percentage of initially treated patients in migrating population may be that most patients with TB may choose to stay at the place of their registered permanent residence or go back to the place of their registered permanent residence after retreatment.

3 Surveillance of TB

Surveillance of TB is to describe the epidemic of TB and its changes as well as to assess the prevention and control strategies of TB based on systematic analysis of consecutive systematic long-term collection of data. Surveillance of TB is intended to provide important reference for predicting the prevalence of TB and formulating effective strategies and measures to prevent and control TB.

3.1 Surveillance of TB Prevalence

Data about the infection, incidence, morbidity, and mortality of TB is acquired via routine report of TB prevalence, epidemiological survey, study of typical epidemic, study of implementation, and site of surveillance.

Routine Report of TB Prevalence

On September 20, 1978, the Ministry of Health in China issued Regulations of Acute Infectious Diseases in P. R. China, which classified acute infectious diseases into class A and class B, and tuberculosis fell into none of the categories. On July 20, 1982, the Ministry of Health in China issued the National Tuberculosis Control Planning in 1981–1990, which required improvement of the registry and reporting system of TB in the regions and areas with TB control agencies within 2–3 years. On May 10, 1984, the Ministry of Health in China issued the Interim Regulations for Prevention and Control of Tuberculosis, which stipulated the implementation of registry and reporting policy of TB for knowledge about its epidemic changes. On February 21, 1989, the Standing Committee of the National People's Congress issued the Law of People's Republic of China on Prevention and Treatment of Infectious *Diseases*, in which tuberculosis was categorized into class C of the notifiable infectious diseases. On February 28, 1996, the CDC of the Ministry of Health in China issued the Notice on Further Reinforcement for Prevention and Control of Tuberculosis, in which TB was listed as one of the class B infectious diseases. Revisited by the Standing Committee of the National People's Congress on August 28, 2004, the Law of People's Republic of China on Prevention and Treatment of Tuberculosis was implemented on December 1, 2004, in which TB was enlisted as one of class B notifiable infectious diseases. Since early 1980s of the twentieth century, the epidemic of TB had been reported by using paper cards. In 2004, the Infectious Diseases Reporting Management System was developed and the epidemic of TB has been reporting on-line.

In early 1980s of the twentieth century in Shenzhen, the epidemic of TB was reported by using paper cards. In 1995, the Disease Control Information Management System of Shenzhen was developed by the Center for Disease Control in Shenzhen, which was revisited and upgraded in 1998 and 2000. In 2002, an internet on-line reporting system of infectious diseases (including tuberculosis) was established and cases of infectious diseases (including tuberculosis) have been reporting on-line by health-care institutions in Shenzhen since then. And Shenzhen is one of the earliest cities with internet on-line reporting system of infectious diseases in China. Since then, the TB control agencies can obtain the real-time report about detection and death of tuberculosis for rapid response to sudden outbreak of TB. In addition, early detection, early report, and early control can be achieved. Since 2004, the National Infectious Diseases Reporting Information Management System has been applied by health-care institutions in Shenzhen for real-time on-line reporting of infectious diseases.

Basis of Reporting

Tuberculosis is one of the 39 notifiable infectious diseases and is managed as one of the class B infectious diseases. According to the Law of People's Republic of China on Prevention and Treatment of Infectious Diseases [29], the Technical Guideline for National Infectious Diseases Information Reporting Management [30], and the Diagnosis of Pulmonary Tuberculosis [31], the cases of pulmonary tuberculosis should be reported via internet on-line reporting system within specified period of time.

Data of Reporting

The onset and death of pulmonary tuberculosis should be reported. The reported data includes the name, gender, date of birth or chronological age, valid ID No., company or organization, emergency contact telephone number, and residence of the patient. The relationship between the patient and the reporting health care institution should be reported as one of the followings: (1) in the same county or district; (2) in the different county or district but in the same city; (3) in the different city but in the same province; (4) in the different province; (5) the patient lives in Hong Kong or Macao of China; (6) the patient is a foreigner. The detailed address of residence of the patient should be reported. And the categorization of population of the patient should also be reported as one of the followings: (1) nursery children; (2) children taken care of at home; (3) students (university, middle school, or primary school); (4) teachers; (5) child care workers or house maids; (6) workers in catering or food industries; (7) workers in commercial service; (8) health care workers; (9) workers working in factories; (10) peasant workers; (11) farmers; (12) herdsmen; (13) fishing population; (14) office staffs; (15) the retired population; (16) housewives or unemployed; and (17) the others including unspecified. In addition, the categorization of the case should be reported as one of the followings: (1) suspected cases; (2) clinically diagnosed cases; and (3) definitively diagnosed cases. The classification of TB should be reported as one of the followings: (1) rifampicin resistant; (2) smear positive; (3) culture positive only; (4) bacteriologically negative; (5) sputum undetected; and (6) simplex tuberculous pleurisy. In addition to the above data, the date of onset, the date and time of diagnosis, the date of death, the name of reporting health-care institution, the name of reporting clinician, the date of reporting, and the close contacts of the patient should also be reported.

Quality Control

Based on the quality assessment function of the Infectious Diseases Reporting Information Management System, the timely reporting rate, timely review rate, duplicate reporting rate, and the other indices of pulmonary TB reporting in each district and the city of Shenzhen are assessed monthly. The reports are exported monthly for statistical data of the completeness of ID card No. and the completeness of telephone numbers. The quality of pulmonary TB reporting is assessed regularly in each health-care institutions in Shenzhen. The staffs working in the TB control agencies are trained regularly about the knowledge and technical procedures of pulmonary TB reporting. The pulmonary TB reporting management of the health-care institutions in Shenzhen is assessed on-site quarterly based on the Quality Assessment Standards on Public Health-care Service in Shenzhen and the Responsibilities of Public Health-care Service in Shenzhen. The pulmonary TB reporting management in one randomly chosen health-care institution is assessed on-site each year by an experts committee organized by the Health Commission of Shenzhen.

Commonly Selected Indices in Quality Assessment

Annual Infection Rate of TB

The annual infection rate of TB is the frequency of natural Mtb infection within a certain population in one region during 1 year, which is represented by %.

Annual infection rate of TB (%) = Total number of natural Mtb infections during 1 year/average annual population of the year × 100

Reporting Incidence of TB

The reporting incidence of TB is the reporting frequency of TB within a certain population in one region during a certain period of time (commonly a year), which is represented by 1/0.1 million.

Reporting incidence of TB (per 0.1 million) = number of reported cases of TB/average annual population of the year × 100,000

Reporting Mortality of TB

The reporting mortality of TB is the frequency of deaths from TB within a certain population in one region during a certain period of time (commonly 1 year), which is represented by 1/0.1 million.

Reporting mortality of TB (per 0.1 million) = number of reported deaths from TB/average annual population of the year × 100,000

Percentage Increase/Decrease of Reported Cases of TB

The percentage increase/decrease of reported cases of TB is the percentage increase/decrease of reported cases of TB during a certain period of time (1 year or 1 month) compared to the number during the previous period of time (1 year or 1 month).

Percentage increase/decrease of reported cases of TB (%) = [reported cases of TB during a certain period of time (1 year or 1 month) − reported cases of TB during the previous period of time (1 year or 1 month)]/reported cases of TB during the previous period of time (1 year or 1 month) × 100

TB Reporting Rate

TB reporting rate is harvested by survey on-site. It is the percentage of internet on-line reporting cases of TB within one region or one health-care institution during a certain period of time in the total number of diagnosed cases of TB during the same period of time, which is represented by %.

TB reporting rate (%) = internet on-line reporting cases of TB/total number of diagnosed cases of TB × 100

Timely Reporting Rate of TB

The timely reporting rate of TB is the frequency of timely reporting cases of TB in the total number of internet on-line reported cases of TB within one region or one health-care institution, which is represented by %. Timely reporting of TB refers to completion of internet on-line reporting of TB within 24 h after the diagnosis. The range of its quality assessment includes primary reporting data, revisited reporting data, and deleted reporting data.

Timely reporting rate of TB (%) = number of timely reporting cases of TB/number of internet on-line reported cases of TB × 100

Missed Reporting Rate of TB

The missed reporting rate of TB is harvested by survey on-site. It is the frequency of missed reporting of TB during a certain period of time in one region or one health-care institution in the total number of registered TB cases in the same region or health-care institution, which is represented by %.

Missed reporting rate of TB (%) = number of missed reporting/number of registered TB cases × 100

Timely Review Rate of TB Reporting

The timely review rate of TB reporting is the frequency of timely review of the internet on-line reporting of TB cases in one region during a certain period of time, which is represented by %. The timely review refers to review of the internet on-line reporting of TB within 24 h after the reporting by the county/district-level TB control agency. The range of quality assessment of timely review includes primary reporting, revisited reporting, and deleted reporting. For the reviewed reporting of a case, if the diagnosis is changed, the reporting should be re-reviewed for statistics.

Timely review rate of TB reporting (%) = number of timely reviewed reporting/total number of reviewed reporting × 100

Duplicate TB Reporting Rate

The duplicate TB reporting rate is the frequency of duplicate TB reporting in the total number of internet on-line reporting of TB in one region during a certain period of time, which is represented by %. The quality assessment is based on daily checking and screening of duplicate report in the reporting cases with present address in the county/district by the county/district-level TB control agency.

Duplicate TB reporting rate (%) = number of duplicate report/total number of reports with present address in the county/district × 100

Completeness of Valid ID No.

The completeness of valid ID No. is the frequency of complete valid ID No. in the reported cases of TB in one region within a certain period of time (1 month, one quarter or 1 year), which is represented by %. The valid ID No. in standard format indicates complete valid ID No. And the statistics excludes the patients from Hong Kong, Macao, and Taiwan of China, infants aged no more than 31 days, under-reviewing reports, and deleted reports.

Completeness of valid ID No. (%) = number of complete valid ID No./total number of reported cases × 100

Population Distribution

The population distribution of TB is described by age, gender, occupation, and family history.

Age
Age is the most important factor in description of population distribution. The description of age distribution of TB is commonly based on age groups. The incidence and mortality of TB in each age group are then calculated. The age distribution of TB cases can also be statistically analyzed based on percentage of each age group in a certain population.

Gender
The occurrence of and deaths from a disease always show gender difference. The incidence of TB is higher in males than in females. The gender distribution of TB cases can also be statistically analyzed based on percentage of males and females in a certain population.

Occupation
The occurrence of and deaths from a disease are closely related to the occupation, no exception to TB. Description of occupational distribution of TB provides reference for the prevention and control of TB.

Family History
Contacts between family members are close and TB is more frequently spread within family members.

Regional Distribution
The international distribution of TB can be described based on country or continent, while the national distribution of TB can be described based on province, city, autonomous region, county/district, or smaller administrative unit. Such geographic divisions facilitate data collection and are therefore commonly applied. However, the distribution of TB shows variance within the same administrative region due to different control strategy, population density, population mobility, and natural environment.

Chronological Distribution
The onset of TB is not seasonal. It has been reported that the onset of TB reaches the peak during winters and springs in the cold north of China, which is closely related to poor ventilation and close contacts during winters and springs.

Epidemiological Data of TB in 2007–2016 in Shenzhen [32, 33]

Based on the Infectious Diseases Reporting Information Management System, the cases from 2007 to 2016 with the present address in Shenzhen were collected for epidemiological analysis. And the epidemiological data of TB in 2007–2016 in Shenzhen is reported as follows.

Occurrence of TB
During 2007–2016, totally 54,760 cases of TB are reported, including 27,030 smear-positive cases, 1345 culture positive only cases, 26,310 bacteriological negative cases, and 75 sputum undetected cases. The average annual reporting rate is 53.1 per 0.1 million. During the 10 years, there have been no epidemics or outbreaks of TB in Shenzhen, with all the reported cases as sporadic occurrence. The reporting incidence of TB has generally decreased, with minor fluctuations during the 10 years. The reporting incidence of TB has increased from 2008 to 2010, with more detected patients (Fig. 2.1). The reason is that the 5th round of globally funded program for prevention and control of TB in migrating population is initiated in Shenzhen. More funding has been invested to reinforce detection and management of patients with TB and propagation for prevention and treatment of TB during the 3 years.

Chronological Distribution
The monthly statistical report shows no significant seasonal variance in the reported cases of TB. Because of the traditional Chinese custom of family reunion during the Spring Festival, the migrating population significantly decreases in Shenzhen in the beginning and end of a year. The reported cases of TB during the beginning and end of a year decrease accordingly. Due to the backflow of the migrating population into Shenzhen after the Spring Festival and entry health examination for the newly employed, the reported cases of TB reach peak from March to May each year. Therefore, the

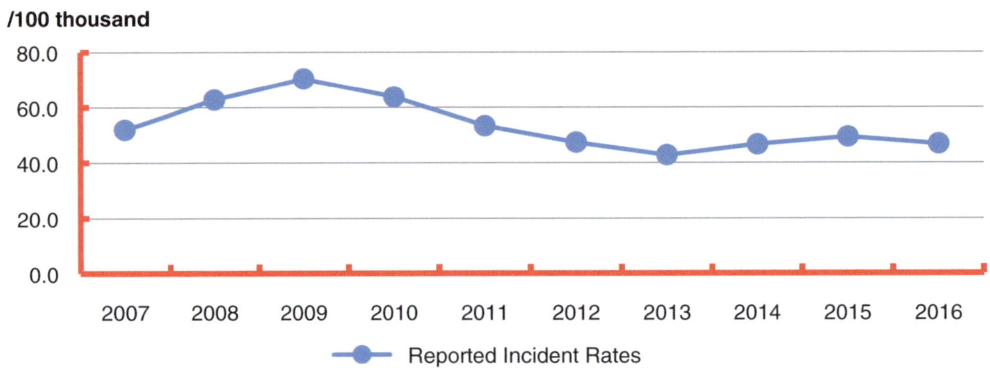

Fig. 2.1 TB reported incident rates from 2007 to 2016

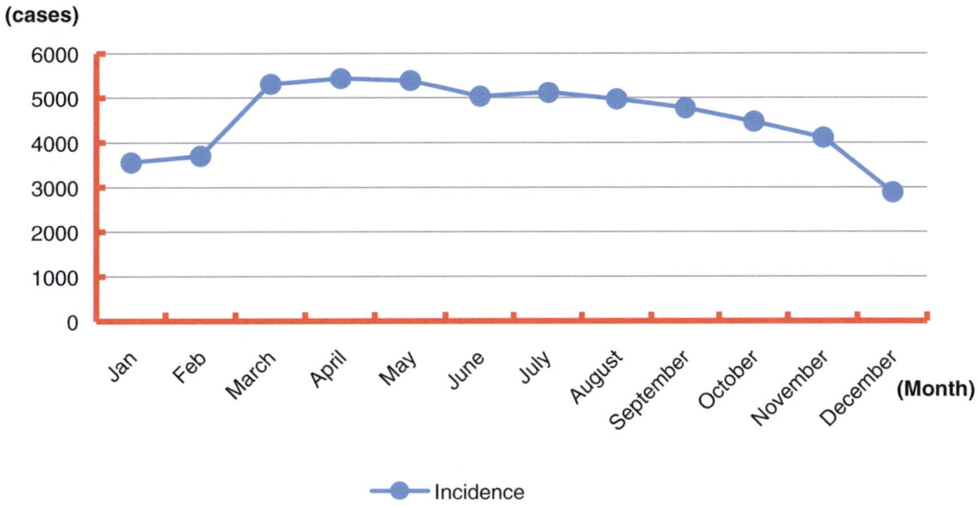

Fig. 2.2 TB distribution from 2007 to 2016

Table 2.1 TB distribution in Shenzhen from 2007 to 2016

Districts in Shenzhen	Population (/10,000)	Reported incident rate (year/100,000)
Luohu	929.65	65.8
Futian	1326.24	43.2
Nanshan	1105.72	80.4
Baoan	3395.42	51.8
Longgang	2019.03	48.6
Yantian	213.99	38.8
Guangming	368.82	52.4
Pinshan	236.11	46.3
Longhua	654.80	40.4
Dapeng	60.25	20.7
Total	10,310.03	53.1

chronological distribution of TB shows high occurrence during the middle of a year but low occurrences in the beginning and end of a year (Fig. 2.2).

Regional Distribution

Before the year 2009, there had been six administrative districts in Shenzhen. For more efficient management, Guangming New district and Longhua New district were divided out from the Baoan district; and Pingshan New district and Dapeng New district were divided out from the Longgang district after the year 2009. From 2007 to 2016, the average annual reporting incidence of TB is the highest in Nanshan district of Shenzhen, being 80.4 per 0.1 million, followed by Luohu district, being 65.8 per 0.1 million. The other districts with average annual reporting incidence of TB from high to low are Guangming New district, Baoan district, Longgang district, Pingshan New district, Futian district, Longhua New district, Yantian district, and Dapeng New district (Table 2.1). By statistical chi-square test, the average annual reporting incidence of TB in different districts shows statistical significance ($\chi^2 = 2583.1$, $P < 0.01$).

The reporting incidence of TB shows great district variance in Shenzhen. The factors influencing the district variance may include geographic climate, air quality, population density, percentage of the migrating population, industries distribution as well as reporting and referral quality of healthcare institution. Dapeng New district and Yantian district are coastal districts with great mountain areas, small population, low population density, and good air quality. The reporting incidence of TB in these two districts is low. In Nanshan district and Baoan district, there are industrial zones. In Nanshan district, there is new and high technology zone. In Nanshan district and Luohu district, there are villages in the city and old residential areas. Such zones, areas, and villages in the city are characterized by large migrating population, dense population, and poorly ventilated occupational environment in some industries. In such high-risk areas of TB infection, the reporting incidence of TB is high accordingly.

Gender and Age Distribution

From 2007–2016, the reported cases of TB in Shenzhen have amounted to 35,758 males (65.3%) and 19,002 females (34.7%), with a gender ratio of 1.9:1. Concerning to age distribution, there has been a curve with high middle and low ends. In children aged under 14 years; a total of 191 cases are reported, accounting for 0.3%. The number of reported cases rapidly increases since the age of 15 years, reaches a peak at the age of 20–29 years, and rapidly decreases since the age of 30 years. There are totally 24,766 reported cases of TB in the age group of 20–29 years, accounting for 45.2%. And in the age group of ≥65 years, the number of reported cases obviously decreases to 2041, accounting for 3.7% (Fig. 2.3). By statistical chi-square test, the age group percentages between males and females show significant difference (χ^2 = 929.4,

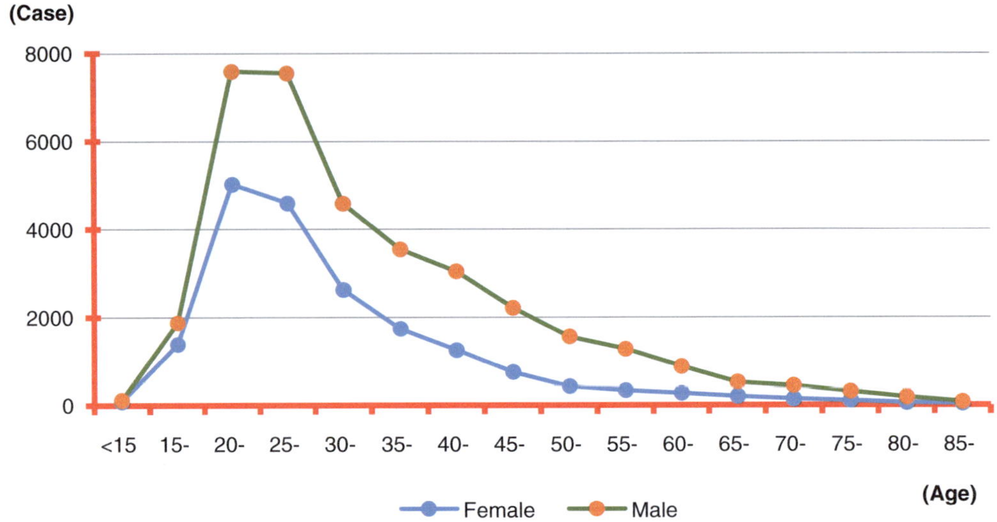

Fig. 2.3 Distribution of reported TB incidences according to sex and age

$P < 0.01$). The number of male patients is significantly higher than that of female patients, which is in accordance with the data released from the national epidemiological sampling survey in 2010. The higher incidence of TB in males may be attributed to more intense physical labor and higher mobility to increase the family income due to more personal, familial, and social responsibilities as well as more unhealthy personal habits such as smoking and alcoholism.

The data of age distribution of TB in Shenzhen in 2007–2016 is not in accordance with the data released from the national epidemiological sampling survey in 2010. The reported cases in Shenzhen in 2007–2016 reach the peak in the age group of 20–34 years (58.4%) rather than the peak in the age group of ≥65 years according to the national survey in 2010. This discrepancy may be attributed to the high percentage of migrating population in Shenzhen (75%). The patients with TB in the migrating population are mainly young people working in Shenzhen.

Occupation Distribution

Exception for those who failed to report their detailed occupation and the category of the other occupations, the top 5 occupations that the reported cases of TB in Shenzhen in 2007–2016 are mainly involved include workers (37.6%), domestic service and unemployed (32.7%), commercial service (5.4%), office staffs (4.9%), and the retired (2.4%) (Table 2.2). The reported cases of TB are mainly involved in the occupations of workers as well as domestic service and the unemployed, accounting for about one third, respectively. The workers are mainly migrating population with low or unstable income, more intense physical labor, and compromised immunity. They are susceptible to endogenous infection. In addition, they are also exposed to exogenous infection due to their crowded housing with poor hygiene and high mobility. Some migrating population working in domestic service is temporarily at rest due to their infection of diseases.

Table 2.2 Occupational distribution of TB patients in Shenzhen from 2007 to 2016

Occupation	Reported cases	Proportion (%)
Worker	20,569	37.6
Housework/unemployed	17,882	32.7
Others	3763	6.9
Business	2969	5.4
Government	2657	4.9
Unknown	1708	3.1
Retirement	1334	2.4
Student	1083	2.0
Laborer	906	1.7
Food service	665	1.2
Farmer	475	0.9
Public servant	220	0.4
Teacher	179	0.3
Medical workers	171	0.3
Sailor/long-distance pilots	96	0.2
Scattered children	38	0.1
Childcare children	10	0.0
Childcare workers/nannies	25	0.0
Herdsman	4	0.0
Fisherman	6	0.0
Total	54,760	100.0

There are totally 40,032 registered cases of TB in Shenzhen in 2007–2016, including 36,034 cases in the migrating population (90%). Due to the special composition of population in Shenzhen and predominant percentage of patients in the migrating population, the patients with TB in the migrating population are the key population that receives close attention for prevention and control of TB. The local governments of Shenzhen should further increase the funding investment and implement more effective measures to prevent and control of

TB targeting on the migrating population. The patients should be provided with more free-in-charge physical examinations, medications, and hospitalizations. In addition, the patients should also be provided with allowances for foods and transportations. Based on these measures, the disease burden can be alleviated for the patients and their compliance to therapies can be improved. The cure rate can thus be increased.

Epidemiological Survey of TB [34–36]

To understand the prevalence of TB and implementation of strategies for its prevention and control in China, five national epidemiological sampling surveys were conducted in 1979, 1984–1985, 1990, 2000, and 2010, respectively. Based on the technical procedures of the national surveys, almost synchronous epidemiological sampling surveys have been conducted in Shenzhen in 1985, 1987 (provincial survey), 1990, 2000, and 2010. In the five national epidemiological surveys, Shenzhen was a city for epidemiological sampling. And the sampling method in the surveys in Shenzhen, stratified random cluster sampling with equal ratio, was the same as the national surveys.

Data for Collection

In the epidemiological surveys of TB in Shenzhen, questionnaire survey was conducted in the sampling populations. The data included PPD test, X-ray examination, sputum smear and culture, drug sensitivity test, their knowledge about TB, their health condition, patients with TB or non-patients with TB, drug resistance of Mtb, and socioeconomic status.

Quality Control

Before the surveys were conducted, a detailed plan of survey, sampling design, and detailed procedures of survey were formulated. A team for epidemiological sampling survey was established and the members received training. The formulated procedures of survey were strictly observed during the survey. The subjects were well-informed about the survey and the questionnaires were printed with uniform formats and directions. The finished questionnaires were reviewed and the missed information was timely completed. According to the standards and requirements, the primary data and database were checked and accepted. After reviewed, the data was double typed into the software adopted by the national epidemiological sampling survey, with a review rate of above 95%.

Indices of the Survey

Morbidity of TB

Morbidity of TB is the percentage of patients with active TB in the surveyed population at a certain time point, which is represented by per 0.1 million.

Morbidity of TB (per 0.1 million) = number of patients with active TB/total number of surveyed population × 100,000

Morbidity of Smear-Positive TB

Morbidity of smear-positive TB is the percentage of patients with smear-positive TB in the surveyed population at a certain time point, which is represented by per 0.1 million.

Morbidity of smear-positive TB (per 0.1 million) = number of patients with smear-positive TB/total number of surveyed population × 100,000

Morbidity of Bacteriologically Positive TB

Morbidity of bacteriologically positive TB is the percentage of patients with bacteriologically positive TB in the surveyed population at a certain time point, which is represented by per 0.1 million.

Morbidity of bacteriologically positive TB (per 0.1 million) = number of patients with bacteriologically positive TB/total number of surveyed population × 100,000

Gender/Age Morbidity of TB

Gender/age morbidity of TB is the percentages of patients with active TB in different gender/age groups in the corresponding gender/age groups of surveyed population at a certain time point, which is represented by per 0.1 million.

The curves based on gender/age morbidity of TB demonstrate difference of TB morbidity between males and females, distribution of TB morbidity in different age groups, and the age group with peak morbidity of TB.

Residence Morbidity of TB

Residence morbidity of TB is the percentages of patients with active TB in different residence groups (local residents and migrating population) in the corresponding residence groups of surveyed population at a certain time point, which is represented by 0.1 per million.

Regional Morbidity of TB

Regional morbidity of TB is the morbidity rates of TB calculated based on certain geographic division, such as urban and rural morbidity of TB, east, middle, and west morbidity of TB, provincial, and city morbidity of TB.

Morbidity Decrease Range of TB

Morbidity decrease range of TB is the proportion of the morbidity difference between two consecutive epidemiological surveys of TB in the morbidity of previous epidemiological survey of TB, which is represented by %.

Morbidity decrease range of TB (%) = (morbidity of present epidemiological survey − morbidity of previous epidemiological survey)/morbidity of previous epidemiological survey × 100

Average Annual Decline Rate of TB

Average annual decline rate of morbidity is the percentage of average annual decline of TB morbidity based on morbidity of two epidemiological surveys, which is represented by %.

$$\text{Average annual decline rate of morbidity} = \left(1 - \sqrt[n]{\text{morbidity of present epidemiological survey / morbidity of previous epidemiological survey}}\right) \times 100$$

In the above formula, n represents the interval years between the two epidemiological surveys.

Drug Resistance of Mtb

Resistance of Mtb to single or multiple anti-tuberculosis drugs that is confirmed by laboratory tests can be defined as drug resistance of Mtb. Drug resistance of Mtb can be classified into the following four types:

(1) Single-drug resistance. It is defined by resistance of Mtb to one anti-tuberculosis drug.
(2) Polydrug resistance. It is defined by resistance of Mtb to more than one anti-tuberculosis drugs.
(3) Multidrug resistance. It is defined by resistance of Mtb to at least isoniazid and rifampicin.
(4) Extensive drug resistance. It is defined by resistance of Mtb to at least isoniazid and rifampicin plus any fluoroquinolones plus at least 1 injectable from capreomycin, kanamycin, and amikacin.

Core Information Awareness Rate of TB

The subjects chosen by random sampling are asked about five core information about TB and the general awareness rate and total awareness rate are calculated based on the collected data.

General awareness rate (%) = total number of correct answers/(the number of subjects × 5) × 100

Total awareness rate (%) = number of subjects with all correct answers/total number of subjects × 100

Predicted Morbidity of TB

The prediction to epidemics of TB is complex due to the complex factors influencing the epidemic of TB. But the future morbidity of TB can be predicted based on the morbidity, annual decline rate of morbidity, and interval years of epidemiological surveys. The formula is as follows:

$$P1 = (1 - S)^n \times P2$$

In this formula, $P1$ represents the future morbidity; S represents the annual decline rate of morbidity; n represents the interval years; and $P2$ represents the morbidity of present epidemiological survey.

Recent Three Epidemiological Surveys of TB in Shenzhen

In 1991, 2000, and 2010, in addition to completion of the assigned tasks in the national and provincial epidemiological surveys of TB, one epidemiological survey site was randomly selected in each district of Shenzhen according to the sampling of national surveys. In this way, epidemiological surveys of TB in Shenzhen were conducted. The results indicated that the epidemic of TB in Shenzhen has been effectively controlled. In 1991–2000, the morbidity of TB in local residents has decreased by 62.8%, with an annual decline rate of 10.4%; the morbidity of smear-positive TB has decreased by 55.8% with an annual decline rate of 8.7%. Meanwhile, the morbidity of TB in the migrating population has decreased by 42.1% with an annual decline rate of 5.9%; the morbidity of smear-positive TB has decreased by 38.6% with an annual decline rate of 5.3%. During 2000–2010, the morbidity of TB in local residents has decreased by 50.8% with an annual decline rate of 6.9%; the morbidity of smear-positive TB has decreased by 70.6% with an annual decline rate of 11.5%. Meanwhile, the morbidity of TB in the migrating population has decreased by 10.6% with an annual decline rate of 1.1%; the morbidity of smear-positive TB has decreased by 19.5% with an annual decline rate of 3.3% (Table 2.3).

Predicted Morbidity of TB in Shenzhen in 2020

Multiple factors influence the prediction of morbidity of TB, which is, therefore, complex. Based on the epidemiological survey of TB in Shenzhen in 2010 and the calculating formula, the morbidity of TB in Shenzhen in 2020 is predicted. The result indicates that control of TB in the migrating population should be paid close attention in the near future (Table 2.4 and Fig. 2.4).

3.2 Surveillance on Detection, Treatment, and Management of TB

In 1982, annual statistical report of registered patients of active TB was approved by the National Statistical Bureau of China. Since then, the national statistical report of TB has been reported each year. It requires timely data col-

Table 2.3 TB epidemiological study results in 1991, 2000, and 2010

Registered residence type	Patient type	Prevalence (1/100,000)[a]			2000 vs 1991		2010 vs 2000[b]	
		1991	2000	2010	Falling rate (%)	Yearly falling rate (%)	Falling rate (%)	Yearly falling rate (%)
Residence	Active TB	336	125	78	62.8	10.4	50.8	6.9
	Smear-positive TB	118	52	19	55.8	8.7	70.6	11.5
Migrating population	Active TB	417	241	219	42.1	5.9	10.6	1.1
	Smear-positive TB	131	80	66	38.6	5.3	19.5	3.3

[a]For 1984, 1991, and 2000, the prevalence rate was calculated based on the whole population. For 2010, the prevalence rate was calculated based on the 15-year-old and over population, and the prevalence rate was the statistical result at that time

[b]When calculating the decrease of prevalence rate and yearly falling rate in 2010 and 2000, the prevalence rate in 2010 and 2000 was standardized according to the population structure, and the comparison results were the change magnitude of the standardized rates, which was not calculated directly from the patient's third to fourth column of data

Table 2.4 Predictive prevalence of smear-positive TB in 2020 in Shenzhen

Registered residence type	Patient type	Predictive prevalence in 2020 (/100,000)
Residence	Active TB	38.2
	Smear-positive TB	5.7
Migrating population	Active TB	196.5
	Smear-positive TB	47.1

lection and analysis of TB nationwide, which has guided the prevention and control of TB. In April 1992, TB control program in China was initiated in 12 provinces and autonomous regions based on the World Bank loan and local counterpart funding. Since then, 1 monthly report about the program development and 8 quarterly reports on detection of patients, treatment management, treatment outcomes, and drugs management were added. During implementation of the TB control program in China, the Guangdong Reporting Management System was developed by the Guangdong TB Control Institute. In the system, patient management card was added. After the information about treatment and management of patients was input into the system, patient-related statistical reports were automatically generated. In 2005, the National Tuberculosis Management Information System was developed and has been improved since then. The surveillance information management of TB and the prevention and treatment planning information management of TB have been integrated into it. The data can be real-time on-line reported. In implementing the national reporting system and Guangdong reporting system, a reporting system of Shenzhen was designed to assess the management quality in detecting, treating, and managing patients of TB. Monthly, quarterly, and yearly data from each district of Shenzhen was reported to the Shenzhen managing office of TB control program. In 2011, the Shenzhen Directly Observed Treatment Management System was developed for real-time supervision of the patients. In 2018, the data of health management service for patients with TB was integrated into the system.

The surveillance of TB detection, treatment, and management includes two parts, namely the surveillance of TB information management and surveillance of TB prevention and treatment planning information management. The surveillance of TB detection, treatment, and management plays an important role in the modern TB control strategies. It is the important basis in formulating TB control strategies and measures, assessing TB prevention and treatment, and predicting prevalence of TB. In addition, it is also an important part in national planning of TB prevention and treatment.

Basis of Surveillance

The surveillance of TB detection, treatment, and management is based on the National Technical Guideline for Implementation of TB Prevention and Treatment Planning [37].

Information for Surveillance

Information of TB Detection, Treatment, and Management

The information of TB detection, treatment, and management includes personal data of TB patient, detection, reporting, treatment and management of suspected/defined cases of TB and suspected/defined drug-resistant cases of TB, and health management service of TB patient. The register of initially present patient, register of laboratory tests, register of drug-resistant cases, first home follow-up record form, follow-up service record form, and primary medication records are applied for surveillance.

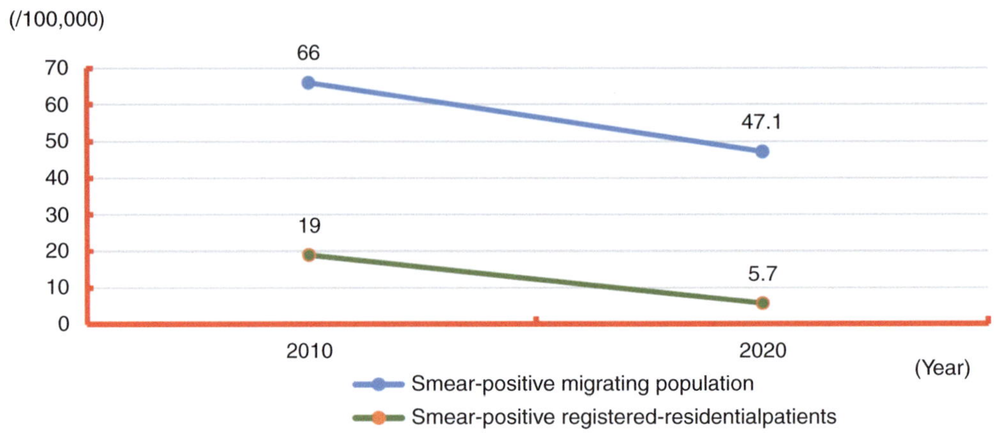

Fig. 2.4 Predictive smear-positive TB decreasing trend in 2020

Information of Planning Management

The information of planning management includes coverage planning, 5-year planning, supply and use of drugs, reagents, and equipments, planning of training, supervising and health promoting, planning and use of funding, and basic data of institution personnel. The register of drug dispensing, financial accounts, and records of related activities are applied for surveillance.

Quality Control

Primary Data Review

To secure the data quality, the primary data and manually input data in the Tuberculosis Management Information System are reviewed for completeness, accuracy, and promptness. The primary data for review includes longitudinal data register of suspected/defined TB cases, register of initially present patient, register of sputum smear test, register of TB patient, case history of TB patient, register of suspected drug-resistant TB patient, register of drug-resistant TB patient, case history of drug-resistant TB patient as well as the quarterly, semi-annual, and annual report of manual data input.

Management for Data Quality Control

The primary data and manually input data in the TB Management Information System are reviewed monthly in the district TB control agency. The data management in the district TB control agency is supervised regularly by the Shenzhen Chronic Diseases Prevention and Control Center. The shortcomings in district data management can thus be timely detected and improved. The staffs responsible for district data management receive training and technical guidance from the Shenzhen Chronic Diseases Prevention and Control Center. The requirements and legal responsibilities in data management are emphasized in the training and technical guidance. In addition, the staffs should be educated for their awareness about the importance of data management and for their sense of responsibility to secure the promptness, accuracy, and authenticity of data reporting.

Promptness of Data

It is required by the TB Management Information System that the data should be timely input. The update longitudinal data about suspected/defined TB cases should be input into the system within 24 h. The case history of defined TB patient should be input into the system within 24 h after the diagnosis. The data collected in follow-up of TB or drug-resistant TB patient should be input into the system within 24 h after the data collection. The data about drug resistance surveillance and suspected drug-resistant case should be input into the system within 24 h after the data collection. The quarterly data input report should be input in the first 5 days of the first month following each quarter. The annual data input report should be input before January 30th of the following year.

Quality Statistics of the TB Management Information System

The quality statistics function in the TB Management Information System can also be used for data quality control. The quality of data input by district TB control agency is assessed monthly by Shenzhen Chronic Diseases Prevention and Control Center. Supervision of data input by district TB control agency is conducted quarterly by Shenzhen Chronic Diseases Prevention and Control Center based on the General Assessment Standards for Public Health-care Service in Shenzhen and the Performance Assessment Standards of Chronic Diseases Control System in Shenzhen. The information management by the district TB control agency is assessed on-site at the end of each year by an experts committee organized by the Health Commission of Shenzhen.

Dynamic Surveillance

According to the reported data by the district institution for TB control, the completion rate of each TB control task is dynamically monitored. The shortcomings can be timely detected for the following supervision.

Indices for assessment

DOTS (Directly Observed Treatment, Short-Course) Coverage

DOTS is the modern strategy for TB control. DOTS coverage is the percentage of counties/districts that implement DOTS in the total number of counties/districts of a city within a certain period of time.

DOTS coverage (%) = number of counties/districts that implement DOTS/total number of counties/districts × 100

Professionals Employment Rate for TB Control

Professionals employment rate for TB control is the percentage of professionals employment for full-time work in a TB control agency based on *the National Guidelines for Implementation of TB Control Planning* and the need of local TB control.

Professional employment rate for TB control (%) = actual number of professionals full-time working in a TB control agency/total number of professionals that a TB control agency should employ × 100

According to the National Guidelines for Implementation of TB Control Planning, at least 15 full-time working professionals should be employed in a city TB control institution and the number should be appropriately added according to the specific number of its counties and districts. In a city with more than 10 counties and districts, one full-time working professional should be added for every additional one county/district. If a city institution takes additional responsibilities of a county/district institution, corresponding additional full-time working professionals should be employed according to the need of actual work. In a county or district TB control institution, at least eight full-time working professionals should be employed and the number can be added according to the actual population of the county/district. In a county or district with a population of more than 0.4 million, one full-time working professional should be added for every additional 50,000 population.

Per Capita Funding for TB Control

Per capita funding for TB control is the per capita funding for TB control based on the total investment of local government to TB control and the total population administered by the local government during a certain period of time.

Per capita funding for TB control (¥) = total funding investment of local government to TB control/total number of the administered population by the local government

Sputum Detection Rate in Initially Present Patients

Sputum detection rate in initially present patients is the percentage of suspected TB patients who received sputum smear test in a TB control agency in the total number of suspected TB patients in the TB control agency during a certain period of time.

Sputum detection rate in initially present patients (%) = number of suspected TB patients who received sputum smear test/total number of suspected TB patients × 100

Detection Rate of Sputum Smear-Positive Patients

Detection rate of smear-positive patients is the percentage of sputum smear-positive patients of TB in the total number of suspected TB patients who received sputum smear test.

Detection rate of sputum smear-positive TB patients (%) = number of sputum smear-positive TB patients/total number of suspected TB patients who received sputum smear test × 100

Screening Rate of Suspected Drug-Resistant TB Patients

Screening rate of suspected drug-resistant TB patients is the percentage of suspected drug-resistant TB patients who received drug sensitivity test in the total number of suspected drug-resistant TB patients who should receive drug sensitivity test during a certain period of time in a region. The suspected cases of multidrug resistance and the suspected cases of drug resistance should be separately calculated.

Screening rate of suspected drug-resistant TB patients (%) = number of suspected drug-resistant TB patients who received drug sensitivity test/number of suspected drug-resistant TB patients who should receive drug sensitivity test × 100

Screening rate of suspected multidrug-resistant TB patients (%) = number of suspected multidrug-resistant TB patients who received drug sensitivity test/number of suspected multidrug-resistant TB patients who should receive drug sensitivity test × 100

Suspected cases of multidrug-resistant TB (high-risk cases) refer to retreated patients with smear-positive TB, new smear-positive TB patients who are still positive after treatment for 2–3 months, chronic TB patients, and smear-positive patients with close contacts to multidrug-resistant TB patients.

Suspected cases of drug-resistant TB refer to bacteriologically positive TB patients including all the smear-positive TB patients and only culture-positive TB patients.

Referral Rate of Suspected/Defined TB Cases

Referral rate of suspected/defined TB cases is the percentage of referrals of suspected/defined TB cases that TB control agencies received from non-TB-control agencies in the total number of internet reporting suspected/defined TB cases by non-TB-control agencies within a certain period of time in a certain region.

Referral rate of suspected/defined TB cases (%) = referrals of suspected/defined TB cases that TB control agencies received from non-TB-control agencies/total number of internet on-line reporting suspected/defined TB cases by non-TB-control agencies × 100

Total Management Rate of Suspected/Defined TB Cases Reported by Non-TB-Control Agencies

Total management rate of suspected/defined TB cases reported by non-TB-control agencies is the percentage of referral patients by non-TB-control agencies who received appropriate management by TB control agencies in the total number of suspected/defined patients that should be referred to TB control agency (number after exclusion of duplicate report—inpatients of TB—reported but discharged within the same period of time).

Total management rate of suspected/defined TB cases reported by non-TB-control agencies (%) = number of referred patients who received appropriate management/ number of suspected/defined cases that should be referred and managed × 100

The number of suspected/defined cases that should be referred and managed = reported number of patients after exclusion of duplicate report − inpatients + reported but discharged within the same period of calculation

Detection Rate of New Smear-Positive Patients

Detection rate of new smear-positive patients is the percentage of detected and registered new smear-positive patients in the estimated smear-positive patients within a certain period of time (commonly a year) in a region.

Detection rate of new smear-positive patients (%) = number of detected and registered new smear-positive patients/estimated the number of smear-positive patients × 100

Estimated number of smear-positive patients = total population of a region × incidence of smear-positive TB (per 0.1 million)

Completion Rate of Detecting New Smear-Positive Patients

Completion rate of detecting new smear-positive patients is the percentage of detected and registered new smear-positive patients in the planned number of detected and registered new smear-positive patients within a certain period of time (commonly 1 year) in a region.

Completion rate of detecting new smear-positive patients (%) = number of detected and registered new smear-positive patients/planned number of detected and registered new smear-positive patients × 100

Registry Rate of Active TB Patients

Registry rate of active TB patients is the percentage of detected and registered active TB patients in the average annual population within a certain period of time (commonly 1 year) in a region.

Registry rate of active TB patients (per 0.1 million) = number of detected and registered active TB patients/average annual population × 100,000

Registry Rate of New Smear-Positive Patients

Registry rate of new smear-positive patients is the percentage of detected and registered new smear-positive patients in the average annual population within a period of time (commonly 1 year) in a region.

Registry rate of new smear-positive patients (per 0.1 million) = number of detected and registered new smear-positive patients/average annual population × 100,000

Management Rate of TB Patients

Management rate of TB patients is the percentage of managed TB patients in the internet on-line reported TB patients within a certain period of time (commonly 1 year) in a region.

Management rate of TB patients (%) = number of managed TB patients/number of internet on-line reported TB patients × 100

Etiologically Positive Rate of TB

Etiologically positive rate of TB is the percentage of registered etiologically positive TB patients in the total number of registered TB patients within a certain period of time (commonly 1 year) in a region.

Etiologically positive rate of TB (%) = number of registered etiologically positive TB patients/total number of registered TB patients × 100

Medication Coverage

Medication coverage is the percentage of TB patients receiving medication therapy in the total number of registered TB patients within a certain period of time in a region.

Medication coverage (%) = number of TB patients receiving medication therapy/total number of registered TB patients

Screening Rate of Individuals with Close Contacts to Etiologically Positive TB Patient

Screening rate of individuals with close contacts to etiologically positive TB patients is the percentage of individuals receiving screening examination due to close contacts to etiologically positive TB patients in the registered individuals with close contacts to etiologically positive TB patients within a certain period of time in a region.

Screening rate of individuals with close contacts to etiologically positive TB patients (%) = number of individuals receiving screening examination due to close contacts to etiologically positive TB patients/number of registered individuals with close contacts to etiologically positive TB patients × 100

Referral Rate of Registered TB Patients

Referral rate of registered TB patients is the percentage of the referrals in the registered TB patients during a certain period of time in a region.

Sputum Negative Conversion Rate After 2–3 Months Treatment

Sputum test negative conversion rate after 2–3 months treatment is the number of sputum test negative conversions after 2–3 months treatment in the total number of registered smear-positive TB patients during a certain period of time in a region. The rates in initially treated patients and the retreated patients are respectively calculated.

Sputum test negative conversion rate after 2 months treatment (%) = number of sputum test negative conversion after 2 months treatment/total number of registered smear-positive TB patients × 100

Sputum test negative conversion rate after 3 months treatment (%) = number of sputum test negative conversion after 3 months treatment/total number of registered smear-positive TB patients × 100

Cure Rate of TB

Cure rate of TB is the percentage of patients that are cured or finished the therapeutic course in the registered TB patients during a certain period of time in a region.

Cure rate of TB (%) = number of cured and those finished the therapeutic course/total number of registered TB patients × 100

Cure Rate of Smear-Positive TB

Cure rate of smear-positive TB patients is the percentage of cured smear-positive TB patients in the total number of registered smear-positive TB patients in a certain period of time in a region. The rates of initially treated patients and retreated patients are respectively calculated.

Cure rate of smear-positive TB patients (%) = number of cured smear-positive TB patients/total number of registered smear-positive TB patients × 100

Cure Rate of Multidrug-Resistant TB

Cure rate of multidrug-resistant TB is the percentage of multidrug-resistant TB patients who are cured or finished the therapeutic course in the registered multidrug-resistant TB patients.

Cure rate of multidrug-resistant TB (%) = number of multidrug-resistant TB patients who are cured or finished the therapeutic course/total number of registered multidrug-resistant TB patients × 100

Observation Rate of Medication

Observation rate of medication is the percentage of patients receiving direct observation for medication in the registered patients during a certain period of time in a region.

Observation rate of medication (%) = number of patients receiving direct observation for medication/total number of registered patients × 100

Loss Rate

Loss rate is the percentage of lost patients in the registered patients during a certain period of time in a region.

Loss rate (%) = number of lost patients/total number of registered patients × 100

Standard Management Rate of TB Patients (Including Multidrug-Resistant TB Patients)

Standard management rate of TB patients is the percentage of patients receiving standard management in the total number of patients who should receive standard management during a certain period of time in a region. Based on the standard management, the TB patients should be initially home visited within the required time period, followed by monthly follow-ups according to the standard requirements.

Standard management rate of TB patients (%) = number of patients receiving standard management/total number of patients who should receive standard management × 100

Regular Medication Rate of TB Patients (Including Multidrug-Resistant TB Patients)

Regular medication rate of TB patients is the percentage of number of patients receiving regular medication in the registered TB patients during a certain period of time in a region. Regular medication refers to the actual medications during therapeutic course account for above 90% of the required medications.

Regular medication rate of each TB patient (%) = number of patients receiving required times of regular medication/total number of registered TB patients × 100

Core Information Awareness Rate for TB Control

Core information awareness rate for TB control is the percentage of patients who know about core information of TB control in the population who receive the survey.

Core information awareness rate for TB control (%) = number of patients who know about core information of TB control/total number of the population receiving the survey × 100

Analysis of Data from Shenzhen TB Control Program

In 1993, the migrating population was firstly recruited into the TB control program in Shenzhen. The measures of uniform goal and systematic management were implemented. That is to say, the migrating population and the local residents of Shenzhen shared the same policies and managing mode. The registry and management of TB patients were assessed based on the classification of local residents and the migrating population. The World Bank loan for TB control program in China, Guangdong TB control program, the global funding TB control program, and China TB control planning program were successively initiated. Since 1999, surveillance on drug resistance of Mtb has been conducted each year. Since 2003, drug-resistant TB has been included into the program. In more than 20 years, TB epidemics in Shenzhen have been effectively controlled based on innovations and improvements in policies formulating and their implementation.

Population Structure

Shenzhen is a typical city of migrants. In 1979 when the city was founded, the population of local residents was as large as 0.3141 million. And the population of local residents has been increasing nearly 40 times to 12.5238 million in the year 2017. Meanwhile, Shenzhen is a city with the largest migrating population in China, accounting for above 75% of the total population in Shenzhen. During 1993–2017, the population in Shenzhen has been rapidly increased (Fig. 2.5, Table 2.5).

Funding for TB Control

In 1993–2017, the TB control program in Shenzhen has received great financial support from the city and district governments. One-time full specified funding has been invested each year, with a gradual increase of per capita funding. In the 25 years, a total of more than ¥313 million has been invested into TB control program in Shenzhen, which secured the successful implementation of the program (Fig. 2.6).

Overall Management Rate

In 2004, all the health-care institutions in Shenzhen were required to real-time on-line report the data of TB patients into the Infectious Diseases Reporting Information Management System. The city and district level TB control agencies began then to trace the suspected/defined cases of TB that were not managed based on the data in the system. In addition, the treatment and management of TB began to be assessed according to the Overall Assessment Standards of Public Health-care Service in Shenzhen. Since then, the management rate of TB patients in the local residents of Shenzhen has been remained to be high, and the management rate of TB patients in the migrating population of Shenzhen has been gradually increasing (Fig. 2.7).

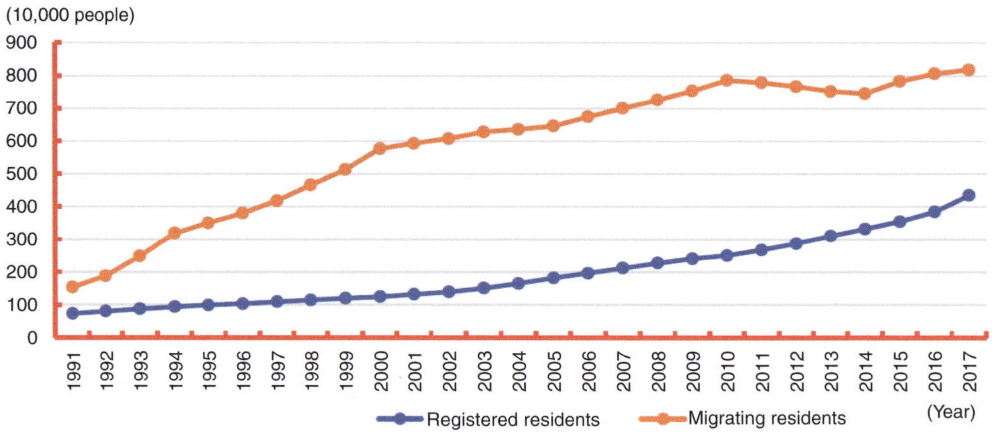

Fig. 2.5 Annual population of Shenzhen

Table 2.5 Human resources investment

Year	Education					Professional title				
	High school/technical secondary school or below	Junior college	College	Graduate	Total	None	Junior	Medium grade	Senior	Total
1993	17	5	8	0	30	0	17	12	1	30
2001	40	14	33	2	89	9	35	26	19	89
2005	43	32	45	6	126	16	51	29	30	126
2010	32	42	78	22	174	29	61	36	48	174
2017	20	54	112	37	223	39	70	55	59	223

Human resources investment: professionals with high education and high professional titles increase year by year

Fig. 2.6 Annual and per capita investment of TB control program

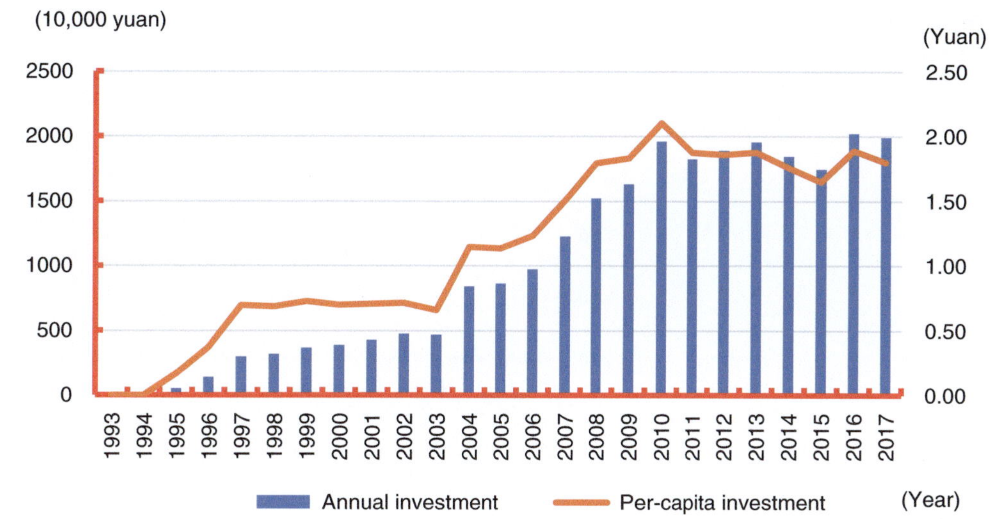

Fig. 2.7 Suspected TB reported by non-TB control facilities/TB overall in-place rate

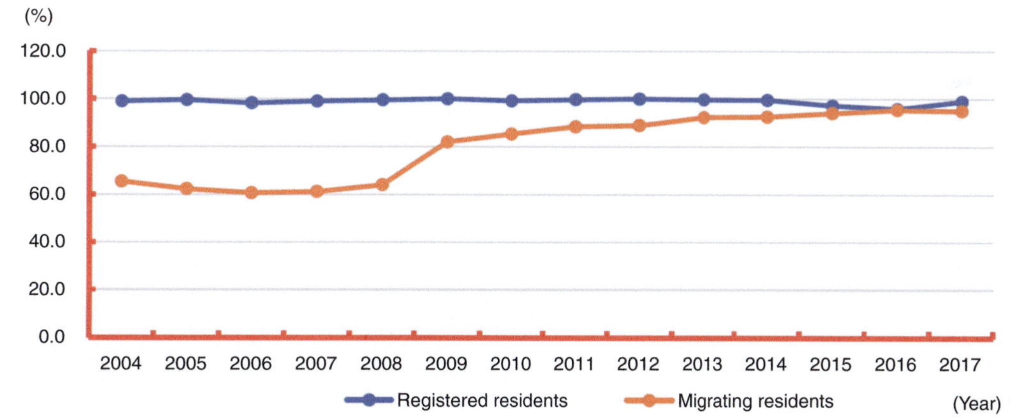

Health Examination for the Suspected Cases of TB

During 1993–2017, a total of 346,120 suspected cases of TB have received free-in-charge health examinations (Fig. 2.8).

Registry Rate of New Smear-Positive TB Patients

In 1993, the World Bank loan for China TB control program was initiated in Baoan district of Shenzhen. In 1996, registry and management of TB covered both local residents and population with temporary residence in Shenzhen. The curve of registry rate of new smear-positive TB patients has remained steady. In 2004, the registry and management of TB additionally covered the migrating population. In 2006, the global funding for TB control in migrating population program was initiated in China and the funding for TB control in migrating population was reinforced. Since then, the detection and management of TB patients have been reinforced and propagation of TB control has been strengthened. In addition, the patients with TB have been provided with allowance for transportation and well-nourishing foods. Based on these efforts, the registry rate of new smear-positive TB patients has been sharply increased. In 2017, the patients with TB receiving treatment and management in Shenzhen Hospital Specialized in Tuberculosis were registered and managed in the TB planning program. And the registry rate of new smear-positive TB patients increased slightly. Along with control of TB epidemic in Shenzhen, the overall registry rate of new smear-positive TB patients has been decreasing (Fig. 2.9).

Referral Rate of Registered TB Patients in Shenzhen

Treatment and management of TB patients in specialized TB control institutions have been paid close attention by the Health Commission of Shenzhen. In 1996, the Procedures for Treatment and Management of TB patients in Specialized TB Control Institutions of Shenzhen was issued, and the document was revisited and issued in 2008 and 2014. The requirements and procedures issued by national, provincial, and city documentations have been strictly observed by health-care institutions in Shenzhen and the suspected/defined cases of TB have been referred to the specialized TB control institutions. Most of the TB patients registered in the TB control agency of Shenzhen have been referred from the health-care institutions. The high referral rate reflects the importance of collaborative efforts (Fig. 2.10).

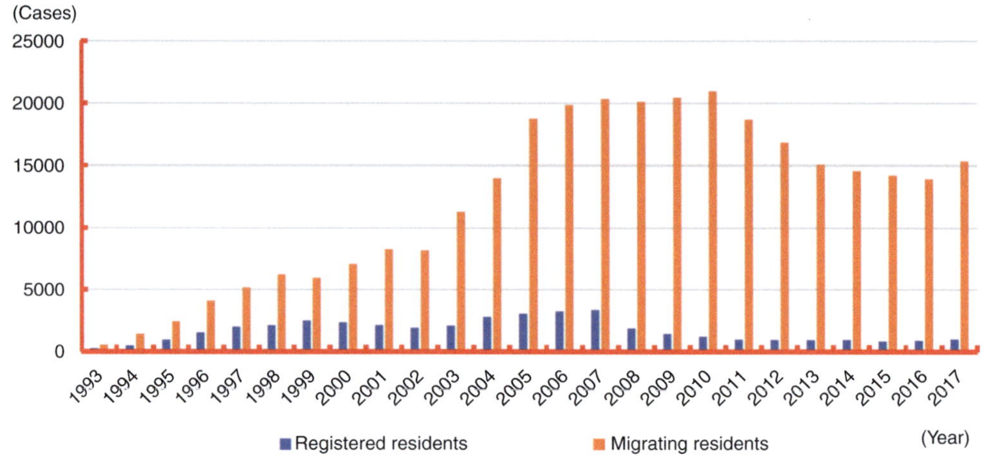

Fig. 2.8 Annual free screenings for suspected TB patients by Shenzhen TB control program

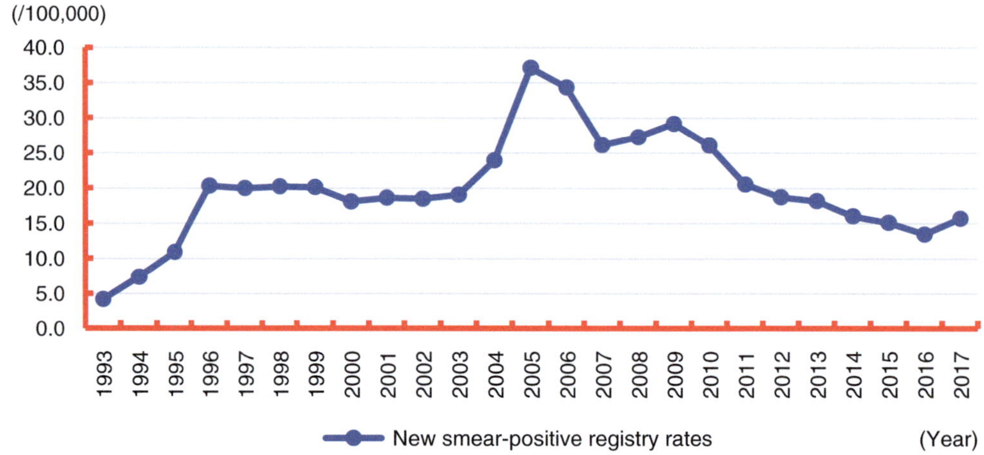

Fig. 2.9 Annual new smear-positive registry rates reported by TB control program

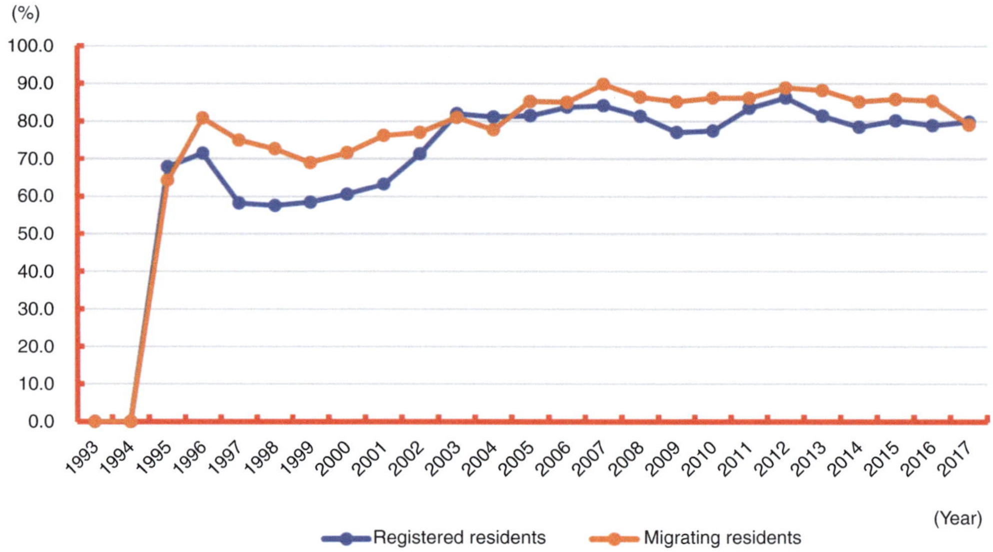

Fig. 2.10 Annual ratios of patients who has been transferred to overall reported TB patients

Treatment and Outcome of the Registered TB Patients

The cure rates of new smear-positive TB patients in the local residents and migrating population have remained high (Fig. 2.11).

Surveillance on Drug Resistance of Mtb

Since 1999, surveillance on drug resistance of Mtb has been an annually routine work. Based on observations and studies for consecutive 19 years, the drug resistance rate of Mtb and its developing tendency in Shenzhen have been well under-

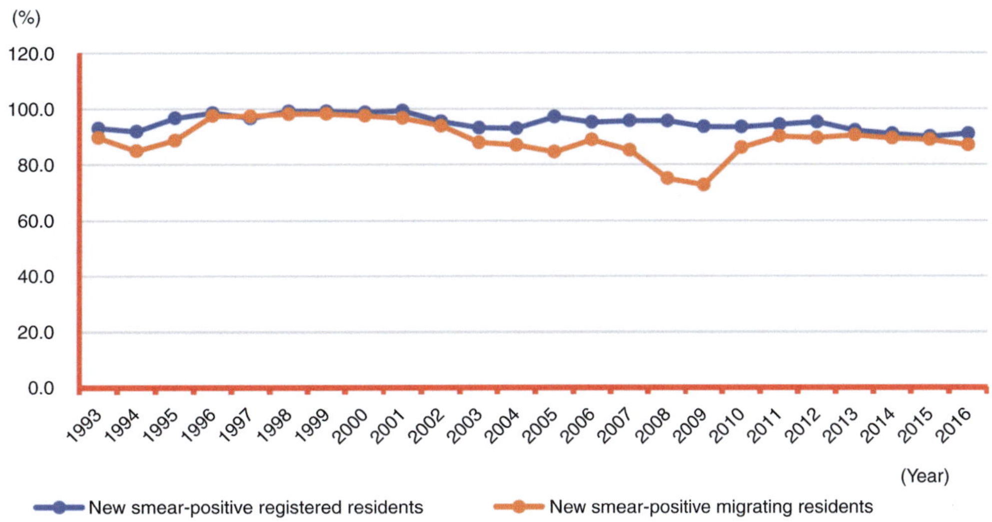

Fig. 2.11 New smear-positive patients' cure rates reported by Shenzhen TB control program (%)

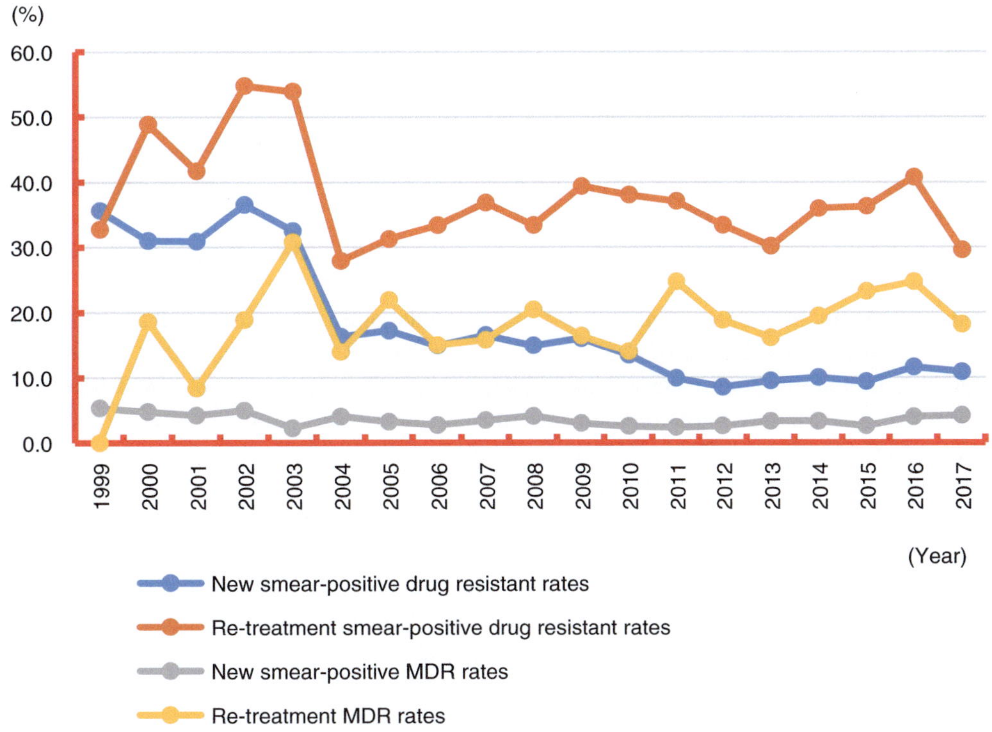

Fig. 2.12 Trends of Shenzhen drug-resistant and MDR rates

stood. The knowledge provides scientific basis for assessing TB control planning and improving TB control in Shenzhen. In addition, it is the important reference for related policies making (Figs. 2.12 and 2.13)

3.3 Data Analysis and Application

Data Analysis

Regular Analysis of TB Epidemic

Based on the statistics and TB report output functions in the Infectious Diseases Reporting Information Management System as well as appropriate application of epidemiology and statistics, the population distribution of TB and the factors influencing it can be described. In addition, the outcome of TB control measures can be assessed.

Dynamic Surveillance of TB Epidemic

Based on the internet on-line reported data, the epidemic of TB can be dynamically monitored. Agglomerated cases of TB can be paid more close attention for possible outbreak of TB. Its population distribution, epidemiological history, and possible tendency of prevalence can be analyzed and predicted.

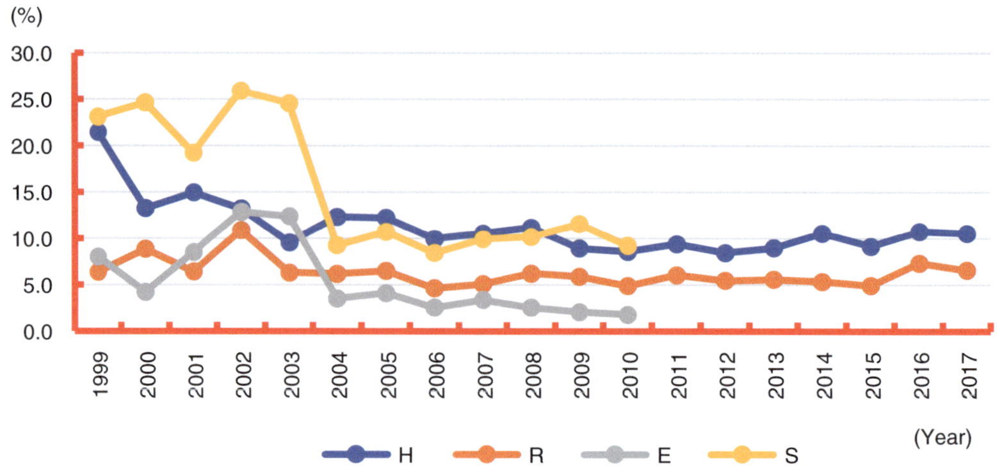

Fig. 2.13 Shenzhen TB drug-resistant frequency

Detection and Management of TB Patients

Based on the statistic and reports output functions in the Tuberculosis Management Information System, the referrals of suspected/defined TB cases, the case history of TB patients, the suspected cases of drug-resistant TB, and the case history of suspected drug-resistant TB patients can be analyzed and traced. Based on the quarterly and annual reports, the detection of TB patients can be analyzed, such as referral of suspected/defined TB cases and their follow-ups, source and laboratory tests results of the initially present patients, population categories of TB patients, and gender and age distribution of the new smear-positive TB patients. In addition, the management of the registered TB patients can be analyzed. The data includes management of the quarterly registered TB patients, the sputum test negative conversions after 2–3 months treatment in the previous quarter, and the cure rate and regular medication rate of registered TB patients in the same quarter of previous year. The planning implementations can also be analyzed, including technical training, drug supply, supervision and health management of TB patients, and health education. Based on the annual report, the funding investment and its expenditure, the equipment and professionals in TB control institutions, and registry and treatment of TB patients can be analyzed.

Figures and the Illustrations

In the data analysis, texts should be presented with figures and tables. The present prevalence of TB should be the focus of analysis and the developing tendency should be predicted. The measures of TB control and their outcomes should be assessed based on data analysis. And measures and recommendations targeting on the shortcomings should be proposed.

Feedbacks Based on Data Analysis

Based on data analysis, the results should be feedbacked to the superior TB control institution, the health-care administrative department of the same level, and the inferior TB control institutions in the form of briefs, reports, and epidemic analysis meetings.

3.4 Preservation of Data and Its Safety Management

Data Preservation

Paper and electronic Infectious Diseases Reporting Cards and the related records should be well preserved for 3 years.

The primary records in TB control institutions about the diagnosis and treatment of local residents and migrating population living in the same region should be well preserved for 15 years.

The electronic data should be regularly backed up, and the backup data should be preserved at a safe place to avoid damage and loss.

The reported data of TB, the case history, the suspected cases of drug-resistant TB, and the case history of drug-resistant TB as well as the generated monthly, quarterly, and annual reports should be regularly output and preserved.

Safety Management of the Information System

A full-time working staff should be specified in a TB control agency to manage the TB information data and the documentation of the information according to the national guidelines.

A TB control agency is responsible for maintenance of its TB management information system. Institutional regulations should be formulated to guarantee the safety of account. And the national information system should be logged in via VPN and digital certificate.

Based on the principle of user responsible, the user of the information system should not transfer or release the operational account and password to other individuals. When the account/password is released or embezzled, a new password should be applied based on the approval by the team leader.

The registry and review regulations should be formulated to manage the institution and working staffs working in TB information reporting and management. The reporting data of TB cases should not be abused to threaten the national security, social welfare, and legal rights of other individuals. The personal privacy data should not be released.

4 Effects of Migrating Population in a Region on the Regional Epidemic of TB

Currently, TB control in migrating population is a common issue worldwide. The migrating population flows from villages, industrially under-developed regions and regions with high incidence rate of TB into cities, industrially well-developed regions and regions with low incidence rate of TB. In the well-developed countries and regions, the prevalence of TB is low. When migrating population flows into cities, their immunity to fight against diseases is compromised due to poor housing conditions, more intense physical labor and high mental stress. Therefore, the probability of TB infection increases. In addition, migrating population with TB are commonly subject to delayed diagnosis and treatment, unwillingness to inform the clinicians about their conditions, failures to complete DOTs therapy, and arbitrary retrieval of the medication after the symptoms are improved. Therefore, TB in migrating population constitutes greater threat to the health of other populations. The increasingly larger migrating population presents challenges to the TB control in the influx region, especially in the economically well-developed regions. TB in migrating population causes its interpersonal spread to the local residents and the other individuals of migrating population, with consequent increase of its prevalence in the influx regions.

In China, 80% patients with TB live in rural areas and migrating population commonly has their registered permanent residence in rural areas. Therefore, migrating population is the high-risk population of TB infection. And TB in migrating population has been the main risk factor deteriorating the epidemics of TB in Beijing, Shanghai, Qingdao, Ningbo, Suzhou, and other economically well-developed regions. In 1993–2002, the numbers of newly registered active TB patients and smear-positive TB patients have remained steady in local residents of Beijing, showing a decrease of 6% and 8%, respectively. However, the numbers have sharply increased in the migrating population, with an increase of 344.2% and 237.8%, respectively [38]. In 1995–2006, the number of registered active TB patients has decreased by 22.78% and the number of bacteriologically positive TB patients has increased by 18.08% in local residents of Shanghai. Meanwhile, the numbers of registered active TB patients and bacteriologically positive TB patients have increased by 211.47% and 650.92%, respectively [39]. In 1995–2004, the ratio of active TB case between the migrating population to the local residents in Huangdao district of Qingdao has increased from 23.3% to 116.9%, and the ratio of smear-positive TB cases has increased from 21.7% to 150.0%. The cases of TB patients in migrating population have rapidly increased, with higher average annual increase rate and new registry rate than those in the local residents [40]. In 2013–2015, a total of 12,109 cases of TB have been reported in Ningbo of China, with a gradual decrease of the incidence. However, the percentage of TB patients in migrating population has increased. A study has demonstrated that population density and large migrating population are the important factors influencing outbreak of TB [41]. In 2008–2013, the morbidity rate of TB in the migrating population of Suzhou has been 21.6% higher than that in the local residents, which has increased the incidence of TB in the total population of Suzhou by 10.5%. In addition, the high incidence of TB in the migrating population has slowed the decrease of TB incidence in the total population of Suzhou by 4.4%. The contribution rates of TB incidence in the migrating population to the incidence in total population of Suzhou have been positive value, which has increased the incidence of TB in the total population of Suzhou by 0.3–42.3% [42]. In 2007–2010, the number of active TB patients in the migrating population of Sunan region in China has increased by 77.0%, with an average annual increase of 21.0%. Meanwhile, the number of active TB patients in local residents of Sunan region in China has decreased by 32.9%. In addition, the total number of TB patients in the three cities of Sunan region has more slowly decreased than that in the other regions of Jiangsu province, but with a more rapidly decreased number of TB patients in the local residents of the three cities. The increase of TB patients in the migrating population is the main reason for the slower decrease of TB patients in Sunan region [43].

According to the data released by WHO, the incidence of TB has been decreasing worldwide, with the most rapid decrease in the European Union. Although there is national variance in the number of TB patients in the European Union, the data shows the same underlying epidemiological trend. The prevalence of TB in the European countries is epidemiologically characterized by a gradual decrease of TB incidence in the local residents but a gradual increase of TB incidence in the migrating population. TB mostly commonly occurs in populations with recent migration or younger age groups. In the population of migration and previously treated TB patients, the percentage of drug-resistant TB (DR-TB) remains high. The incidence of TB is even higher in migrants with poor housing, especially in densely populated cities [44].

The migrants from countries with high morbidity of TB may present great challenge to the TB control in the influx regions. Hollo et al. studied the effects of population migration in the European Union/Economic Area on the national distribution of TB. The study has demonstrated that a total of 527,000 cases of TB have been reported in 29 countries in the European Union/Economic Area during 2007 to 2003, including 117,000 cases (22.2%) from the population migrating from other countries. And the cases from the countries in the European Union/Economic Area other than the 29 countries account for only 2.4% [45]. In 2014, a total of 58,000 cases of TB were reported in the 29 countries in the European Union/Economic Area (except for Italia and Liechtenstein), with a morbidity rate of 12.8 per 0.1 million and the patients from the migrating population accounted for 27%. In the reported cases in France, Germany, Spain, and Britain, 75% was from migrating population [46]. The contribution of TB in migrating population to the economic burden in the European Union/Economic Area has been increasing. Measures for prevention and control of TB targeting the migrating population are needed for progress towards eradicating TB [47].

In the high-income countries, an important variance has been covered by the overall morbidity rate of TB. The variance is the decrease variance of TB morbidity rates in local residents and migrating population. In the local residents, the morbidity rate of TB remains the same or has been decreasing, while in migrating population, it has been increasing or more slowly decreasing. According to the data from 134 countries and regions worldwide, the population of migration in the high-income countries is one of the important factors slowing the decrease of TB incidence. A study has demonstrated that the number of TB cases has decreased by 50% in the local residents of high-income countries in the Europe and America but the number has increased in the migrating population of the same region in 2000–2013. In nearly half of OECD high-income countries, the number of TB cases in migrating population has been increasing. In 2013, the cases of TB in migrating population accounted for 52.0% in the high-income countries of Europe and America and the morbidity rate of TB in the migrating population was 8.7–18.4 times as high as that in the local residents [48].

A descriptive data about population and TB cases in 21 European countries in 1996–2005 demonstrated that the reported morbidity rate of TB has increased only in Britain, Norway, and Sweden. Considering the fact that about three-fourths of TB cases were in migrating population of these countries, the increase may be attributed to the large population of migrants from countries with high morbidity rate of TB [49]. In Britain, the morbidity rate of TB in migrating population is 23 times as high as that in the local residents, and the overall morbidity rate has increased from 78 per 0.1 million in 2000 to 94 per 0.1 million in 2004. During the same period of time, the morbidity rate of TB in the local residents of Britain has remained steady and low [44].

The increasing incidence rate of TB has existed in Italy, Spain, and France. In large cities, the percentage of TB cases in migrating population has been even higher. The impacts of migrants to prevalence of TB in a country are directly related to the incidence of TB in the migrating population. Compared to the other countries in the European Union, the increasingly more migrants from countries with high prevalence of TB may significantly affect the overall incidence of TB in a country [44]. In Italy, TB has gradually been a disease specifically affecting the migrating population. A descriptive data from Umbria of Italy (with low incidence rate of TB but high percentage of migrating population) in 1999–2008 indicated that in the total 590 cases of TB, 254 cases (43%) are from migrating population. In 2008, the morbidity rate of TB in the migrating population of Umbria was 39.7 per 0.1 million but only 3.8 per 0.1 million in the local residents [50]. In Murcia Autonomous Region in Spain, a total of 162 cases of TB have been reported in 2004–2009. A cohort study on these 162 cases indicated that there are 110 cases of migrants, accounting for 67.9%, with an incidence rate of 43.4–101.2 per 0.1 million. In addition, occurrence of TB in the local residents is related to smoking, amount of alcohol use, and intravenous drug abuse. However, the main risk factor of TB infection in the migrants is overcrowded housing [51].

In 2001–2005, 349 strains of Mtb have been isolated in the western part of Sweden, with 26% from the local residents. The migrants from countries with high incidence of TB strongly impact the prevalence of TB in the western part of Sweden [52].

In the USA, a genome analysis on 546 cases of Mtb culture-positive TB from northern part of Manhattan in 1990–1999 showed that the morbidity rate of TB in the USA has decreased during the 10 years. However, the morbidity rate only decreased among the local residents. In the migrating population, TB was mainly caused by reactivated infection after incubation, while in the local residents, TB was mainly caused by recent spread of Mtb [53]. A data analysis based on the National Tuberculosis Surveillance System of the USA in 1994–2007 showed that in 18,659 reported cases of TB under the age of 18 years, 5806 cases (31%) were born in another country. The morbidity rate of TB in children and adolescents born in another country was 10–20 times as high as that in peers born in the USA. In the children and adolescents born in another country whose data of entry into the USA was known, more than 20% was diagnosed with TB within 3 months after their entry into the USA [54]. The effects of new comers (born in another country with entry into the USA for no more than 1 year) on the prevalence of TB in the USA have been assessed. The study indicated that the new comers of non-immigrant tourists into the USA constitute a heavy burden of TB [55].

In Canada, the morbidity rate of new active TB in the population born in Ontario province has more rapidly decreased than that in the migrating population in 1961–1971. In the year 1971, the local residents and the migrating population accounted for 77% and 22% of the overall population in Ontario, but the cases of TB were equal in number. During 1961–1971, the migrant population in Ontario changed, with more from countries and regions with high TB morbidity rate but less from countries and regions with low TB morbidity rate. The percentage of recent migrants in TB patients of migrating population increased from 25% in 1961–1966 to 40% in 1967–1971 [56].

Generally speaking, the increasingly larger migrating population necessarily aggravates the epidemic of TB in their influx countries and regions. However, it remains controversial that the migrating population with high incidence of TB may cause its spread to the local residents with low incidence of TB.

A molecular epidemiological study has been conducted for the effects of migrants on prevalence of TB in Rhode Island of the USA. The study demonstrated that the recent spread of TB is limited among individuals of migrating population, but its spread between migrating population and local residents should not be neglected. The genome analysis of Mtb showed that 80% cases of Mtb infection are from migrating population in a mixed population with local residents and migrating population [57]. However, another study was conducted for the effects of migrants on TB infection in children and adolescents born in Montreal of Canada. The study indicated that tuberculin reaction in schools, workplaces, and neighborhoods is not related to the contact index to migrating population from countries and regions with high prevalence of TB. No evidence has been found to prove that the infected high-risk population spreads TB to the common healthy populations in schools and workplaces [58]. A prospective study has been conducted in 749 defined cases of culture-positive TB and the individuals with close contacts to them in a federal state of Germany. The study indicated that the influx of population from regions with high prevalence of TB has no great impact on the prevalence of TB in the local residents. The reason might be effective implementation of TB screening plan before their entry into the federal state of Germany and/or low mixing degree of the migrating population with the local residents [59].

References

1. Zhuo ZW. Report on population migration and migrating population in China across the century. Beijing: Population Institution, Renmin University of China; 2003. p. 89.
2. Wu X. Rural community in cities: areas inhabited by the migrating population. Urban Plan. 2001;12:25–30.
3. Hugo GJ. Migration as a survival strategy: the family dimension of migration. In: Population distribution and migration. New York: United Nations, Department for Economic and Social Affairs, Population Division; 1998. p. 49–65.
4. Li Y, Wang Y. Studies on factors influencing tuberculosis. Foreign Med Sci. 2005;22:53–7.
5. Pons JEPA. Testing the new economic geography: migrations and industrial agglomerations in Spain. J Reg Sci. 2007;47:289–313.
6. Nigg C. Medical problems in migrants. Praxis. 2003;92(15):689–96.
7. Bwire R, Nagelkerke N, Keizer ST, et al. Tuberculosis screening among immigrants in The Netherlands: what is its contribution to public health. Neth J Med. 2000;56(2):63–71.
8. Han Q. Urban development and problems in Latin America. Res Latin Am. 1999;2:44–9.
9. Zhang JT. Modern development of Latin America and the problems. J Hebei Univ. 2000;1:11–5.
10. Zhao HY. Migration of rural population during industrialization in Latin America and Africa. J Cap Univ Econ Bus. 2007;1:111–5.
11. Hugo G. Changing patterns and processes of population mobility. In: Population and human resource. Canberra: Australian National University; 1997. p. 68–100.
12. Zhu Y. Foreign studies on non-permanent migration of population and the implications to the issues of migrating population in China. Pop Res. 2004;28:52–9.
13. Zhong D. Prevalence of tuberculosis in migrating population and developments in its control strategies. Prevent Contr Dis. 2011;38:4277–82.
14. UN. Total international migrant stock. New York: United Nations, Department of Economic and Social Affairs; 2015.
15. Lönnroth K, Mor Z, Erkens C, et al. Tuberculosis in migrants in low-incidence countries: epidemiology and intervention entry points. Int J Tuberc Lung Dis. 2017;21(6):624–36.
16. Stewart RJ, Tsang CA, Pratt RH, et al. Tuberculosis--United States 2017. Atlanta: MMWR Morb Mortal Wkly Rep; 2018.
17. Odone A, Tillmann T, Sandgren A, et al. Tuberculosis among migrant populations in the European Union and the European Economic Area. Eur J Pub Health. 2015;25(3):506–12.
18. Zhong D, Zhang YH, Fu YY, et al. Research development on prevalence of tuberculosis in the migrating population and the control strategies. Mod Prevent Med. 2011;20:4277–8.
19. Xie RQ, Cheng JQ, Yang YZ, et al. Social support to patients with tuberculosis in the migrating population. Chin J Behav Med Sci. 2006;5:437–9.
20. Jia L, Li X, Li J, et al. Geographic distribution of registered TB patients in the population living at the place other than their registered permanent residence in China. Chin J Anti-tuberc. 2012;34(11):712–20.
21. Du X, Liu EY, Cheng SM. Analysis of new smear positive TB patients in registered migrating population of 2010 in China. Chin J Anti-tuberc. 2011;33(8):461–5.
22. Chen J, Wei XL, Li HD. Factors influencing treatment and management of tuberculosis in the migrating population of Shanghai. Chin J Anti-tuberc. 2009;31(6):337–40.
23. Yang SB, Li Q, Miao ZP. Surveillance of pulmonary tuberculosis in the migrating population in Zhejiang province in 2001-2002. Chin J Anti-tuberc. 2004;26(3):170–2.
24. Wu QF, Lv DL, Guan HY, et al. Epidemiological study of pulmonary tuberculosis in 2007-2016 in Shenzhen. J Trop Med. 2018;1:86–9.

25. Liu XQ, Jiang SW, Li XX, et al. Provincial distribution of active pulmonary tuberculosis in the migrating population in 2010. J Dis Surveill. 2013;28(7):521–7.
26. Zhong J, Mai JE, Luo YL, et al. Prevalence of pulmonary tuberculosis in Haizhu district of Guangzhou. Chin J Anti-tuberc. 2006;28(1):25–7.
27. Zhao P, Li HM, Yang ZB, et al. Epidemiological study on pulmonary tuberculosis in the migrating population in Chaoyang district of Beijing in 1996-2006. J Dis Contr. 2008;12(1):83–5.
28. Bi HS. Treatment and management of tuberculosis in the migrating population in Baoan district of Shenzhen. Wuhan: Huazhong University of Science and Technology; 2015.
29. Health Commission of P. R. China. Law of People's Republic of China on Prevention and Treatment of Infectious Diseases (No. 17th Presidential Order of the People's Republic of China) issued on Aug 28, 2004. http://www.nhfpc.gov.cn/zwgk/falv/200804/b357d2f993ce422eb054f4f971884eba.shtml.
30. Center for Disease Control of China. Notice on Publication of 2016 Technical Guideline for National Infectious Diseases Information Reporting Management (No. [2016] 106 issued by CDC of China).
31. Health Commission of P. R. China. Health-care Occupational Standards of People's Republic of China: the Diagnosis of Tuberculosis. November 9, 2017. http://www.nhfpc.gov.cn/zhuz/s9491/201712/a452586fd21d4018b0ebc00b89c06254.shtml.
32. Wu QF, Lv DL, Guan HY, et al. Epidemiological analysis of tuberculosis in Shenzhen during 2007 to 2016. J Trop Med. 2018;18(1):86–9.
33. Statistics Bureau of Shenzhen and Shenzhen Survey Team of the National Statistics Bureau of China. 2016 statistical annuals in Shenzhen. Beijing: China Statistics Press; 2016. p. 53–5.
34. Health Ministry of People's Republic of China. Complied data about the national epidemiological sampling survey on tuberculosis in 2000. Beijing: People's Medical Publishing House; 2000.
35. Wang Y. Complied data about the 5th national epidemiological sampling survey on tuberculosis. Beijing: Military Medical Science Press; 2011.
36. Technical Guidance Team of the 5th National Epidemiological Sampling Survey on Tuberculosis and the Management Office of the 5th National Epidemiological Sampling Survey on Tuberculosis. Report of the 5th national epidemiological sampling survey on tuberculosis in 2010. Chin J Anti-tuberc. 2012;34(8):485–508.
37. Disease Prevention and Control Bureau of Health Ministry & Health-care Administration Department of Health Ministry & Center for Disease Control of China. The 2008 technical guideline for implementation of tuberculosis prevention and treatment planning. Beijing: Peking Union Medical College Press.
38. An YS, Zhang LX, Tu DH. Effects of migrating population on the prevalence of tuberculosis in Beijing. Chin J Anti-tuberc. 2004; 6:4–8.
39. Xia Z, Mei J, Ni HL, et al. Effects of migrating population on tuberculosis control in Shanghai. Shanghai Prevent Med. 2008;20(2):67–8.
40. Liu CX. Effects of migrating population on prevalence of tuberculosis in Huangdao district of Qingdao in 1995-2004. 2005.
41. Yang TC, Hong H, Chen T, et al. Sociological factors influencing prevalence and spatial distribution of tuberculosis in influx cities by migrating population. Chin J Amphixenosis. 2017;9:800–4.
42. Mu WM, Wang FX, Jiang J. Effects of migrating population on prevalence of TB in Suzhou. Mod Prevent Med. 2016;6:1047–50.
43. Zhu LM, Xu WG, Peng H, et al. Demographic analysis of patients with tuberculosis in Sunan region of China and effects of migrating population on its prevalence in the region. Chin J Dis Contr. 2011;11:975–7.
44. Khyatti M, Trimbitas RD, Zouheir Y, et al. Infectious diseases in North Africa and North African immigrants to Europe. Eur J Publ Health. 2014;24(suppl 1):47–56.
45. Hollo V, Kotila SM, Kodmon C, et al. The effect of migration within the European Union/European Economic Area on the distribution of tuberculosis, 2007 to 2013. Euro Surveill. 2016;21(12):30171.
46. van der Werf MJ, Zellweger JP. Impact of migration on tuberculosis epidemiology and control in the EU/EEA. Euro Surveill. 2016;21(12):30174.
47. Kodmon C, Zucs P, van der Werf MJ. Migration-related tuberculosis: epidemiology and characteristics of tuberculosis cases originating outside the European Union and European Economic Area, 2007 to 2013. Euro Surveill. 2016;21(12):30164.
48. Pareek M, Greenaway C, Noori T, et al. The impact of migration on tuberculosis epidemiology and control in high-income countries: a review. BMC Med. 2016;14:48.
49. Gilbert RL, Antoine D, French CE, et al. The impact of immigration on tuberculosis rates in the United Kingdom compared with other European countries. Int J Tuberc Lung Dis. 2009;13(5):645–51.
50. Buonora N, Chiavarini M, Salmasi L, et al. Impact of immigration on burden of tuberculosis in Umbria: a low-incidence Italian region with high immigrants rates. J Prev Med Hyg. 2013;54(1):29.
51. Molina-Salas Y, de Las MLM, Romera-Guirado FJ, et al. Influence of migration on tuberculosis in a semi-urban area. Arch Bronconeumol. 2014;50(8):325–31.
52. Svensson E, Millet J, Lindqvist A, et al. Impact of immigration on tuberculosis epidemiology in a low-incidence country. Clin Microbiol Infect. 2011;17(6):881–7.
53. Geng E, Kreiswirth B, Driver C, et al. Changes in the transmission of tuberculosis in New York City from 1990 to 1999. N Engl J Med. 2002;346(19):1453–8.
54. Menzies HJ, Winston CA, Holtz TH, et al. Epidemiology of tuberculosis among US- and foreign-born children and adolescents in the United States, 1994-2007. Am J Public Health. 2010;100(9): 1724–9.
55. Liu Y, Painter JA, Posey DL, et al. Estimating the impact of newly arrived foreign-born persons on tuberculosis in the United States. PLoS One. 2012;7(2):e32158.
56. Ashley MJ, Anderson TW, Le Riche WH. The influence of immigration on tuberculosis in Ontario. Am Rev Respir Dis. 1974;110(2):137–46.
57. Vanhomwegen J, Kwara A, Martin M, et al. Impact of immigration on the molecular epidemiology of tuberculosis in Rhode Island. J Clin Microbiol. 2011;49(3):834–44.
58. Menzies D, Chan CH, Vissandjee B. Impact of immigration on tuberculosis infection among Canadian-born schoolchildren and young adults in Montreal. Am J Respir Crit Care Med. 1997;156(6):1915–21.
59. Barniol J, Niemann S, Louis VR, et al. Transmission dynamics of pulmonary tuberculosis between autochthonous and immigrant sub-populations. BMC Infect Dis. 2009;9:197.

Strategy of TB Control in Migrating Population

3

Hong-yun Guan, Sheng-yuan Liu, Yu-zheng Fan, Wei-guo Tan, and Wei-ye Yu

1 Strategies of TB Control

1.1 Strategies of Global TB Control

Directly Observed Treatment, Short-Course (DOTS) During 1995–2005

Active detection and treatment of patients with TB is the most effective intervention with the lowest cost-benefit ratio in TB control. During the 1970s and 1980s in the twentieth century, Karel Styblo from the International Union Against Tuberculosis and Lung Disease proposed the strategy of directly observed treatment (DOT) [2]. In 1991, the goal of global TB control was proposed in the World Health Assembly. Specifically, the goal was to diagnose 70% smear-positive TB patients and to cure 85% definitively diagnosed TB patients before the year 2000. Meanwhile, active participation by countries worldwide in TB control was called for [3]. In 1994, the WHO announced that DOT strategy shows the lowest cost-benefit ratio in TB control. And DOT strategy was recommended by the WHO as the strategy for global TB control [4]. In 1995, the promotion of DOTS strategy was initiated by the WHO [5], which includes the following measures:

(1) Commitment of the government on TB control planning;
(2) Sputum smear examination as the main way for detection of patients with communicable TB;
(3) Whole-course supervision on the treatment and management of smear-positive TB patients;
(4) To establish a free-in-charge anti-tuberculosis drug supply system;
(5) To establish a TB registry, reporting, and surveillance system.

Commitment of the government to support TB control is a necessary condition for coordination of various resources and sustainable development of TB control plans. Microscopic examination of sputum smear section is the way with the lowest cost-benefit ratio in screening of suspected TB patients. In DOTS, the directly observed treatment should be at least observed during the strengthening period for appropriate medication for patients with TB. The anti-tuberculosis drug supply should be sufficiently planned and implemented. The recording and reporting system is mainly applied to systemically assess the progress and outcome of the therapy. By adopting DOTS, the patients can be secured regular medications as outpatients and the cure rate has been improved with fewer relapses. Therefore, the spread of drug-resistant TB has effectively interfered. Meanwhile, the DOTS strategy has advantages of low cost to recover labor productivity, which plays an important role in improving and controlling epidemics of TB. However, DOTS has some disadvantages, such as insufficient connotation in the commitment of the government, low detection rate of sputum smear test, failure to exclude non-Mtb infection, failure to diagnose drug-resistant TB, supply only first-line anti-tuberculosis drugs, and incomplete surveillance system.

1.2 DOTS-Plus

To actively interfere multidrug-resistant TB, DOTS-Plus strategy was firstly proposed in the WHO conference that was held in Cambridge, Massachusetts in April 1998. The key contents of the strategy include [6]:

(1) Sustained commitment of the government in TB control, which is the foundation of the other four basic elements;
(2) Timely and accurate diagnosis of drug-resistant TB via qualitatively secured culture and drug sensitivity tests;

H.-y. Guan (✉) · S.-y. Liu · Y.-z. Fan
Shenzhen Nanshan Center for Chronic Disease Control, Shenzhen, Guangdong, China

W.-g. Tan · W.-y. Yu
Department of Tuberculosis, The Shenzhen Center for Chronic Disease Control, Shenzhen, Guangdong, China

W.-y. Yu et al. (eds.), *Tuberculosis Control in Migrating Population*, https://doi.org/10.1007/978-981-32-9763-0_3

(3) Reasonable application of second-line anti-tuberculosis drugs and standardized medications;
(4) Reliable and continuous anti-tuberculosis drug supply;
(5) Establish a system for registry and reporting of drug-resistant TB.

The focus of DOTS-Plus is the application of second-line anti-tuberculosis drugs to interfere the spread of MDR-TB. The focuses of DOTS-Plus and DOTS are different. Individualized therapy rather than standardized therapy is commonly applied for patients with MDR-TB. Laboratory tests include sputum culture and drug sensitivity tests in addition to sputum smear test. Reliable and low-cost second-line anti-tuberculosis drugs supply is secured. Necessary scientific research can be conducted to improve the TB control planning. And supports from local governments as well as international organizations and developed countries are necessary [7]. Based on these differences, DOTS-Plus strategy is believed to be an effective supplementation to DOTS strategy.

Stop TB Strategy During 2006–2015

To realized the Millennium Development Goals (MDG) and significantly reduce the global TB burden, a new TB control strategy was proposed in 2006 by the WHO and its global partners in TB control. The standpoint of the strategy is the emphasis of TB as a public health issue and a serious social problem due to the emergence of MDR-TB and TB in patients with HIV/AIDS. In response to these new challenges, the new strategy is focused on the leading role of policies to accelerate TB control with new technology, new drugs, and new vaccines. The collaborative efforts of departments and sections, social participation, and personal responsibilities are also emphasized in the new strategy.

Vision

The vision of the new strategy is a world with no tuberculosis.

Overall Goal

In the year 2015, MDG can be realized with significant decrease of global TB burden. Meanwhile, the significantly progressing science and technology serve to eradicate TB.

Objective

The objective of the new strategy is as follows:

(1) To increase the accessibility of health-care service for patients with TB and to provide high-quality health-care service for TB patients with well-developed diagnosis and treatment.
(2) To reduce physical and mental sufferings as well as economic burden of TB.
(3) To protect the susceptible populations of TB from TB infection and to decrease the incidences of co-infection of TB and HIV/AIDS and MDR-TB.
(4) To develop new detection and therapy for TB and to promote their timely and effective application.

Specific Goals

(1) The detection rate of patients with communicable TB reaches 70% and the cure rate 85%.
(2) By the end of 2015, the morbidity and mortality of TB decrease by 50% and the incidence stops increasing based on the data in 1990.
(3) By the end of 2050, the average annual incidence rate is lower than 1 per million, which is considered a successful eradication of TB.

The Key Points of the Strategy Include the Followings [8]

(1) DOTS is extended for higher-quality DOTS. The measures include sustained funding by the governments, detection of patients via qualitatively secured bacteriological examinations, standardized medication therapy, supervised medication and humane supports, sustained effective supply of anti-tuberculosis drugs, and timely effective dynamic surveillance of TB control.
(2) The stop TB strategy is formulated to overcome challenges of TB/HIV and MDR-TB. The institutions for TB control and HIV/AIDS control make strengthened collaborative efforts and the cases of TB in imprisoned population, refugee population and other high-risk populations are paid close attention for control of TB.
(3) The stop TB strategy is implemented along with reform of health-care system. The reforms of health-care system include health-related policies making, human resources management, financial management, health-care service providing, and information system management. In addition, measures for reform of TB control system are implemented. The innovative experience in other fields is adopted to innovate the health-care system and TB control system. The care for TB patients is integrated with the health-care of respiratory system to effectively promote the health of lungs.
(4) All the health-care service providers are mobilized to participate in the TB control. The collaborative efforts are made via collaborative modes of public–public and public–private (PPM). The international standards for care of TB are formulated.
(5) The roles of community and patients themselves in the health care of TB are exerted via initiation, communication, and social mobilization.
(6) The scientific research on TB is promoted in aspects of applied research and collaborative research to develop new technology, new drugs, and new vaccines against TB.

Table 3.1 End TB goal

Index	Milestone		Target	
	2020	2025	SDG 2030	End TB 2035
Compared to 2015, the mortality of TB decreases (%)	35	75	90	95
Compared to 2015, the morbidity of TB decreases (%)	20% (<85/100,000)	50 (<55/100,000)	80 (<20/100,000)	90 (<10/100,000)
Families experience catastrophic cost due to TB (%)	0	0	0	0

End TB Strategy During 2016–2035

In 2016, global TB control stepped into an era with sustainable development and the end TB strategy began to play its role in TB control. The strategy strengthened its emphasis on actions and responsibilities of the governments, more extensive social participation, protection, and promotion of human rights, ethics, and equity, as well as implementation of national strategy based on global collaboration. "After 2015, the global TB control strategy is intended to end the global prevalence of TB. The goal is to decrease the mortality of TB by 95% and to decrease the new cases of TB by 90% during 2015–2035. Meanwhile, it should be ensured that no family has catastrophic expense on TB."

Vision

The vision of end TB strategy is a world with no TB and TB no longer causes death, disease, and sufferings.

Overall Goal

The overall goal is to end TB across the world.

Principles

The government is responsible for management, supervision, surveillance, and assessment.

A strong alliance is established among the government, social organizations, and communities.

The human rights, ethics, and equity should be protected and promoted.

The national strategies and goals can be adjusted and applied based on global collaborations.

Key Points of the Strategy

The comprehensive treatment and prevention should be patient-centered. The early diagnosis of TB includes widespread use of drug sensitivity test as well as systematic screening of individuals with close contacts to the patients and high-risk populations. All the patients including patients with DR-TB should receive treatment and supportive service should be simultaneously provided. Collaborative efforts for TB control and HIV/AIDS control should be made and the complications should be managed. Preventive therapies should be provided for the high-risk populations. And the populations should receive vaccination to fight against TB.

Strong policies and supportive system are implemented. Sufficient resources should be politically committed into the treatment and prevention of TB. Communities, social organizations, and public/private health-care service providers should participate in the control of TB. The health-care formulary should cover all the populations. A managing framework should be established for case reporting, dynamic population registry, quality management and appropriate use of anti-tuberculosis drugs, and infection control. Measures for social protection, alleviation of poverty, and other measures targeting on determinants of TB prevalence should be planned and implemented.

Scientific research and innovation should be strengthened. The new tools, and new interfering measures and strategies should be developed and rapidly applied based on scientific research and technological innovation.

Scientific research should also be conducted to optimize the implementation of policies and measures and to promote innovations.

Implementation Plans

In the end TB strategy, three milestones in 2020, 2025, and 2030 are planned. It is proposed that the incidence of TB decreases by 20%, 50%, and 80% in 2020, 2025, and 2030, respectively, based on the data of 2015. And the goal of end TB should be finally realized in 2035 (Table 3.1).

1.3 TB Control Strategy in China

Active Introduction of DOTS During 1991–2000

In 1991, the Health Ministry of China formulated the National TB Control Planning (1991–2000), in which the goal of TB control was proposed. In the planning, DOTS strategy was appraised and introduced to increase the detection rate and cure rate of TB and to control the prevalence of TB in China. To accelerate the implementation of DOTS in China, the World Bank Loan for TB Control program was initiated in 13 provinces, autonomous regions, and province-level municipalities in China in 1992–1999. The coverage of DOTS strategy reached up to 560 million population in China. In 1993, the Finance Ministry and the Health Ministry of China initiated the Reinforcement and Promotion of TB Control program by using the Central Disease Control Funding. The implementation of DOTS strategy was then extended to cover a population of 140 million.

In 1991–2000, the TB control in China has achieved great progress. The coverage of DOTS strategy has increased from less than 10% to 66%, with an increase of detection rate from 5% to 28% [9]. However, the TB control in China has faced many challenges and barriers. The coverage of DOTS strategy has increased slowly, with an increase by 6% during the 5 years from 1995 to 2000. The coverage of DOTS strategy in the western area of China has been in urgent need of extension to effective control the prevalence of TB.

Promotion of DOTS During 2001–2005

According to the situation, difficulties, and challenges in TB control in China, the General Office of the State Council of China issued the National TB Control Planning (2001–2010) in 2001. In the planning, the main principles, overall goal, organizational guarantee, and measures for TB control were clearly proposed. By the end of 2005, the DOTS strategy had been implemented in all the 31 provinces, autonomous regions, and province-level municipalities in Chinese mainland.

During 2001–2005 when the DOTS strategy was implemented in Chinese mainland, the main measures for TB control included the followings.

Strengthened Commitment of the Government to Secure the Funding for TB Control

In the TB control planning formulated by different levels of governments, the principles of TB control include leadership of the government, collaboration of multiple sections, extensive social participation as well as predominant funding by governments with supplementary funding from other social resources.

An Improved Health-Care Service System for TB Control

A health-care service system for TB control was established and improved. The system consisted of the managing institution for TB control and professional health-care institutions. The professional health-care institutions include TB control agency, all the health-care institutions, and community-based health-care service network or community health-care service centers.

Increased Detection Rate and Management Rate of TB Patients

The measures of TB symptoms-based clinic presentation, recommendation, referral, and trace were implemented for detection of TB patients. The suspected cases of TB were prescribed to receive free-in-charge sputum smear test and chest X-ray. The individuals with close contacts with smear-positive TB patients were screened. Pilot work for sputum smear test in health-care clinics of towns was conducted. The patients received mainly standardized medication treatment as outpatients. DOTS was conducted by clinicians for patients with TB and the medication compliances of the patients were improved. Collaborative efforts of health-care institutions and TB control agencies were made, and the other health-care institutions made referrals according to the requirements. The diagnosis and treatment of TB were strengthened in the health-care institutions specialized in TB control, and community-based TB control was conducted. Laboratory tests including sputum smear test, sputum culture, and drug sensitivity test were performed. And biological safety management and infection control were strengthened. The anti-tuberculosis drug supply and management system were established and improved to secure continuous supply of anti-tuberculosis drugs. Fixed-dose compounds were gradually promoted for application.

Responses to the Three Challenges

The migrating population was fitted into the TB control planning. And prevention and control of MDR-TB, TB in population with HIV/AIDS, and TB in jails were gradually implemented.

Strengthened Health Education

Guidance and communication for social mobilization were conducted. And collaborative efforts for health education were made and their effects were assessed.

Strengthened Surveillance and Assessment

Based on the TB Management Information System, data of TB was collected, analyzed, and assessed. Field epidemiological surveys were conducted for deep understandings about effects of TB control planning.

Active Scientific Studies

The scientific studies on implementation of TB control planning were conducted to find the priority fields in TB control. And the research achievements were promoted for wider application.

Emphasized Implementation of Stop TB Strategy in 2006–2015

During 2006–2015, China has been ranked second in the total number of TB cases across the world. The TB cases in China were predominantly DR-TB, with increasing number of co-infection of TB and HIV/AIDS. However, the health-care service system for TB control was insufficiently developed for the actual demand of TB control in China. In addition, the people in China had insufficient knowledge about the threats of TB. Under the severe situations, the stop TB strategy was uniformly implemented in the whole country. And the specific measures are as follows:

(1) The leadership by governments, collaboration of multiple sections, funding, and system construction were strengthened.
(2) The reporting and referral of TB patients were further implemented. Early detection of TB patients was

conducted via screening of individuals with close contacts to patients with TB and high-risk populations. Sputum smear test and chest X-ray were performed in the designated health-care institutions.

(3) The diagnosis and treatment of TB were standardized. The anti-tuberculosis drugs in standardized therapy and follow-up reexaminations were provided free-in-charge. The management technology was explored and the fixed-dose compounds were promoted for wider application to improve the effects of patients management.
(4) The coverage of MDR-TB treatment was further increased. The suspected cases of TB were timely detected for drug sensitivity and the diagnosis was timely defined in the health-care institution for TB control. The suspected and defined cases of TB were managed in basic health-care institutions according to the requirements to effectively stop the spread of drug-resistant Mtb.
(5) The detection, registry, and management of TB patients in the migrating population were further implemented. Collaborative management of TB patients was performed by the referral-out and the referral-in health-care institutions.
(6) The diagnosis, treatment, and management of TB-HIV/AIDS patients were collaboratively performed. The bidirectional screening and humane care were conducted to improve the quality of life of the patients and to decrease the mortality rate.
(7) Health education for TB control was strengthened to spread the core information about TB control.
(8) Scientific research was promoted and the scholarly attention was focused on the new technologies, new drugs, and new vaccines against TB. The scientific studies provided technical support to explore the effective measures for TB control.
(9) International collaborations were strengthened for absorption and promotion of new technologies worldwide.

In 2010, the morbidity rate of smear-positive TB patients was 66 per 0.1 million, with a decrease by 61%, compared to the data in 2000. The MDG was realized in China in advance. During 2011–2015, the prevalence of TB in China decreased gradually, and 4.27 million patients with active TB received treatment and management. The cure rate remained to be above 85%. The data indicated that the national 12th 5-year planning for TB control has been realized.

Active Exploration of End TB Strategy Since 2016

TB control in China is an important work in the national 13th 5-year planning of China. In February 2017, the General Office of State Council of China issued the National 13th 5-year Planning for TB Control. In the planning, the system for TB control, namely the leadership of the government, collaboration of multiple sections, coordination of the whole society, and participation of the mass, was required to be further improved. A comprehensive service system should be further improved, including TB control agencies, designated health-care institutions, and community-based health-care institutions. All of the institutions should have well-coordinated definitive responsibilities. The performance of TB control should also be further improved, including early detection, standardized treatment, consecutive prevention and treatment, and rehabilitations of TB. The health-secure policies should be further improved to further decrease the economic burden of TB patients and their families. The number of new cases and death cases of TB should be further decreased. The incidence rate of TB should be controlled under 58 per 0.1 million. And the incidence rate of TB in the seriously affected areas should be reduced by 20%, compared to the data in 2015. The specific measures for TB control are as follows:

(1) A graded comprehensive system for TB diagnosis and treatment should be improved. The TB control agencies, designated health-care institutions, and community-based health-care institutions should have specific responsibilities. And the institutions should well-cooperated and well-coordinated when necessary.
(2) Detection of TB patients should be strengthened via multiple routes and ways. The screening of suspected TB patients in the present patients should be strengthened. Active screening of TB in high-risk populations should be conducted. Screening of TB patients should be enlisted into routine health examination. Meanwhile, suspected cases of DR-TB should receive screening and diagnosis of TB for early detection of the spreading source.
(3) The guidelines for the diagnosis and treatment of TB should be strictly observed. And the health-care quality control should be strengthened. Diagnosis and treatment of TB should be enlisted into the health-care quality system to promote standardized diagnosis and treatment of TB.
(4) In the health management, patients with TB should be seamlessly transited. And new technologies should be applied for accessible health-care service to improve the compliance of the patients.
(5) Health-care formulary and humane care should be promoted. The mode of payment for health-care service should be innovated. TB, including MDR-TB, should be gradually enlisted as the special disease category for outpatients. The patients with TB in poverty should be timely aided to avoid catastrophic expenses on TB.
(6) The high-risk populations, including school students, migrating population, patients with co-infection of TB

and HIV/AIDS, and imprisoned population should be paid close attention for TB control to avoid clustering epidemic of TB.

(7) The supply of anti-tuberculosis drugs should be secured. The procedures for purchase of anti-tuberculosis drugs should be improved to secure the quality of drugs, reasonable price of the drugs, and sufficient supply of the drugs.

(8) Based on the national health insurance informatization project, the procedures of TB patient management should be performed by using information technology. Data about patients with TB should be shared via internet among TB control agencies, designated health-care institutions, community-based health-care institutions, and health insurance management institutions.

2 Progresses of TB Control in Migrating Population

Internationally, migrant population refers to individuals migrate into another country for permanent residence or large-scale organized migration of population. Migration is not necessarily accompanied by transition of the nationality. It includes temporary migration of population and migration of population with transition of the nationality. In China, migrating population refers to the population that migrates to a place that is not their registered permanent residence, namely the separation of the individual from his/her registered permanent residence [10]. Along with economic and cultural development as well as increased interpersonal communications, the migrating population presents serious challenge to the TB control in their influx countries and regions.

2.1 TB Control in Migrants

TB in migrants is an extensively existing problem worldwide. In 2010, the number of migrants amounted up to 214 million. The high-income countries in Europe, Asia, and North America are the main influx countries of the migrants [11]. According to the data from 134 countries and regions worldwide, migrant population in the high-income countries is an important factor impeding the decrease of TB incidence [12]. Similar results have been harvested in some other high-income countries [13–16].

TB Control in the Migrant Population in the USA

The migrant population in the USA increased from 7.5% in 1986 to 13.7% in 2015, including about 11 million illegal migrants. During 1993–2015, the incidence rate of TB in the population with their birth place in the USA decreased from 7.4 per 0.1 million to 1.2 per 0.1 million. And it is far lower than that in the population with their birth place other than the USA. The average annual incidence rate of TB in the population with their birth place in the USA was 1.2 per 0.1 million, while it was 15.1 per 0.1 million in the population with their birth place other than the USA. The patients with TB in the migrant population in the USA are mainly from five countries, including Mexico, Philippines, India, Vietnam, and China. The incidence rate of TB in migrant population from Asia is the highest in all populations in the USA [17]. In 1992, the incidence of TB in New York city was three times as high as that in 1978, and the patients with TB in the migrant population in the USA accounted for up to 58% in 1999 [18].

In 2015, the prevalence of TB in the USA increased again after a decrease. Based on data analysis, the reasons for the increase include the followings:

(1) The national funding for TB control was decreased or suspended. Due to the low prevalence of TB in the USA, the health-care management system for TB control in the USA was weak with limited performance of laboratory tests. The anti-tuberculosis drugs and professionals in TB control remained insufficient and no enough experience was summarized in the treatment of complications of TB.

(2) The high-risk populations of TB were insufficiently managed. The management and treatment of TB in drug abusers, prisoners, and homeless population presented challenge to the TB control system of the USA. The patients with TB in the USA commonly suffered from the complications of diabetes, which caused much more difficulty for the treatment. And the management of these patients was challenging.

(3) Diagnostic examination and medication therapies were insufficiently innovated. Due to the fact of low incidence of TB, more rapid diagnostic examinations and more effective medication therapies were necessary.

(4) The patients with incubated TB infection were inappropriately treated. Due to the low incidence of TB in the USA, the clinicians were less alert to the onset of TB and their experience in rapid diagnosis and exclusion was insufficient.

Targeting on the increased prevalence of TB in the USA, the TB control strategy in the USA was further improved [19]. The measures included the following:

(1) The weakness in management and control of TB were strengthened. Anti-tuberculosis drugs and therapies for the complications were timely supplied.

(2) The patients with DR-TB were effectively treated. In the USA, the cases of DR-TB were extremely rare. But once detected, effective therapies were immediately

administered. And the individuals with close contacts with the patients with DR-TB were timely found and screened.

(3) Scientific research and technological innovations for TB control were supported. The development of new drugs and new vaccines was supported. These provided basis to achieve the goal of end TB.
(4) The TB control in the USA was integrated with other global health-care programs. TB control in patients with HIV/AIDS, pregnancies, and pediatric patients with TB was emphasized.
(5) The cost of TB treatment was resolved. Under the financial shortage of the government, construction of the health-care service system for TB control was strengthened. And the health-care service system for TB control in the USA was well coordinated with other international TB control institutions (such as the Global Funding Organization). On August 25, 2015, the Center for Diseases Control (CDC) of the USA issued the goal of national TB control planning in 2020. The goal is to end TB in the USA via prevention and treatment of TB. In addition, the planning is intended to control TB worldwide via collaborative efforts with other countries and international partners and thus to enhance the health of populations and their quality of life [20].

TB Control in Migrant Population in Other Countries

Along with the increasing number of migrants, the cases of TB in migrants and population with birth place in another country have obviously increased in many industrially developed countries. However, the cases of TB in the local residents have obviously decreased. The prevalence of TB showed an X-shaped tendency in the two different populations. In the end of 1980s of the twentieth century, the registry rate of TB increased after a decrease in Holland, Switzerland, Sweden, and Denmark [21]. In 1994–2003, the reporting rate of TB decreased from 48.5 per 0.1 million to 23.3 per 0.1 million in Madrid, Spain. However, the percentage of migrant TB patients increased from 2.6% to 33.7% during the same period of time in Madrid, Spain [22]. A 10-year longitudinal study on 24,610 refugees (mainly from south-east Asia) in Sydney, Australia in 1984–1994 demonstrated that the incidence of TB in the population was 74.9 per 0.1 million but the percentage of defined cases by routine follow-ups was only 29.6% [23]. The study indicated that active detection facilitates the early detection of TB patients in the refugees.

In Peru, Switzerland, and some other countries, DOTS strategy was implemented to decrease the prevalence of TB via strong leadership and funding of the government. In 1993–2000, the registry rate of TB in Peru decreased annually by 6% [24, 25]. In 1951, TB control was managed according to laws and regulations in Japan. A national epidemiological survey for prevalence of TB has been conducted every 5 years in Korea. In addition, the funding for TB control, human resources for TB control, and a surveillance network system were secured and strengthened. Consequently, the epidemic of TB showed a steady decrease. Studies in several countries indicated that DOTS strategy obviously alleviated the economic burden of TB for individual patients and their families and it is the strategy with the highest ratio of cost-benefit in the control of TB [26].

2.2 TB Control in the Migrating Population in China

In China, the migrating population flows from villages to cities, from economically under developed region to the economically well-developed region, and from middle-west of China to the eastern coastal region of China. In the field of TB control, the migrating population in China flows from region with high prevalence of TB to the region with low prevalence of TB. According to the *2016 Development Report of the migrating Population in China*, the migrating population was enlarged to 247 million in the year 2015 in China, accounting for 18% of the total population, equivalent to one migrating individual in every six Chinese citizens. The migrating population is a vulnerable population to TB infection due to their low income, low-level education, insufficient knowledge about TB control, poor housing conditions, and high unemployment rate after diagnosis of TB. In the migrating population, the outcomes of TB control are unfavorable due to their high mobility, high prevalence of TB, and difficult management after the diagnosis.

Stage of Scattered Pilot Work (1991–2005)

The migrating population is the high-risk population of TB and thus the emphasized population in TB control in China. TB control in migrating population is a challenge in TB control in many large cities of China [27]. Shenzhen is the first city promoting TB control in the migrating population in China. In 1993, the government of Shenzhen firstly applied funding for management and treatment of TB in the population with Shenzhen as their temporary residence. In the application, the funding for TB management in migrating population, integration of migrating population into the TB control program along with local residents, and application of DOTS strategy were firstly proposed. A study by Zhong et al. [28] introduced the implementation of DOTS strategy in Shenzhen. The health-care institutions for TB control in Shenzhen charged treatment deposit from the patients for their compliance to the directly observed treatment. After the therapeutic course was finished, the deposits were returned back to the patients. The measure implemented in Shenzhen achieved favorable outcomes. Another study by Tan et al.

[29] showed that integration of migrating population into the regional TB control program is feasible and necessary. With effective measures, the patients with TB in migrating population can achieve the same therapeutic outcomes with the local residents. In 2003, TB control in migrating population was integrated into the TB control planning and management program. Since then, the detection, registry, treatment, and management of TB patients in migrating population were effectively conducted. In 2004, the *Implementation Procedures for Cost-reduced or exempted Treatment for Bacteriologically Positive TB Patients* was formulated and issued in Shanghai. Funding was invested by the government of Shanghai to reduce or exempt cost in anti-tuberculosis drugs and diagnostic examinations for local residents and migrating population with temporary residence in Shanghai for at least 6 months.

Wei et al. [30] reported the control of TB in the migrating population in Beijing. In the report, it is recommended that the government should provide funding for TB control to reduce or exempt cost in anti-tuberculosis drugs and improve compliance of the patients to the medication therapy. Chen et al. [31] reported the management of TB patients in migrating population in Zhejiang province of China. It was believed that TB control in migrating population is a public health issue and the government should strengthen funding for TB control to guarantee regular medication treatment of the patients. In some provinces or regions, TB control in migrating population has been integrated into the TB control planning, but the outcomes of management and treatment are unfavorable due to high mobility of patients and poor coordination between provinces or regions. TB control in migrating population remained in the stage of scattered pilot work.

Stage of Comprehensive Promotion (2006–2010)

In October, 2006, the 5th round of global funding for TB control in migrating population in China was initiated in 307 counties/districts of 124 cities in China. The program was implemented in China for 5 years, targeting on the migrating population in China with exception of migrating population to anther district of the same city and patients presented in health-care institution for once. In the program, the detection, treatment, and management of TB patients in migrating population were conducted. Allowances for transportation and well-nourished foods as well as psychological support were provided. Cooperations among NGOs and health education for TB control were promoted. The construction of human resources for TB control was strengthened and the health-care service for TB control was prolonged. The measures were intended to reduce the incidence and mortality rates of TB in migrating population.

By the end of June, 2008, 56,910 cases of initially treated TB patients had been registered in the global funding for TB control in migrating population program in China. Meanwhile, 15,166 cases of active TB had been detected, including 6629 cases of new smear-positive TB patients. The patients receiving treatment accounted for up to 99.7%, the supervised treatment rate was up to 91.4%, and the cure rate was above 80% [32]. The implementation of the program provides valuable experience for developing a scientific and reasonable TB control strategy that is situated to the domestic conditions of China [32].

Stage of Overall Planning (2011–)

In 2011, TB control in migrating population was integrated into *the National TB Control Planning (2011–2015) of China*. In the planning, detection, registry, referral, and management of TB patients in migrating population were required to be carefully implemented. The trans-regional management mechanism of TB patients in migrating population was required to be implemented. The humane care and social support for patients with TB in migrating population were strengthened. The measures, practice, and experience targeting on TB control in migrating population were actively explored to improve TB control in migrating population. In the planning, the information feedback rate of TB patients in trans-regional migrating population was required to reach 90% in 2015 and the cure rate of TB in migrating population was required to reach 80%.

In 2013, the Health Ministry of China issued the Management Procedures for TB Control, which required localized management of TB patients in migrating population and the same cost exemption as the local residents. The referral-out and referral-in designated health-care institutions were required to well coordinate for standardized medication treatment of the patients. In 2017, *the National 13th 5-year Planning for TB Control* was issued. In the planning, the localized management, trans-regional information transition, and trans-regional direct payment by the essential health-care formulary for TB control in migrating population were emphasized again. In addition, health education in migrating population was also emphasized and the awareness rate of the core knowledge about TB control in migrating population was required to be increased.

3 TB Control at the Port

3.1 Prevalence of TB at the Port

The port is the cross-border harbors, stations, airports, and channels for individuals, commodities, materials, and transportation vehicles [33]. Along with the rapid development of globalization and increase of international communications, the population flow and commodity flow have been increasing year by year. According to the data from the Exit Entry Administration of the Public Security Ministry in China, the cross-border individuals and transportation vehicles have been continuously increasing. In 2017, the population exiting and entering Chinese mainland amounted up to 598 million, with an increase by 4.76% compared to data of the previous year. The population exiting and entering Chinese mainland in 2017 included 292 million residents of Chinese mainland, 221 million residents of Hong Kong, Macao, and Taiwan of China as well as 58.3636 million foreigners. In addition, in 2017, the transportation vehicles exiting and entering Chinese mainland amounted up to 30.9766 million, with an increase by 6.84% compared to data of the previous year. The transportation vehicles included 29.5246 million motor vehicles, 0.9257 million planes, 60,000 trains, and 0.4663 million ships. In such a large flowing population, there is an underlying great threat of TB epidemic, including MDR-TB and EDR-TB. The ports for exiting and entering Chinese mainland are facing higher possibilities of TB or even DR-TB outbreaks.

According to the data released by the Inspection and Quarantine System of China, in 2001–2004, a total of 1179 million crossing-border individuals were inspected, including 4505 cases of TB patients. In 2005–2009, health examination for infectious diseases surveillance was performed for 6,129,714 crossing-border individuals and 2553 cases of active TB were detected, with workers accounting for 45.52%. In 2010, health examination was performed for infectious diseases surveillance in 1,191,789 crossing-border individuals and 458 cases of active TB were detected. The detected cases of TB at the ports in China were as follows:

- In 2005–2015, 118 cases of active TB were detected at the ports in Henan province, with a detection rate of 48.70 per 0.1 million [34].
- In 2005–2011, 2019 cases of active TB were detected at the ports in Shandong province, with a detection rate of 33.86 per 0.1 million, and the patients were predominantly workers [35].
- In 2011–2016, 16 cases of active TB were detected at the ports in Yangzhou, and all of the patients were workers [36].
- In 2009–2015, 494 imported suspected cases of TB were detected at the ports in Shanghai, including 88 cases of sputum culture positive TB patients. A study indicated that the imported TB epidemic shows a tendency of increase [37].

TB control at the ports of foreign countries is also challenging. A meta-analysis of 15 studies on screening of TB before entering a country was conducted by Aldridge et al. The analysis indicated that the detection rate of TB before entering a country is 19.7 per 0.1 million in emigrants from a country with an incidence of TB ranging from 50 per 0.1 million to 149 per 0.1 million, with a confidence interval of 95% (10.3 per 0.1 million, 31.5 per 0.1 million). The detection rate of TB before entering a country is 335.9 per 0.1 million in emigrants from a country with an incidence of TB being above 350 per 0.1 million, with a confidence interval of 95% (283.0 per 0.1 million, 393.2 per 0.1 million) [38]. In Australia, the individuals applying to enter the country during July 2009 to June 2010 received health examination before their entering into the country. The data indicated that the detection rate of TB was 137 per 0.1 million and the detection rate of MDR-TB was 1.06 per 0.1 million. And the patients were mainly from Philippines (21.8%), India (16.8%), Vietnam (16.2%), and China (8.3%) [35]. Studies have demonstrated that the infection rate and morbidity rate of TB in emigrants from countries with high incidence of TB are commonly higher than the rates in local residents of the immigrated country. These immigrants negatively impact on the TB control in the immigrated country [36–38]. The surveillance data in 2017 from the USA indicated that the incidence of TB in population born in foreign countries was 15 times as high as the incidence in population born in the USA. And the highest incidence of TB was in population born in Asian countries (27 per 0.1 million), which was followed by the population of non-Spanish black people (22 per 0.1 million) [39]. A survey in Britain in 2013 indicated that the incidence of TB had gradually increased [40], with 75% of the patients from the population born in foreign countries [41]. A survey in Japan indicated that in 2005–2014, the percentage of TB patients in population born in foreign countries increased from 3.5% to 5.8%. Compared to the decreased reporting incidence of TB in Japan, the incidence of TB in population born in foreign countries increased from 40.7 per 0.1 million to 56.2 per 0.1 million during 2007 to 2016 [42].

TB control at the crossing-border ports has been an international challenge and the governments of countries all over the world have paid close attention on TB control at the crossing-border ports. Entrance of TB patients and individuals carrying Mtb is even forbidden by the government of some developed countries. According to article 99 in the Implementation Procedures of the Frontier Health Quarantine Law of the P. R. China., revisited on February 6, 2016, foreigners with serious psychiatric disorders, communicable TB, or another infectious disease that may constitute major threat to the public health should be prevented from entering the country.

3.2 TB Control Strategy at the Ports in Developed Countries

An international study has demonstrated that screening of TB is an effective way for TB control in the countries with low prevalence of TB [43]. The TB screening strategies in immigrants include screening of TB before entering the country, screening of TB when entering the country, and screening of TB after entering the country. Because screening of TB is not one of the mandatory conditions when and after entering the country, the coverage of screening is, therefore, incomplete. On the contrary, screening of TB is one of the mandatory conditions for entering the country and its coverage is complete. To prevent import of communicable TB, screening strategy and surveillance policy for TB control before entering the country were formulated in some developed countries, including Australia, Austria, Canada, Israel, Jordan, New Zealand, Britain, and the USA [44]. Take the USA and Britain as examples, the TB control strategies at the ports in developed countries are introduced hereafter.

The commonalities of TB control at the ports in the USA and Britain include: (1) foreword shift of TB screening to the time point of before entering the country; (2) formulation of scientific TB screening strategy and highly feasible technical guidance; and (3) establishment of health assessment institution and employment of clinicians in the emigrated countries [45]. The specific strategies for TB control at the ports are as follows.

The United States of America

The TB control strategy and technical guidance were formulated by the division of global migration and quarantine (DGMQ) in the Center for Disease Control (CDC) of the USA and related experts. In the technical guidance, highly feasible operational procedures concerning screening, diagnosis, treatment, and follow-up are described in detail. Complete procedures for screening of TB include case history, physical examination, interferon γ release assay (performed when necessary), chest X-ray (performed when necessary), sputum smear test, and sputum culture. Being different from the procedures in Britain, all the applicants for immigration into the USA are required to receive screening of TB. Based on the incidence of TB in the emigrated country and the age group of the applicant, different screening protocols are implemented. In addition, the applicants for immigration into the USA are categorized and managed based on the results of the screening. The applicants categorized into class A are forbidden to enter the USA (Table 3.2).

Table 3.2 Tuberculosis screening strategy at US ports

Target population	Population category	Screening projects	Action after screening
Applicant's country has TB morbidity <20/100,000	Below 15 years old	1. Physical examination 2. Medical history 3. IGRA:people with TB symptoms/HIV infected 4. Chest X-ray:people with TB symptoms/HIV infected 5. Sputum smear, sputum culture, and DST:people with TB symptoms/HIV infected	According to screening results 1. Not TB 2. Type A TB 3. B0 TB (already completed standard treatment) 4. B1 TB (culture-negative) 5. B2 Extrapulmonary TB 6. B3 LTBI 7. B4 Close contacts Different actions are needed according to screening results. Type A TB patients are forbidden to enter the country
	15 years old or above	1. Physical examination 2. Medical history 3. Chest X-ray 4. Sputum smear, sputum culture, DST: suspected TB patients suggested by chest X-ray or people with TB symptoms/HIV infected	
Applicant's country has TB morbidity≥20/100,000	Below 2 years old	1. Physical examination 2. Medical history 3. TST: people with TB symptoms/HIV infected 4. Chest X-ray: people with TB symptoms/HIV infected 5. Sputum test: people with TB symptoms/HIV infected	
	2–14 years old	1. Physical examination 2. Medical history 3. IGRA 4. Chest X-ray: IGRA positive or people with TB symptoms/HIV infected 5. Sputum test: suspected TB patients suggested by chest X-ray or people with TB symptoms/HIV infected	
	15 years old or above	1. Physical examination 2. Medical history 3. Chest X-ray 4. Sputum smear, sputum culture, DST: suspected TB patients suggested by chest X-ray or people with TB symptoms/HIV infected	

Table 3.3 Tuberculosis screening strategy at UK ports

Target population	Population category	Screening projects	Action after screening
(1) Duration will exceed 6 months and applicant is from WHO's high TB prevalence country (2) As required by the UK Immigration Office	Adult	1. Symptoms screening 2. TB contact history 3. Physical examination (decided by physicians) 4. Chest X-ray 5. Sputum test: active TB/old TB patients suggested by chest X-ray or people with TB symptoms	1. If there is no active TB/old TB suggested by chest X-ray and physicians eliminate active TB's possibility clinically, applicants can continue to apply for entry permission 2. Active TB patients need to be transferred to local special hospitals by physicians 3. After the treatment is completed, active TB patients can apply for entry permission again
	Pregnant women	1. Symptoms screenings 2. TB contact history 3. Physical examination (decided by physicians) 4. Chest X-ray: considering the risk of radiation, pregnant women have three options: (1) X-ray after childbirth, (2) sputum culture, (3) double-shielded X ray detection 5. Sputum test: active TB/old TB patients suggested by chest X-ray or people with TB symptoms or pregnant women who have not taken X-ray	
	11 years or below	1. Symptoms screenings 2. TB contact history 3. Physical examination (decided by physicians) 4. If children have TB/active TB symptoms, TB history or TB contact history, they should take chest X-ray or sputum bacteriological detection 5. If children have chronic respiratory disease, physicians should recommend X-ray and sputum test if needed 6. If there is active TB/old TB suggested by chest X-ray, children should take sputum test	

Britain

During the recent decades, screening of TB before and after entering the country has been adopted in applicants of immigration. Since April 1, 2014, screening of TB was performed before entering the country. And the screening coverage of TB has been extended to applicants of immigration from 67 countries with high incidence of TB. Before April 1, 2014, only those applicants for permanent residence in Britain should receive screening of TB. But since April 1, 2014, all the applicants for stay in Britain for above 6 months should receive screening of TB in the designated health-care institutions before the visa is approved. The detected cases with definitive diagnosis of TB should be referred to the local hospital specialized in TB control for treatment. And the specific medication therapy and follow-ups are not specified in the screening protocol (https://www.gov.uk/government/publications/uk-tuberculosis-technical-instructions) (Table 3.3).

3.3 Development and Prospects of TB Control at the Ports in China

Present Mode and Measures for TB Control at the Ports

The institutions responsible for entry–exit inspection and quarantine are the functional section for surveillance of infectious diseases at the ports in China, related policies making and their implementation in China. To guarantee the health of exiting personnel and prevent import and export of TB, the TB control strategy at the ports in China, to prevent import and spread of TB in the country, has been implemented by the institutions responsible for entry–exit inspection and quarantine. During recent years, many effective TB control modes are explored and established during the implementation of the TB control strategy. For instance, a system of electronized application, organizational mechanism, prevention and control mechanism, guarantee mechanism, and collaboration mechanism have been established for infectious diseases control by Beijing Inspection and Quarantine Bureau. A system of port inspection, laboratory test, and collaborative efforts for rapid control was established for infectious diseases control at the ports by Guangdong Inspection and Quarantine Bureau. A 3 plus 4 mode for infectious diseases control at the ports was established by Guangxi Inspection and Quarantine Bureau. The 3 indicates collaboration of 3 institutions, namely the local government, the institution responsible for inspection and quarantine at the port, and the institution responsible for inspection and quarantine of the adjacent country. And the 4 indicates epidemiological data collection of infectious diseases at the ports, assessment of the epidemic, reporting of the epidemic, and management of the epidemic.

In addition to the effective working modes, multiple government documents have been issued since 2002 targeting on the TB control at the ports in China. In 2002, the Requirements for TB Surveillance in Entry and Exit Populations and the Standards for Laboratory Detection of Tuberculosis in the Entry–Exit Inspection and Quarantine System were issued. In 2003, the Operational Procedures for Surveillance of Tuberculosis at the National Ports and the Operational Procedures for Detection of Tuberculosis at the Ports in China were issued. In 2012, the new version of the Operational Procedures for Surveillance of Tuberculosis at the National Ports was issued. The documents specified the surveillance, screening, diagnosis, management, detection, and quarantine of communicable TB at the ports in China. Different TB screening protocols are formulated targeting on different populations, such as common exit population, entry population from countries with high incidence of TB, and exit population to the countries requiring detection of TB. And *the Diagnostic Standards of Tuberculosis* (the National Standards WS 288) was adopted for the diagnosis of TB. But treatment and management of the suspected and defined cases of TB were not specified in these documents (Table 3.4).

Goal and Strategy of TB Control at the Ports in China

To end prevalence of TB worldwide is the common goal of end TB strategy by the WHO and sustainable development of the UN from 2016 to 2025. The specific goals of end TB strategy include death cases of TB decrease by 90% and incidence of TB decrease by 80% in 2030 based on the data in 2015. TB control in migrating population is a difficulty in realizing the abovementioned goals. On the background of accelerating globalization and increasingly close international communications, the TB control mode needs to be innovated, the technology applied in TB control needs to be improved, and the collaborative efforts are needed for TB control. The goal of TB control at the ports is to further decrease international prevalence of TB and the specific measures include as follows.

To Improve TB Control at the Ports

Being different from the screening of TB before entering the country implemented in the USA, Canada, and Australia, the screening of TB when entering the country is implemented in China. If the entry population is defined with communicable

Table 3.4 Tuberculosis screening strategy at China ports

Types	Target population	Monitor and screening	Manage after discovery of cases	Close contacts	Sterilization
Entry	Immigrant, Chinese labor personnel, foreign students Transportation staff Inhabitants of a border area, catering practitioners	X-ray, sputum smear and sputum culture	Refer suspected/confirmed cases to hospitals; move transportation staffs to other job spots	When discovering infectious TB patients, register and monitor the close contacts	Sterilize the transportation after discovery of patients
	Overseas for over 1 year	Chest X-ray; suspected TB patients suggested by X-ray take sputum smear and sputum culture test	Refer suspected/confirmed cases to hospitals		
	HIV	TB monitoring	Refer suspected/confirmed cases to hospitals		
Departure	Chinese living overseas for over 1 year, overseas Chinese, Hong Kong, Macao, and Taiwan compatriots	TB detection according to whether applicants come from TB epidemic areas	Refer suspected/confirmed cases to hospitals		
	Chinese labor personnel, Transportation staff	Chest X-ray, sputum smear and sputum culture	Move suspected/confirmed cases from their jobs		
	Foreign nationals coming to China for more than 1 year, foreign residents to settle in China, employment, foreign scholars, family visits	TB detection according to whether applicants come from TB epidemic areas	1. Don't issue Health Certificate to suspected patients 2. Arrange departure for confirmed cases		

TB after their entry into China, they are highly infectious during the required period of exit. The management and control of TB in such population is a challenge in TB control of China. A study has demonstrated that screening of TB before entering the country plays a key role in the control of TB in the country [46]. Therefore, the screening of TB in the entry populations should be extended forwards to the time when the TB screening certificate is obtained in the exit country. In addition, appropriate screening time and screening standards of TB as well as detailed operational guideline should be formulated based on the facts and related policies in China.

In addition to screening of TB, the screened suspected/defined cases of TB should be managed based on the respective grading and categorization. A comprehensive assessment should be performed based on the laboratory test of the sputum specimen, diagnostic imaging, infectivity of the suspected/defined cases, and the possible consequences. Based on the assessment, the condition should be graded for corresponding management. The extended TB control forwards and afterwards at the ports would actually stop international spread of TB.

To Strengthen the Laboratory Construction

For rapid entry and exit, the screening of TB requires high positive rate within a short period of time. However, the presently applied laboratory tests for TB are sputum smear test and sputum culture, which are not efficient enough. Along with the development of laboratory tests for detection of TB, bacteriological tests should be combined with rapid biological examinations, such as molecular biological examinations and immunological assays, for more efficient screening of TB at the ports in China.

Immunological Assays

The immunological assays include interferon γ release test and Mtb antibody detection. In the Mtb antibody detection, the serum tuberculin antibody is detected, with a sensitivity of 53.2–68.8% and a specificity of 83.5–100%. The serum antibody titer in patients with TB is positively related to the clinical stages of the illness. Along with improved condition after treatment, the level of serum antibody correspondingly decreases, which can be applied as an indicator for the prognosis of TB. In the interferon γ release test, the production of interferon γ produced by T cells due to stimulation of Mtb specific antigen is detected. It is an assistant laboratory test to detect Mtb infection and active TB. And the interferon γ release test shows higher specificity and sensitivity than PPD test within a shorter period of time. However, it requires more advanced technology and costs much more than PPD test.

Molecular Biological Examination

The molecular biological examinations for TB include polymerase chain reaction (PCR) and Xpert Mtb/RIF test. PCR is a method for in vitro elective amplification of specific DNA segment. With two strands of DNA segments to be amplified as the template and two strands of artificially synthesized oligonucleotide primers as mediator, the target DNA sequence is exponentially amplified via enzyme-driven DNA replication. And a conclusion can be drawn according to the size of amplified segments. PCR is a laboratory test with high specificity and sensitivity but consumes shorter period of time. Xpert Mtb/RIF is based on fully automatic semi-nested real-time PCR. With rpoB gene as the target gene, Mtb infection and rifampicin-resistant TB can be detected within 2 h by Xpert Mtb/RIF. It is valuable in rapid detection of TB.

The immunological assays and molecular biological examinations provide basis for TB control at the ports. Application of different TB control mode and laboratory tests for TB control at the ports should be based on the specific conditions of the ports. In the economically well-developed regions, IGRA, PCR, Xpert Mtb/RIF, and sputum smear test can be applied for preliminary screening of TB and sputum culture for definitive diagnosis of TB. But in the economically under-developed regions, PPD and sputum smear test can be applied for preliminary screening of TB and sputum culture for definitive diagnosis of TB.

To Strengthen the Health Education for TB Control at the Ports

According to *the Diagnostic Standards of Tuberculosis* (WS288-2017), the diagnosis of TB should be based on a comprehensive analysis of pathogenic examinations, epidemiological history, clinical manifestations, diagnostic imaging of lungs, and other assistant detections. However, some travelers entering or exiting a country untruthfully declare their health status or refuse to cooperate to the health examination for more rapid customs formalities. Therefore, the health education for TB control at the ports should be strengthened by the institution for entry–exit inspection and quarantine to increase the awareness about prevention of TB in the entry–exit populations. Based on the health education, their cooperation to surveillance and examinations for TB control can be improved.

At the site of inspection and quarantine, brochures, bulletin board, broadcasting, electronic display screen, and other media can be applied to spread the knowledge about TB control, health quarantine, and related laws and regulations. The health education should be especially emphasized in high-risk populations of TB, such as workers. The health education via multiple ways facilitates to spread knowledge about health quarantine and TB control before entering or exiting a country. The well-educated population thus actively and truthfully declares their health status, which alleviates the contradictions between rapid customs formalities and strict quarantine inspection.

To Strengthen Internationally Collaborative Efforts in TB Control

Concerning the internationally collaborative efforts, the WHO International Port Cooperation Center and the WHO International Travel Health Cooperation Center were established in July 2014. Their branches in Chinese mainland have been managed by the National Bureau of Quality Inspection in China, which has effectively strengthened the international collaboration on the health inspection and quarantine at the ports of China [47].

Concerning the domestic collaborative efforts, the institutions responsible for entry–exit inspection and quarantine have strengthened their collaborations with the Transportation Ministry, the Public Security Ministry, the Commerce Ministry, the Religious Affairs Bureau, the Health Commission, and the mass media. The collaborative efforts have been made to optimize the working procedures, improve the service, and improve the techniques for TB control at the ports. The collaborative efforts with the mass media have increased the social impact of entry–exit inspection and quarantine and improved the communication about epidemic of TB.

Generally speaking, the surveillance and supervision of TB is an important but difficult job at the ports, which requires advanced technology [48]. Due to the severe epidemic of TB across the world, the TB control mode should be consecutively optimized by the institutions responsible for health inspection and quarantine at the ports. The TB control mode at the ports of some developed countries should be adopted as the reference. The technological support should be strengthened. Concerning the techniques of TB control at the ports, information management should be actively promoted for intelligent health inspection at the ports. Management based on grading and categorization should also be actively promoted. In addition, detailed technical guideline and operational procedures should be formulated to apply limited human resources and materials to the management of high-risk populations. Based on the well-coordination on control of infectious diseases, the coordination can be further extended for real-time information interaction about TB control for high efficiency of customs formalities. All of these prospects are based on emphasis and supports of the governments.

4 TB Control Mode in Shenzhen, China

Shenzhen is the city with the largest migrating population in China and even across the world. The prevalence of TB in the migrating population constitutes a challenge to effective control of TB in Shenzhen. An epidemiological survey on prevalence of TB in Shenzhen was conducted in 1991. The study showed that the morbidity of smear-positive TB patients in local residents of Shenzhen was 118 per 0.1 million, while in the migrating population, 131 per 0.1 million. The morbidity of active TB in the local residents of Shenzhen was 336 per 0.1 million, while in the migrating population, 417 per 0.1 million. The prevalence of TB in the migrating population was obviously higher than that in the local residents. The cases of TB in the migrating population accounted for above 75% in the total cases of TB in Shenzhen. And the migrating population was one of the important risk factors for prevalence of TB in Shenzhen [49]. The migrating population in Shenzhen is characterized by rapid alternation and the life cycle has an obvious turning point at the age of 25 years. Some cured TB patients in the migrating population return to the place of their registered permanent residence. And some individuals flow from their registered permanent residence into the migrating population in Shenzhen, who might be new cases of TB in the future.

4.1 Development of TB Control Mode in Shenzhen

Stage of Pilot Work and Exploration in 1993

In May 1993, TB control program was firstly initiated in Baoan district, as the first model district for migrating population management across the country. In the program, the free-in-charge policy for TB control was implemented in both local residents and the migrating population. And the DOT strategy was officially initiated in the program under the principle of uniform target and systematic management. In 1993, the government of Shenzhen issued an application for funding of TB management and treatment in the migrating population in Shenzhen. This was the first government commitment to TB control funding for the migrating population. With the financial support from the government, systematic measures were implemented for TB control in the migrating population in Shenzhen. Targeting the characteristics of the migrating population, the implemented measures included reasonable and unrestricted selection of health-care institution for medication, deposit management, directly observed medication with no vacations, trans-district referrals, categorization of the registry information, incentive mechanism, privacy protection, and convenient medication.

Stage of Gradual Promotion in 1994–2002

The pilot work in Baoan district of Shenzhen achieved success. With Baoan district as a model, the TB control program was actively initiated and arranged by the governments of other districts. In March 1994, DOT strategy was officially initiated in Longgang district of Shenzhen. And in June 1995, DOT strategy was successively initiated in Nanshan district, Futian district, Luohu district, and Yantian district. With district as working unit, the coverage of DOT strategy reached up to 100%. In the TB control program, smear-positive TB patients and smear-negative TB patients with serious symptoms from both local residents and the migrating population received free-in-charge treatment and management. The TB control mode in Shenzhen consisted of the following aspects.

Responsibilities of the Government

The migrating population was firstly integrated into the TB control plan formulated by the government to promote TB control strategy in the total population in China. A leadership team for TB control was established. And the standard of funding for TB control in the migrating population is the same as that in the local residents in Shenzhen. The government departments of finance, human resources, social security, labor, and health have been coordinated to secure the implementation of the program. A three-level network for TB control has been established and improved. More health-care professionals have been employed for TB control and a system for promotion of their professional titles in TB control was supplemented. And the TB control professionals have been privileged in transfer of their working position. And the salary of TB control professionals was increased by 8% and the bonus was no less than other professionals working in infectious diseases control. The policies of free-in-charge health examination and treatment were widely propagated in the migrating population in Shenzhen.

A Detection System of Sporadic Reporting and Group Diagnosis

Due to strengthened social publicity, the suspected cases of TB were referred to the localized TB control agency. The suspected cases of TB in any health-care institutions were timely reported via internet on-line reporting system and referred with a triplicate referral sheet. If the suspected cases of TB did not present in the referral-in TB control agency, the suspected cases were timely traced. The diagnosis of TB was performed in district- and above level TB control agencies and the other health-care institutions were not approved for the diagnosis of TB. In 1996, *the Procedures for Centralized Management of Tuberculosis in Shenzhen* was issued. The document specified the procedures for reporting, referral, tracing, management, and treatment of TB in the migrating population in Shenzhen. And corresponding rewarding and punishment measures were also formulated.

A system of Categorized Treatment and Management

Since 1993, the DOT strategy has been implemented. Based on the principles of within 15-min walking of the patients and per 10,000 population, health-care institutions were designated as the institution for DOT. The medication of the patients has been directly observed. The anti-TB drugs have been successively supplied and dispensed via internal channel.

A system of categorized treatment and management was established for the migrating population in Shenzhen. The smear-positive TB patients who were willing to stay at Shenzhen for treatment received free-in-charge DOT. And the smear-positive TB patients who returned to their registered permanent residence for treatment were referred to the TB control agency at the place of their registered permanent residence. The smear-negative TB patients received treatment and management in the TB control agency at their own expenses. To secure the completion of DOT management in the patients with TB in the migrating population, treatment guarantee deposits were charged from the patients. After the completion of DOT management, the deposits were returned back to the patients. By this way, their compliance of medication was secured.

In addition, health education about TB control was strengthened in the migrating population. The clinicians of initial treatment and direct observation conducted health education about TB control to improve their compliance of medication.

Assessment of DOT Management

DOT management was assessed in ways of grading categorization, routine assessment, and specialized assessment. The indices for assessment included patient detection, referral and tracing, diagnosis and treatment, patient management, laboratory tests, observed medication, health education, funding, material resources, and drug supply. In *the Protocol for Assessment of TB Control Program in Shenzhen*, it has been specified that the indices for assessment of TB control program in the migrating population include sputum detection rate in initially treated patients, detection rate of smear positive in initially treated patients, positive rate of sputum detection in initially treated patients, and detection rate in patients with chest X-ray abnormality.

Stage of Comprehensive Improvement in 2003–2015

To control MDR-TB, DOTS+ was promoted in Shenzhen in 2003. In October 2006, the Stop TB Strategy was officially initiated in Shenzhen, the only city with simultaneous implementations of the global funding program for TB control in migrating population and the MDR-TB control program in China. Targeting on the three challenges in TB control, a mechanism for comprehensive management, referral and tracing of patients with TB in the migrating population was proposed. The surveillance and detection of MDR-TB were strengthened. And the detected patients with MDR-TB were treated and managed according to the standards. Meanwhile, the detection of patients with co-infection of TB and HIV/AIDS was strengthened. All of the patients with TB received high-quality humane care. The participation of communities in TB control was strengthened. A system for TB control in the total population was established. And the measures were as follows.

Responsibilities of the Government

The migrating population was integrated in *the TB Control Planning in Shenzhen (2001–2010)* and *the TB Control Planning in Shenzhen (2011–2015)*. The Finance Department in Shenzhen was required to gradually increase the funding for TB control. And the funding for TB control was fitted into the annual budget of Shenzhen.

A health-care service system for TB control was gradually improved. Under the leadership of the health administration, a three-level health-care service system for TB control was established. In the system, the Center for Chronic Diseases Control in Shenzhen played the role of guiding the TB control in Shenzhen, with the TB control agencies as the keys and the health-care institutions and hospitals as the basis. All of these institutions had their own specified responsibilities for TB control. Specifically, there were one city-level health-care institution for TB control, 10 district-level TB control agencies, 55 second-level institutions for DOT management, and 1095 third-level institutions for DOT management.

A series of policies concerning TB control in Shenzhen were formulated and issued. In 2014, *the Procedures for Centralized Management of TB in Shenzhen, the Interim Procedures for Electronic Internet On-line Management of TB in Shenzhen*, and *the Notice on Accounts Closure in the Global Funding for MDR-TB Control Program* were formulated and issued. In 2015, the Notice on Management of DR-TB in Shenzhen was formulated and issued, which specified the responsibilities of the city-level and district-level TB control agencies as well as the free-in-charge part in management of DR-TB. In addition, *the Protocol for Assessment of TB Control Program in Shenzhen, the Comprehensive Assessment Standards for Public Health-care Service in Shenzhen*, and *the Responsibilities of and Technical Guideline for Public Health-care Service in Shenzhen* were formulated and issued. Based on the standards, TB control in Shenzhen was assessed each year to improve the performance of the TB control programs.

Detection of Patients by Referral and Registry

Detection of TB in Patients Presenting in the Health-Care Institutions

The new version of *the Centralized Management of TB in Shenzhen* was officially implemented in June 2014. The document further standardized the procedures in detecting, reporting, referring, tracing, treating, and managing suspected cases of TB.

Screening of Individuals with Close Contacts to Bacteriologically Positive TB Patients

Health education was conducted in the district-level TB control agencies. And the individuals with close contacts to bacteriologically positive TB patients were screened.

Timely Detection of MDR-TB

It was stipulated in *the Procedures for Management of DR- and MDR-TB in Shenzhen* that the bacteria strain from suspected cases of DR- and MDR-TB should be sent to the Center for Chronic Diseases Control in Shenzhen within 7 days for identification and drug sensitivity test. The range for screening of MDR-TB was extended from patients with failed re-treatment and patients with chronic excretion of Mtb to smear-positive patients after 3-month treatment, patients with failed initial treatment, and retreated smear-positive patients. Currently, the range for screening of MDR-TB includes all the individuals with close contacts to smear-positive patients, smear negative but culture positive patients, patients with chronic excretion of Mtb, and patients with MDR-TB.

Emphasis on Special Populations in TB Control

(1) Patients with co-infection of TB and HIV/AIDS

In 2005, the Technical Protocol for Screening of Tuberculosis in Patients with HIV/AIDS in Shenzhen was issued by the Health Bureau of Shenzhen. In the document, management of bidirectional referral and screening for TB and HIV/AIDS was further standardized.

(2) Populations in schools

In June 2005, the Notice on TB Control in Schools in Shenzhen was jointly issued by the Health Bureau and the Education Bureau of Shenzhen. In 2009, TB control in schools was integrated into the White Book on Public Health-care Service in Shenzhen. Meanwhile, the Management Planning for TB Epidemic in Schools in Shenzhen was formulated. The TB epidemic in schools in Shenzhen has been managed based on a scientific, standard, and legal principle since then. And TB control strategies and measures have been comprehensively implemented in schools in Shenzhen.

(3) Imprisoned population

Since 2008, TB control in imprisoned population has been gradually strengthened. The health-care institutions for TB control have supplied technical guidance, free-in-charge anti-tuberculosis drugs, reagents for laboratory tests, professional training, and consultant diagnosis for intractable cases. The prisons have been responsible for the detection, diagnosis, treatment, and management of TB as well as health educations in the imprisoned population. During the 12th 5-year in China, the prisoners in Shenzhen received annual health examinations.

Standards for Diagnosis and Treatment of TB

To establish City-Level and District-Level Platform for Diagnosis of TB

The first-level platform for diagnosis of TB was the district-level TB control agency. At the platform, free-in-charge sputum smear test, sputum culture, and chest X-ray were performed for diagnosis of common active TB. The second-level platform for diagnosis of TB was the city-level institution, namely the Center for Chronic Diseases Control in Shenzhen. At the platform, free-in-charge sputum culture, strain identification, and drug sensitivity test were performed for suspected cases of DR-TB. The assistant examinations included chest X-ray, fibrobronchoscopy, CT scanning, and molecular biological examinations. These examinations were for the diagnosis of all types of DR-TB, including single drug-resistant TB, polydrug-resistant TB, multidrug-resistant TB, and extensive drug-resistant TB.

Gradual Promotion of New Diagnostic Technology

The city-level Mtb laboratory in Shenzhen, as the second reference laboratory of Mtb in Guangdong province, was well equipped with new technologies. In 2010, ELISPOT was performed to detect T cells specific to Mtb, and chip analysis for identification of Mtb was also performed. In 2012, gene chip diagnosis, the most advanced technology across the world, was introduced into the laboratory for rapid gene diagnosis of MDR-TB. In addition, gene chip diagnosis for non-Mtb drug sensitivity was established. In 2013, non-Mtb minimum inhibitory concentration (MIC) test was firstly performed, which provides basis for selection of anti-tuberculosis drugs. In 2014, drug-resistant gene detection was performed in all the patients with sputum culture positive in Shenzhen. The new diagnostic technology shortened the time for laboratory diagnosis of TB from traditionally 90 days to presently 6 h. And the time for etiological diagnosis of MDR-TB was greatly shortened.

Standardized Diagnosis and Treatment

According to the Technical Guideline for Implementation of TB Control Planning in China and the Management Guideline for DR-TB Control Planning, FDC standardized therapy was administered for common patients with TB. And based on the results of drug sensitivity test, individualized therapy was formulated for patients with DR-TB and the therapy was adjusted according to the findings in follow-ups during the treatment.

Improved Performance of the Clinicians

In the city-level health-care institution for TB control, cases of TB were regularly discussed and training for diagnostic techniques was regularly performed. The performance of the clinicians was thus improved to reduce the misdiagnosis rate and the miss diagnosis rate.

Management of the Patients

(1) DOT strategy was strictly implemented and medications were innovated based on the mode of Internet plus TB. In 2011, the Electronic Internet Management System of TB was firstly developed in Shenzhen, which was promoted for wider application in 2012. The system was developed by the Founder International Co. Ltd. of China and directed by the Center for Chronic Diseases Control in Shenzhen. The functional modules of the system include observed medication, visiting records, adverse effects, drugs dispensary, follow-up alert, and system management.

(2) A comprehensive management mode was established for trans-regional flowing patients with TB. In 2009, a two-level trans-regional management system was established with district-level TB control agencies and city-level TB control agency. Entrusted management was adopted for the trans-regional flowing patients with TB [50]. The management of the trans-regional flowing patients with TB in district-level TB control agencies was supervised quarterly and assessed annually by the city-level TB control agencies.

(3) Standard procedures for management of MDR-TB were established. DOT strategy was implemented for all of the patients with MDR-TB to secure regular medications. Adverse effects of the drugs were inquired during each medication. The patients were urged to receive follow-up reexaminations. And the health education for TB control was performed via multiple ways to improve the compliance of the patients.

Drugs Supply

In 2008, the brand new version of *the Standards for Management of Anti-tuberculosis Drugs* was implemented. In the document, a drug inventory control system and the monitoring indices were introduced. With application of the system, the financial account and the drugs were efficiently managed to secure successive supply of anti-tuberculosis drugs.

Scientific Research

Basic scientific research as well as application and implementation studies was actively applied and conducted. The important and difficult issues concerning TB control in migrating population, optimization of the medication therapy for DR-TB, and screening of TB in special populations attracted the scholarly attention. The industry, training, research, and application were integrated to improve the scientific and technological strength.

Surveillance and Assessment

The surveillance of TB epidemic [51, 52], surveillance of drug-resistant Mtb [53, 54], and epidemiological sampling survey were routinely conducted for dynamic understanding about the tendency of TB epidemic. The effects of the TB control planning were scientifically assessed, which provided scientific basis for policy making by the government.

Stage of Leaping Forward (Since 2016)

To implement *the Guidance for Promotion of Graded Diagnosis and Treatment System* issued by the General Office of the State Council in 2015 and *the Notice on Pilot Work for Graded Diagnosis and Treatment of Tuberculosis and Comprehensive Service for Tuberculosis Control* issued by the General Office of the National Health and Family Planning Commission in 2016, pilot work for graded diagnosis and treatment of TB and comprehensive service for TB control was implemented in Shenzhen in 2016.

Improved Graded Diagnosis and Treatment System of TB and the Comprehensive Management System of TB for Detection and Management of Patients with TB

Improved Graded Diagnosis and Treatment System of TB and Improved Comprehensive Management System of TB

The responsibilities of the city-level TB control agency, district-level TB control agencies, hospital specialized in TB, general health-care institution, and community health-care service center were specified. The city-level TB control agency, the Center for Chronic Diseases Control in Shenzhen, has been responsible to organize the implementation of *the Protocol for Pilot Work of Graded Diagnosis and Treatment of Tuberculosis and Comprehensive Service for Tuberculosis Control* in Shenzhen. The center has also been responsible for the diagnosis, treatment, management, data collection and analysis, and health promotion of the suspected and intractable cases of TB as well as cases of DR-TB. Laboratory quality control, staffs training, and supervision of TB control in Shenzhen have also been performed by the center. In addition, the center has also been responsible to organize the quality control and assessment on the diagnosis and treatment of TB in Shenzhen. The district-level TB control agencies have been responsible to implement *the Protocol for Pilot Work of Graded Diagnosis and Treatment of TB and Comprehensive Service for Tuberculosis Control* in the corresponding district. The district-level TB control agencies have also been responsible for surveillance of TB epidemic and reporting of TB cases in the district. The common patients with TB have been diagnosed, registered, treated, and managed in the district-level TB control agencies. In addition, the agencies have also been responsible for referral and management of patients with DR-TB. The information management, health promotion in patients with TB, training, and supervision of the staffs have also been conducted in the district-level agencies. All levels and categories of health-care institutions have been responsible for detection, reporting, and referral of suspected and defined cases of TB. All the health-care institutions should refer the suspected and defined cases of TB to the district-level TB control agencies of their residence. Hospitals specialized in TB have been responsible for diagnosis and differential diagnosis of intractable and drug-resistant cases of TB. The specialized hospitals have also been responsible for the quarantine and treatment of patients with serious TB, acute TB, MDR-TB, and smear-positive TB. In addition, the diagnosis, registry, treatment, re-treatment, data collection and reporting, and health education should also be performed in the specialized hospitals. The outpatients in and inpatients discharged from the specialized hospitals should be referred to and the related health-care information should be feedback to the district-level TB control agency of their residence. The outpatients in and inpatients discharged from the specialized hospitals should also be arranged to the community health-care service center of their residence for health management. The hospitals with infectious diseases department have been responsible for quarantine and treatment of common patients with TB and patients with acute TB. And the hospitals with infectious diseases department should also refer the discharged patients to the district-level TB control agency of their residence for further treatment and management. The community health-care service centers have been responsible for referral, assistant tracing, and service management of TB. The signed family doctor service should be provided by the clinicians specialized in chronic diseases and general practitioners in community health-care service center to implement service management for TB control.

Strengthened Detection of Patients with TB

The referral of suspected and defined cases of TB was strengthened in all health-care institutions. Active screening of TB was actively performed for etiologically positive TB patients as well as patients with HIV/AIDS. TB screening was also performed for the elderly aged above 65 years and patients with diabetes in communities. Routine health examinations and annual health examinations were performed in prisons, watch-houses, and institutions specialized in drug abuse quitting [55].

Strengthened Management of all Types of DR-TB

The patients with DR-TB were integrated into the TB control programs. The patients with DR-TB in local residents were treated as outpatients. And drug sensitivity test, diagnosis, treatment, and follow-up examinations were provided free-in-charge. The whole therapeutic course was observed and managed to improve the compliance of the patients.

Promoted Application of New Diagnostic Technology

Application of new diagnostic technology was promoted to improve the etiological diagnosis rate. Drug sensitivity test, non-Mtb strain identification, and rapid diagnosis of DR-TB have been performed in laboratories in the Center for Chronic Diseases Control in Shenzhen and the Third People's Hospital in Shenzhen. There have been also comparatively independent and biologically safe laboratories for diagnosis of TB in the district-level TB control agencies. The sputum smear test, sputum culture, and rapid diagnosis of TB can be performed in these laboratories. In addition, collaborative efforts have been made to approve the price of the new diagnostic technology and the new diagnostic technology for TB has been enlisted in the Essential Health-care Formulary. Thus, rapid diagnosis for TB has been widely applied without additional economic burden for the patients.

Quarantine for Treatment of Communicable TB

Quarantine for treatment of communicable TB was performed to stop the spread of TB. Common patients with smear-positive TB and patients with smear-positive MDR-TB have been free-in-charge hospitalized for treatment. The community-based treatment of communicable TB and infection control have been explored to reduce the spread of TB.

Application of Information Technology in TB Control

The platform of Internet plus TB information management has been established in Shenzhen. The application of information technology in TB control has been accelerated to establish a network integrating HIS system and TB information management system of all the health-care institutions in Shenzhen. The intelligent information management system based on the internet technology has been improved for unified and intelligent management of patients with TB. Based on the network of tele-healthcare and tele-education, technical guidance and training for TB control have been conducted to improve the performance of TB control in basic health-care institutions.

Specified Responsibilities of the Health-Care Institutions for TB Control

The diagnosis and treatment of TB have been standardized in the designated health-care institutions. The responsibilities of the designated health-care institutions have been specified and integrated to the performance assessment. Three high-level talents specialized in engineering have been transferred into Shenzhen to perform basic and application studies in TB control. The cultivation of talents and disciplinary construction in TB control have been accelerated.

Effective Connections of the Essential Health-Care Formulary and Financial Assistance

Coverage of the Essential Health-care Formulary and financial assistance have been well connected to alleviate the economic burden of the patients with TB. A mechanism connecting the Essential Health-care Formulary and financial assistance was explored. And new measures including financial assistance and temporary financial assistance for management of patients with TB were explored to alleviate the economic burden of patients with TB. Allowances for transportation and well-nourishing foods have been provided for the patients with TB for accurate financial assistance to the patients in poverty.

Innovated Management of Patients with TB

Service for patients with TB has been strengthened. Patient-centered intelligent health management was performed for patients with TB. Internet plus DOT was promoted for tele-observed treatment. Classrooms for standard health education have been constructed. And the patients with poor compliance have received more frequent video observations to improve their compliance to the management. Psychological support and humane care have been conducted for patients with TB to alleviate their mental sufferings from TB and improve their confidence to recover from TB.

4.2 Comprehensive Effects of TB Control in Shenzhen

Construction and Improvement of a Comprehensive Service System for TB Control in Shenzhen

(1) A graded diagnosis and treatment system for TB control has been constructed with the leadership of city-level and district-level health-care administrations. And the system has been intended to provide convenient accessibility of TB diagnosis and treatment. In the graded system, the city-level TB control agency played a role in guiding the control of TB in Shenzhen, and the district-level TB control agencies played a key role in the control of TB in Shenzhen. In addition, health-care institutions including general hospitals and community health-care service centers played basic role in the system. And the specialized hospitals were responsible for hospitalization and treatment of patients with serious TB, acute TB, and DR-TB. In such a graded comprehensive health-care service system for TB control, the patients were timely diagnosed and effectively treated.

(2) Two-level diagnostic platform and laboratory quality control system were established. The functions of city-level TB control agency and district-level TB control agencies were specified to construct two-level diagnostic platform for TB. The first-level diagnostic platform of TB is the district-level TB control agencies, which have been responsible for the diagnosis of initially treated and re-treated patients. The second-level diagnostic platform of TB is the Center for Chronic Diseases Control in Shenzhen, which has been responsible for the diagnosis of DR-TB, including DR-TB, MDR-TB, and EDR-TB. The city-level specialized hospitals are responsible for the treatment of inpatients and outpatients with serious TB, acute TB, and DR-TB. A laboratory network and its quality control system were

constructed in city-level and district-level TB control agencies and city-level specialized hospital for graded management and regular quality control. The laboratory in the Center for Chronic Diseases Control in Shenzhen has regularly participated in the proficiency examination in performing drug sensitivity test hosted by the International Reference Laboratory in Hong Kong.

Promoted Application of New Strategies and New Technologies

New strategies and new technologies for TB control have been promoted for wider application in Shenzhen, which was 10 years prior to the proposal of applying new technology by the WHO.

Detection of Patients Via Multiple Ways

Free-in-charge standard sputum detection has been performed for suspected cases of TB in the migrating population in Shenzhen. In the Longhua district of Shenzhen, the TB detection program was implemented for anterior shift of TB detection. Screening of TB has been performed for suspected cases of TB, the elderly aged above 65 years, and patients with diabetes. Rapid detection has been performed for the high-risk populations. By these ways, detection and diagnosis of patients with TB and DR-TB have been improved.

Promotion of New Diagnostic Technology

The new diagnostic technologies were applied, including Hain GenoType MTBDR plus (HAIN), GeneXpert, TB-PCR, tuberculosis specific interferon γ release test (IGRAS), and BD960 device for fast mycobacterial culture. These new technologies shortened the period of time in detecting TB and improved the diagnostic accuracy. The patients with TB thus received timely treatment and the spread of TB was controlled.

Optimization of the Treatment for MDR-TB

In 1999, drug resistance by Mtb was firstly monitored in Shenzhen. Since then, surveillance of drug resistance by Mtb has been performed in Shenzhen for successive 19 years. In 2003, detection, treatment, and management of patients with MDR-TB were implemented in Shenzhen with the cost reduction and exemption policy. And a system for detection, diagnosis and treatment, management, and assessment of MDR-TB was established. In 2015, the management of all types of DR-TB was further standardized. In recent years, the new anti-tuberculosis drug, linezolid, has been applied for MDR-TB and the therapeutic efficacy has been favorable.

Control of the Adverse Effects of Communicable TB

In 2016, free-in-charge hospitalization of patients with MDR-TB and common smear-positive TB was implemented in the Center for Chronic Diseases Control in Shenzhen and the district-level institutions for chronic diseases control. And the inpatients were provided with allowance in Baoan district. Targeting on outpatients with communicable TB, community-based home quarantine and treatment and infection control were explored. Patients surveillance technologies based on GPS and GIS were developed in Nanshan district for home quarantine and treatment as well as daily trajectory of patients with DR-TB. Meanwhile, multiple measures, including lifestyle instruction, infection control, daily activities restriction, regular home visit, and allowance provision, were adopted. The patients with communicable TB were required at least 2 weeks home-stay for quarantine and treatment to decrease its spread to the surrounding population.

Exploration of Incentive Mechanism for Patient Management

The incentive mechanism for patient management was explored to strengthen the public health-care service. To improve the performance of the community in managing patients with TB, management of patients with TB was further innovated. And the health management service in Shenzhen has been greatly improved. In 2017, TB control alliance for patient management was explored in Shenzhen. In the program, the clinicians were mobilized to be the health assistants who directly participated in the health management of the patients with TB. And the job of health management was paid based on the quality assessment of patient management. In this way, the clinicians working in the basic health-care institutions were mobilized for active participation.

Cure Rate of TB Being Up to 91.4% During the Past 22 Years

During 1993–2015, the reported incidence of active TB decreased after reaching a peak. In 1993–1997, the reported incidence of active TB increased from 9.2 per 0.1 million to 45.4 per 0.1 million, which was followed by a decease year by year. In 2005, the reported incidence of active TB was 57.0 per 0.1 million, which reached the peak of 70.3 per 0.1 million in 2009 and decreased year by year then to 49.3 per 0.1 million [56].

During 2005–2015, the management rate of active TB was increasing [57]. In 1993–2015, the reported patients with TB and the suspected cases of TB in Shenzhen amounted 407.1 thousand, including 29.1 thousand local residents and 378.0 thousand migrating population. And the total management rate was up to 80.5%. The management rate of TB in local residents remained steady above 90%. And the management rate of TB in migrating population obviously decreased in 2003–2007, which fluctuated between 60 and 80%, and obviously increased after 2010. In 2015, the total management rate of TB in Shenzhen was above 90%.

During 2010–2015, the registry and management of active TB gradually decreased. In 1993–2015, the registry rate of TB in local residents of Shenzhen decreased after reaching a peak, followed by an increase and then a decrease. The registry rate in local residents of Shenzhen showed an M-shaped change. Since 2005, the number of patients has sharply decreased but the number of population sharply increases, forming an X in 2007. The registry rate of TB in local residents of Shenzhen reached 64.3 per 0.1 million in 2006, followed by a decrease year by year to 7.2 per 0.1 million in 2015. The number of active TB in the migrating population obviously fluctuated, with a peak of 66.9 per 0.1 million in 2009 and a following decrease year by year to 46.8 per 0.1 million in 2015.

During 1993–2015, the cure rate of TB remained high, being above 90%. During 1993–2015, a total of 69,383 cases of active TB were detected, including 12,325 cases in local residents and 57,078 cases in the migrating population. And 66,819 patients received treatment with anti-tuberculosis drugs, with 61,083 cases of cure (including 49,224 patients in the migrating population). And the cure rate was up to 91.4%. The cure rates in the local residents and the migrating population were 96.2% and 90.3%, respectively, which are above the required level by the WHO.

Effective Control of TB Epidemic

Large-scale epidemiological surveys of TB were conducted in 1991, 2000, and 2010 [58]. The results indicated that the morbidity rate of active TB and the morbidity rate of smear-positive TB in Shenzhen decreased in 1991–2010. The morbidity rate of active TB decreased from 336 per 0.1 million in 1991 to 78 per 0.1 million in 2010, with a decrease by 76.8%. The morbidity rate of active TB in the migrating population in Shenzhen decreased from 417 per 0.1 million in 1991 to 220 per 0.1 million in 2010, with a decrease by 47.2%. The morbidity rate of smear-positive TB in Shenzhen decreased from 118 per 0.1 million in 1991 to 19 per 0.1 million in 2010, with a decrease by 83.9% and an average annual decrease by 8.6%. In the migrating population in Shenzhen, the morbidity rate of smear-positive TB decreased from 131 per 0.1 million in 1991 to 60 per 0.1 million in 2010, with a decrease by 54.2% and an average annual decrease by 3.8%.

Enormous Socioeconomic Achievement of TB Control in Shenzhen

The performance assessment of the World Bank loan for TB control program has demonstrated that [59] TB control in Shenzhen was characterized by service equity, health accessibility, obvious effects, and enormous socioeconomic benefits. The health-care service in the control of TB in Shenzhen was provided equally to the local residents and the migrating population. And the same effects of TB control were achieved between local residents and the migrating population in Shenzhen. In the implementation of TB control in Shenzhen, a network for TB control was improved for centralized management of TB. And DOT strategy was implemented with obvious effects. The new patients decreased by 150,000 and the morbidity rate decreased by more than 50%. In addition, the socioeconomic benefits of TB control in Shenzhen were enormous, with direct economic benefits of 14.2 billion yuan and retrieval of GDP loss 3.06 billion yuan.

The assessment of health economics on TB control in Shenzhen has demonstrated that [60] the total cure rate of TB was up to 95.1% during 1993–2004. Cure expenses for one case of active TB were RMB 2857 yuan, *DALY* of 206912 year was directly saved and *DALY* of 89,982 year was indirectly saved. Compared to the traditional therapy, RMB 50.296 million yuan was saved by applying DOTS strategy. And RMB 54.643 million yuan was saved by control of the spreading sources. GDP loss of RMB 7.697126 billion yuan was retrieved. The total personal loss of RMB 4.477576 billion yuan due to TB was avoided. The assessment results indicated that the TB control program in Shenzhen alleviates economic burden of the patients and facilitates avoiding large amount of economic losses, which has obvious socioeconomic benefits.

The performance assessment of *the Tuberculosis Control Planning in Shenzhen (2001–2010)* has demonstrated that [61] DOTS strategy was implemented in Shenzhen with a coverage of 100%. In 2001–2010, a total of 34,024 cases of active TB were detected, managed, and treated. The cure rate of smear-positive TB in the local residents of Shenzhen was 94.79% and the cure rate of active TB in the local residents of Shenzhen was 95.51%, which were significantly higher than the rates in the migrating population in Shenzhen, being 82.91% and 87.25%, respectively. The morbidity rate of smear-positive TB in the local residents of Shenzhen was 19.44 per 0.1 million in 2010, with a decrease by 70.55% compared to the data in 2000. The morbidity rate of smear-positive TB in the migrating population in Shenzhen was 59.96 per 0.1 million, with a decrease by 27.23% compared to the data in 2000. In 2001–2010, the total funding for TB control in Shenzhen was up to RMB 0.150 billion yuan. By implementing TB control in Shenzhen, 136.7 thousand healthy individuals were protected from infection of TB and 13.7 thousand new cases of TB were avoided. The direct and indirect economic benefits were up to RMB 20.245 billion yuan. The investment of RMB 1 yuan for TB control in Shenzhen produced socioeconomic benefits of RMB 134.98 yuan. The assessment results indicated that the implementation of *the Tuberculosis Control Planning in Shenzhen (2001–2010)* achieved great success.

4.3 Advancement of TB Control in Shenzhen

Establishment of a Characteristic System for TB Control in Shenzhen

A network for prevention, control, and management of TB was established in Shenzhen. The network consisted of institutions for chronic diseases control, hospitals for TB control, community health-care service center, community-based institutions for TB control, and health-care institutions in enterprises. Specifically, there was 1 city-level institution for chronic diseases control, 10 district-level institutions for chronic diseases control, 56 hospitals and community-based institutions for TB control, and 1095 community health-care service centers and health-care institutions in enterprises. All of these institutions were organized into a complete network of TB control in Shenzhen. In addition, a funding system for TB control predominantly by local public finance was firstly established in Shenzhen to secure the implementation of TB control measures.

Earliest Attention on TB Control in Migrating Population

In 1991, the migrating population was firstly integrated into the TB control program in Shenzhen, which was 5 years prior to the proposal of TB control in migrating population by the WHO. Since 1993, full coverage of TB control and DOTS strategy were successively implemented in Shenzhen. Such a large-scale full population coverage of TB control program and such a long-term implementation of DOTS strategy have been unprecedented in human history. In 2011, eDOT system (http://218.18.233.234:9080/PHMIS1) was firstly developed in Shenzhen, which has been the only TB management system based on the idea of internet plus TB. With the application of the system, all the reported TB cases are accessible in all the health-care institutions in Shenzhen, which facilitates implementing DOTS strategy [61].

Development of TB Control from Follower to Leading Role

During implementation of DOTS strategy across the world, DOTS strategy was synchronously implemented in Shenzhen. Funding for TB control was emphasized to be the key in the commitments of the government, and the migrating population was firstly integrated into the TB control planning. In 2003, categorized management of MDR-TB was firstly implemented in Shenzhen. In 2006, the global funding for MDR-TB control program was implemented in Shenzhen [62, 63]. Humane care, allowance for transportation and well-nourishing foods, and psychological support were emphasized during the implementation of the program. Since 2011, new diagnostic technologies have been gradually promoted and the cure rate of recruited patients has reached 69.7%, which indicated that Shenzhen has played a leading role in the management and treatment of TB. The achievements in TB control in Shenzhen provide scientific basis and practical experience for national development of new technologies and TB control policies.

Optimal Ratio of Cost to Benefit

The health economical assessment on TB control during 1993–2001 in Shenzhen has demonstrated that TB control in Shenzhen has achievements of service equity, health accessibility, obvious effects, and enormous benefits. Compared to the traditional therapy, RMB 39.37 million yuan have been saved on the cost of smear-positive TB patients by applying the DOTS strategy. The performance assessment on Tuberculosis Control Planning in Shenzhen (2001–2010) has demonstrated that the investment of RMB 1 yuan in TB control in Shenzhen produced socioeconomic benefits of RMB 134.98 yuan.

Basis for National Formulation of TB Control Strategy and Technology Policy

The exploration and practice of TB control in Shenzhen were appraised by the Center of TB control, the National Center for Disease Control (CDC) in China. And the exploration and practice of TB control in Shenzhen provide basis for the national formulation of TB control strategy and technology policy. Based on the Shenzhen experience of TB control in the migrating population, TB control in migrating population was systematically designed and implemented in the pilot work for the global funding program for TB control. The complete system for DR-TB control firstly established in Shenzhen was adopted in the Guideline for MDR-TB Control and training textbooks compiled by the CDC of China. The systematic works for TB control in Shenzhen, including complete TB control system, implementation of TB control measures, policies making, and funding for TB control, provided reference for TB control in other regions of China.

References

1. World Health Organization. Global tuberculosis report 2018. Geneva: World Health Organization; 2018.
2. Styblo K. Dr. Karel Styblo symposium: an emerging global programme against tuberculosis. The Hague, March 15, 1991. Bull Int Union Tuberc Lung Dis. 1991;66(4):139–214.
3. World Health Organization. Forty-fourth world health assembly, resolutions and decisions. Geneva: World Health Organization; 1991.
4. Wang LX, Jiang SW. Development and prospects of the national TB control strategy in China. Chin J Anti-tuberc. 2014;36(8):630–3.
5. Frieden TR, Munsiff SS. The DOTS strategy for controlling the global tuberculosis epidemic. Clin Chest Med. 2005;26(2):197–205.

6. Nie WJ, Chu NH. The 7th interpretation about the partner handbook of the guideline for drug-resistant TB planning management issued by WHO in 2014: treatment of multidrug-resistant TB and extensive drug-resistant TB. Chin J Anti-tuberc. 2015;37(7):800–2.
7. Shen XMJ, Gao Q. DOTS-Plus: a powerful weapon for control of multidrug-resistant tuberculosis. J Shanghai Prevent Med. 2006;18(5):225–6.
8. World Health Organization. The stop TB strategy, building on and enhancing DOTS to meet the TB-related millennium development goals. Geneva: World Health Organization; 2006.
9. Liu JJ. Strategies for tuberculosis control. Health Edu Tuberc Control. 2006;1:11–5.
10. Dai BZ, Zhan SK. TB control and its strategy in migrating population. J Shanghai Prevent Med. 2005;17(3):111–2.
11. Population Division, Department of Economic and Social Affairs, the United Nations. Trends in international migrant stock: the 2008 revision. p. 1–2.
12. Dye C, Lönnroth K, Jaramillo E, et al. Trends in tuberculosis incidence and their determinants in 134 countries. Bull World Health Organ. 2009;87(9):683–91.
13. U.S. Department of Health and Human Services. Centers for disease control and prevention, trends in tuberculosis—United States, 2010. MMWR Morb Mortal Wkly Rep. 2011;60(11):333–7.
14. Menzies HJ, Winston CA, Holtz TH, et al. Epidemiology of tuberculosis among US- and foreign-born children and adolescents in the United States, 1994-2007. Am J Public Health. 2010;100(9):1724–9.
15. Win KMK, Chee CBE, Shen L, et al. Tuberculosis among foreign-born persons, Singapore, 2000-2009. Emerg Infect Dis. 2011;17(3):517–9.
16. Borrell S, Espanol M, Orcau A, et al. Tuberculosis transmission patterns among Spanish-born and foreign-born populations in the city of Barcelona. Clin Microbiol Infect. 2010;16(6):568–74.
17. Salinas JL, Mindra G, Haddad MB, et al. Leveling of tuberculosis incidence United States, 2013-2015. MMWR Morb Moral Wkly Rep. 2016;65(11):273–8.
18. Ho MJ. Migratory journeys and tuberculosis risk. Med Anthropol Q. 2003;17(4):442–58.
19. Bao J. Prevalence of TB and its control strategy in the US. Chin J Anti-tuberc. 2017;39(2):198–201.
20. Centers for Disease Control and Prevention. National TB program objectives and performance targets for 2020. [2016-11-16]. http://www.cdc.gov/tb/programs/evaluation/indicators/default.htm.
21. Raviglione MC, Sudre P, Rieder HL, et al. Secular trends of tuberculosis in Western Europe. Bull World Health Organ. 1993;71(3/4):297–306.
22. Inigo J, Arce A, Rodriguez E, et al. Tuberculosis trends in Madrid, 1994-2003: impact of immigration and HIV infection. Int J Tuberc Lung Dis. 2006;10(5):550–3.
23. Marks GB, Bai J, Stewart GJ, et al. Effectiveness of post-migration screening in controlling tuberculosis among refugees: a historical cohort study, 1984-1998. Am J Public Health. 2001;91(11):1797–9.
24. Suarez PG, Watt CJ, Alarcon E, et al. The dynamics of tuberculosis in response to 10 years of intensive control effort in Peru. J Infect Dis. 2001;184(4):473–8.
25. Frieden TR. Can tuberculosis be controlled? Int J Epidemiol. 2002;31(5):894–9.
26. Baltussen R, Floyd K, Dye C. Cost-effectiveness analysis of strategies for tuberculosis control in developing countries. BMJ. 2005;331(7529):1364.
27. Pantoja A, Lonnroth K, Lal SS, et al. Economic evaluation of Public-private mix for tuberculosis care and control. India, part II. Cost and cost-effectiveness. Int J Tuberc Lung Dis. 2009;13(6):705–12.
28. Zhong Q, Yang YZ. Implementation and prospects of DOTS strategy in TB patients from migrating population in Shenzhen. Chin J Anti-tuberc. 1998;20(2):61–4.
29. Tan WG, Wu QF, Yang YZ. Analysis of TB control in migrating population of Shenzhen [J]. Chin J Anti-tuberc. 2001;23(2):99–102.
30. Wei GF, Zhang YR. Analysis of TB control in migrating population in Shijingshan district of Beijing. J Clin Pneumol. 2002;7(1):33–4.
31. Chen YW, Zhang ZP. Management of TB patients in migrating population in Yin county of Zhengjiang province. Zhejiang Prevent Med. 2000;12(10):23–4.
32. Jiang SW, Wang J, Liu XQ, et al. Development of TB control in migrating population of China. Chin J Anti-tuberc. 2008;30(SI):7–9.
33. Huang JY, Xie QH. Cultural construction at China-ASEAN land border ports. Guangxi Soc Sci. 2018;6:87–9.
34. Li H, Hou RS, Wang JJ, et al. Surveillance of infectious diseases in entry-exit population at the ports in Henan province: data analysis during 2005 to 2014. Port Health Control. 2015;21(4):5–9.
35. Ma S, Chen P, Yang B, et al. Detection of communicable tuberculosis in entry-exit population at the ports in Shandong province: descriptive data, epidemiological analysis and its control strategy. Port Health Control. 2012;4:37–42.
36. Chen L, Wang C, Chen F. Surveillance of diseases in entry-exit population at the ports in Yangzhou: data analysis during 2011-2016. Port Health Control. 2017;22(4):37–9.
37. Wang J, Zhang Q, Fang Y. Surveillance of imported tuberculosis at the ports in Shanghai: data analysis during 2009-2015. J Tuberc Pulm Health. 2016;5(3):222–6.
38. Aldridge RW, Yates TA, Zenner D, et al. Pre-entry screening programmes for tuberculosis in migrants to low-incidence countries: a systematic review and meta-analysis. Lancet Infect Dis. 2014;14(12):1240–9.
39. King K, Douglas PJ, Beath K. Is premigration health screening for tuberculosis worthwhile. Med J Aust. 2011;195(9):534–7.
40. An H, J B, Kg C. Modelling tuberculosis trends in the USA. Epidemiol Infect. 2012;10(140):1862–72.
41. Baker BJ, Winston CA, Liu Y, et al. Abrupt decline in tuberculosis among foreign-born persons in the United States. PLoS ONE. 2016;11(2):e147353.
42. Verhagen LM, van den Hof S, van Deutekom H, et al. Mycobacterial factors relevant for transmission of tuberculosis. J Infect Dis. 2011;203(9):1249–55.
43. Klinkenberg E, Manissero D, Semenza JC, et al. Migrant tuberculosis screening in the EU/EEA: yield, coverage and limitations. Eur Respir J. 2009;34(5):1180–9.
44. Pareek M, Baussano I, Abubakar I, et al. Evaluation of immigrant tuberculosis screening in industrialized countries. Emerg Infect Dis. 2012;18(9):1422–9.
45. Meng CY, Zhou X, Cai L, et al. Tuberculosis screening strategy and result in exit population to five countries at the ports of Shanghai. Chin J Front Health Insp. 2016;5:352–5.
46. Fan XJ, Sun M. Laboratory diagnosis of tuberculosis: a comparative study. Chin J Front Health Insp. 2005;3:160–2.
47. Ruan C. Surveillance and management of infectious diseases in entry-exit population. Ningbo: Ningbo University; 2017.
48. Yang HL, Li L, Wang YL, et al. Problems in surveillance and management of tuberculosis in entry-exit population and the solutions. J Insp Quar. 2016;2:62–4.
49. Yang YZ, Tan WG, Luo YX, et al. Implementation of TB control in migrating population. Chin J Publ Health Manage. 1999;15(2):80–2.
50. Guan HY, Tan WG, Yang YZ, et al. Comprehensive management of trans-regional flowing TB patients in Shenzhen. Chin J Anti-tuberc. 2015;37(5):498–503.
51. Guan HY, Tan WG, Yang YZ, et al. Epidemiological analysis of TB epidemic in students of Shenzhen from 2009 to 2013. J Clin Pneumol. 2016;21(8):1496–9.

52. Wu QF, Yang YZ, Xu L, et al. Analysis of TB epidemic in Shenzhen based on data of reporting and registry in 2006-2010. Guangdong Med. 2011;32(17):2309–10.
53. Wu QF, Tan WG, Yang YZ, et al. Surveillance on drug resistance of mycobacteria tuberculosis in Shenzhen during. J Clin Pneumol. 2010;15(8):1121–3.
54. Lu CR, Tan WG, Zhuo ZP, et al. Epidemic of isoniazid resistant and rifampicin resistant TB in Shenzhen during 1999 to 2015. Electron J Emerg Inf Dis. 2017;2(1):10–3.
55. Wu QF, Tan WG, Luo DQ, et al. TB control in prisons of Shenzhen and its effects. J Clin Pneumol. 2015;20(9):1571–4.
56. Guan HY, Yang YZ, Tan WG, et al. Referral and tracing of suspected cases of TB reported by health-care institutions in Shenzhen in 2011-2016. Chin J Trop Med. 2017;17(8):766–9.
57. Wu QF, Tan WG, Lv DL, et al. Referral and tracing of suspected cases of TB in Shenzhen. Chin J Trop Med. 2013;13(8): 984–6.
58. Guan HY, Yang YZ, Tan WG, et al. Performance assessment of *the Tuberculosis Control Planning in Shenzhen (2001-2010)*. Chin J Anti-tuberc. 2013;35(9):729–37.
59. Cheng JQ, Yang YZ, Zhang D, et al. Performance assessment of the World Bank loan for TB control program in Shenzhen. Chin J Public Health. 2004;20(7):73–5.
60. Wu QF, Xu JJ, Tan WG, et al. Health economical assessment on tuberculosis control in Shenzhen. Chin J Trop Med. 2006;6(5):775–6.
61. Guan HY, Tan WG, Yang YZ, et al. Management and treatment of patients with TB based on eDOT system. Chin J Anti-tuberc. 2017;39(7):702–7.
62. Guan HY, Tan WG, Yang YZ, et al. Detection, treatment and management of 652 cases of MDR-TB in Shenzhen in 2006-2014. Chin J Anti-tuberc. 2017;39(5):518–24.
63. Che XL, Wu QF, Lv DL, et al. Performance assessment of the global funding for MDR-TB control in Shenzhen. Chin J Trop Med. 2017;17(10):988–90.

Prevention, Diagnosis, and Treatment of TB in the Migrating Population

4

Shou-jiang Liu and Wei Wei

1 Key Points for the Diagnosis of TB

The Standards for Classification of Tuberculosis in China (WS196-2017) was implemented on May 1st, 2018 in China. According to the standards, TB can be classified into three types based on its progression: incubated TB, active TB, and inactive TB. And active TB is further classified into active pulmonary TB and active extrapulmonary TB [1].

(1) Primary TB

Clinically active TB caused by human infection of Mtb after its first access into human respiratory tract is known as primary TB. Primary TB can be further classified into primary syndrome and TB of intrathoracic lymph nodes. In children, primary TB also includes caseous pneumonia as well as tracheal and bronchial TB.

(2) Blood disseminating pulmonary TB

Blood disseminating pulmonary TB is caused by once or repeated access of Mtb into the blood flow, which further causes lesions at lungs with corresponding pathological and pathophysiological changes and clinical symptoms. Based on the quantity of Mtb that gains their access into the blood flow, their toxicity, the times of their access, routes of access, intervals of accesses and the immunity of the host, blood disseminating pulmonary TB can be further classified into three types. They are acute blood disseminating pulmonary TB, sub-acute blood disseminating pulmonary TB, and chronic blood disseminating pulmonary TB.

(3) Secondary pulmonary TB

After first infection of Mtb, the Mtb spreading along with blood flow into incubated lesions of TB is re-activated to cause activated lesions of TB. In the other cases, re-infection of Mtb occurs to cause secondary pulmonary TB. Secondary pulmonary TB includes infiltrative pulmonary TB, tuberculoma, caseous pneumonia, chronic fibro-cavitary TB, and lung destruction.

(4) Tracheal and bronchial TB

Tracheal and bronchial TB is TB that occurs at the tracheal and/or bronchial mucosa or submucosa.

(5) Tuberculous pleurisy

Tuberculous pleurisy is pleural inflammation caused by the access of Mtb and their metabolites into high sensitive pleural cavity. Based on its clinical course and pathological manifestations, it can be further classified into dry pleurisy, exudative pleurisy, and tuberculous empyema.

1.1 Standards for the Diagnosis of TB

According to the Diagnostic Standards for Tuberculosis in China (WS288-2017), TB can be classified into suspected cases of TB, clinically defined cases of TB, and defined cases of TB [2, 3].

Suspected Cases of TB Should be Diagnosed Based on One of the Following Conditions

For Adults and Children Aged Above 5 Years

For adults and children aged above 5 years, the demonstrations of chest diagnostic imaging are consistent to active TB.

For Children Aged Under 5 Years

For children aged under 5 years, there are suspected symptoms of TB with one of the followings:

(1) a history of close contacts with patients with sputum smear-positive TB;
(2) moderately positive or above in laboratory tuberculin test;
(3) positive in laboratory interferon γ release test.

S.-j. Liu (✉) · W. Wei
Shenzhen Nanshan Center for Chronic Disease Control, Shenzhen, Guangdong, China

W.-y. Yu et al. (eds.), *Tuberculosis Control in Migrating Population*, https://doi.org/10.1007/978-981-32-9763-0_4

Clinically Defined Cases of TB

Adults

(1) The demonstrations of chest diagnostic imaging are consistent to active TB and the patients present with suspected symptoms of TB such as cough with sputum and hemoptysis.
(2) The demonstrations of chest diagnostic imaging are consistent to active TB. In addition, the tuberculin test is above moderately positive or interferon γ release test shows positive.
(3) The demonstrations of chest diagnostic imaging are consistent to active TB. And the antibody test for Mtb shows positive.
(4) The demonstrations of chest diagnostic imaging are consistent to active TB. And extrapulmonary histopathology demonstrates tuberculosis.
(5) The demonstrations of chest diagnostic imaging are consistent to bronchial TB. And the demonstrations of fibrobronchoscopy are consistent to TB. Such cases can be diagnosed with tracheal and bronchial TB.
(6) The demonstrations of chest diagnostic imaging are consistent to tuberculous pleurisy. And the hydrothorax is demonstrated to be exudates with elevated adenosine deaminase. In addition, the tuberculin test shows above moderately positive or the interferon γ release test shows positive or Mtb antibody positive. Such cases can be diagnosed with tuberculous pleurisy.

Children

The clinical diagnosis of TB can be diagnosed in children based on all of the following findings:

(1) The demonstrations of chest diagnostic imaging are consistent to active TB.
(2) There are suspected symptoms of pediatric TB, including cough, expectoration, hemoptysis, emaciation, and delayed development.
(3) The tuberculin test shows above moderately positive or the interferon γ release test shows positive.

Defined Cases of TB

Diagnosis of Sputum Smear-Positive TB

The diagnosis of sputum smear-positive TB should be based on one of the followings:

(1) Two sputum specimens are detected to be acid-fast bacillus positive.
(2) One sputum specimen is detected to be acid-fast bacillus positive. And the chest diagnostic imaging demonstrates lesions resembling to active TB.
(3) One sputum specimen is detected to be acid-fast bacillus positive. And one sputum specimen is detected to be mycobacteria positive.

Diagnosis of Mycobacterial Isolation and Culture Positive TB

The chest diagnostic imaging demonstrates lesions resembling to active TB. And at least two sputum specimens show smear test negative but mycobacteria culture positive.

Diagnosis of Molecular Biology Positive TB

The chest diagnostic imaging demonstrates lesions resembling to active TB. And molecular biology shows mycobacterial nucleic acid positive.

Diagnosis of Histopathology Positive TB

The histopathology of lung tissue indicates TB.

Diagnosis of Tracheal and Bronchial TB

The diagnosis of tracheal and bronchial TB should be based on one of the followings:

(1) Fibrobronchoscopy demonstrates lesions resembling to TB. And histopathology of lung tissues indicates TB.
(2) Fibrobronchoscopy demonstrates lesions resembling to TB. And pathogenic examination on the tracheal and bronchial excretions shows positive.

Diagnosis of Tuberculous Pleurisy

The diagnosis of tuberculous pleurisy should be based on one of the followings:

(1) The chest diagnostic imaging demonstrates lesions resembling to tuberculous pleurisy. In addition, hydrothorax examination or pleural pathology indicates pathological changes of TB.
(2) The chest diagnostic imaging demonstrates lesions resembling to tuberculous pleurisy. And pathogenic examination of hydrothorax shows positive.

1.2 Epidemiology

History of Contact

The onset of TB after infection of Mtb is related to the toxicity and quantity of infected Mtb. Many studies have demonstrated that individuals with history of contact to patients with TB, especially those with history of close contacts to patients with sputum smear-positive TB show significantly increased infection rate and incidence of TB. Therefore, definitive history of contact to patients with TB, especially to patients excreting Mtb, has important reference value in the diagnosis. In addition, in the history of contact to patients excreting Mtb, if the excreted Mtb can be defined to be drug sensitive or drug resistant, the further assessment would be greatly helped.

Susceptible Population

Currently, it has been believed that onset of TB after infection of Mtb is related to the immunity of the host. Infection of Mtb in individuals with compromised immunity or temporarily compromised immunity is more likely to cause onset of TB. A study has demonstrated that patients with basic pulmonary diseases and subsequent pathological changes of the lung tissues and compromised immunity are vulnerable to infection of Mtb and onset of TB. Clinically, the susceptible populations include patients with long-term use of immunosuppressant, patients with HIV/AIDS, patients with type I or II diabetes, patients with chronic malnutrition, patients with renal deficiency and receiving blood dialysis, patients with pneumosilicosis, and patients with chronic obstructive pulmonary disease (COPD). In addition, patients with malignancy, patients with hypothyroidism, patients with hepatocirrhosis, alcoholics, patients with serious psychiatric disorder, patients with viral infection, and postnatal women are also high-risk populations of TB. Nowadays, clinical practice has indicated that TB shows familial agglomeration. In addition to its spreading routes, some scholars believe that the familial agglomeration of TB may be attributed to genetics, which needs to be proved.

1.3 Clinical Manifestations

Symptoms

Pulmonary TB is an infectious disease of the respiratory tract. And its onset may be slight, serious, chronic or acute, with complex and diversifying clinical symptoms. Along with increasing attention on health by the government and individuals, the screening of individuals with close contacts to patients with TB, epidemiological surveys, and health examinations have been widely conducted. Currently, patients with TB are detected by chest diagnostic imaging.

The clinical manifestations provide important clue for understandings about the occurrence, development, and differential diagnosis of a disease. The clinical symptoms of pulmonary TB vary based on the age, immunity, and nourishment of the patient as well as concurrent disease, quantity, and toxicity of the infected Mtb. Therefore, on clinical encounters, health examinations, and screening of TB, case history and symptoms should be carefully inquired. Although being diversifying and complex, TB has its common symptoms.

Cough and Expectoration

Cough and expectoration for above 2 weeks are the suspected symptoms of TB.

Cough is a protective response of the respiratory tract to invasion of pathogens from the environment. Via coughing and expectorating, the respiratory excretions are expelled out of human body to keep an unobstructed respiratory tract. Cough and expectoration are common respiratory symptoms, which are non-specific to TB. But some patients with TB present with repeated cough and expectoration. Therefore, the cases with cough and expectoration for above 2 weeks, no therapeutic response to symptomatic and anti-infection treatment, routine blood test within normal limits or only elevated total and percentage lymphocytes, and sputum culture for common bacteria negative should be suspected with pulmonary TB [4].

Cough and expectoration are characteristics at different stages of TB:

(1) The early stage of slight TB is characterized by no obvious cough or slight dry cough when the patients get up in the morning or inhale stimulating gas. The cough is occasionally accompanied by small quantity of whitish mucous sputum.
(2) When TB progresses with formation of cavity or caseous pneumonia, persistent severe cough with accompanying expectoration of whitish mucous sputum may occur. In some cases, the sputum is bloody.
(3) In patients with tracheal and bronchial TB, wheezing or frequent coughs due to stimulation commonly occurs with expectoration of whitish mucous sputum.
(4) In the cases of TB complicated by pyopneumothorax or pleural bronchial fistula, the patients present with paroxysmal severe cough with expectoration of purulent sputum or purulent bloody sputum.
(5) In the cases of TB complicated by bronchial lymph nodes TB or lymph node bronchial fistula, wheezing or frequent stimulating coughs occurs.
(6) In the cases of TB complicated by bronchiectasis or other secondary bacterial infection, there are corresponding clinical manifestations. For instances, in the cases of TB complicated by bacterial infection, the patients present with cough and accompanying expectoration of purulent sputum. In the cases of TB complicated by fungal infection, the patients present with cough and accompanying expectoration of jelly-like sputum.

Hemoptysis

Hemoptysis is bleeding of the trachea, bronchus, or lung tissues caused by various factors and the blood is expelled out of human body via cough. Hemoptysis may be caused by respiratory diseases, circulatory diseases, systematic factors, or trauma. Clinically, the common reason of hemoptysis is respiratory diseases. The respiratory diseases that commonly induce hemoptysis include pulmonary TB (especially tracheal and bronchial TB and cavitary pulmonary TB), bronchial dilation and infection, bronchial carcinoma, bronchial adenoma, foreign body in bronchus, acute or chronic bronchitis.

Hemoptysis in patients with pulmonary TB is commonly caused by progression of pulmonary TB to involve the adjacent blood vessels. Patients with cavitary lesion or tracheal and bronchial intimal lesion are more likely to present hemoptysis. The invasion of TB lesions to the vascular vessels causes recurrent hemoptysis. The quantity of blood varies based on the size of involved vascular vessels, artery, vein, or capillary vessels. Generally, in the cases with invasion of TB lesions to capillary vessels or minor veins, the coughed blood is in a small quantity. In the cases with invasion of TB lesions to artery or major vascular vessels, the coughed blood is in a large quantity, which may even obstruct the airway to cause suffocation or cause hemorrhagic shock due to large amount of blood loss. Therefore, the clinicians should be alert to the symptom of hemoptysis.

Fever

Fever is the regulatory elevation of body temperature caused by pyrogen. Clinically, fever is classified into infectious fever and non-infectious fever. According to literature reports, the reason for fever is commonly infectious disease in the developing countries.

Fever is one of the most common symptoms of TB. Fever in patients with TB is characterized by:

(1) Chronic onset. The fever is initially unobvious and the patients can hardly remember the time of its onset.
(2) Tidal fever in afternoons. Fever in patients with TB is typically tidal in afternoons. That is to say, the patients present with low grade or moderate grade fever in afternoons or at dusks, and the body temperature can return to normal by itself. The accompanying symptoms commonly include red cheeks, fatigue, night sweat, and emaciation.
(3) Possibly irregular fever. Fever in patients with TB may be elevated temperature in fatigue or before menstruation in women. During acute progression or systemic dissemination of TB, the patients may present with moderate fever or hyperthermia. However, the patients commonly present with no chill or aversion to cold before onset of fever, with no accompanying herpes simplex at the corner of mouth.
(4) No therapeutic response to anti-infection therapy. Fever in patients with TB shows no therapeutic response to anti-infection therapy. After experimental anti-tuberculosis therapy is administered, the high body temperature commonly returns to normal in 1–4 weeks.

According to literature reports, fever of different degrees occurs in 37–80% cases of pulmonary TB. And fever occurs in 87–100% cases of acute blood disseminating TB and exudative tuberculous pleurisy.

Dyspnea

Dyspnea can be either an objective sign or a subjective feeling. Objectively, it is manifested as changes of respiratory frequency, rhythm, and depth. Subjectively, it is difficulty breathing and inhaling insufficiency. At the early stage of TB or in the cases of slight TB, the patients do not present with dyspnea.

Dyspnea in patients with TB is commonly pulmonary dyspnea, which is common in the following cases:

(1) In the cases with extensive lung lesions, such as fibrotic thick-wall cavity with accompanying bronchial dissemination, lobar or complete atelectasis, compensatory emphysema, large flake of pleural thickening, and diaphragmatic adhesion.
(2) In the cases of tracheal or bronchial luminal stenosis induced by bronchial TB, including compression of lymph nodes adjacent to enlarged bronchus and cicatricial stenosis.
(3) In the cases of tuberculous pleurisy with large quantity of pleural effusion.
(4) In the cases of pediatric primary TB with compression of trachea or bronchus due to para-tracheal or para-bronchial enlarged lymph nodes or lymph node bronchial fistula.
(5) In the cases of TB complicated by other diseases, such as sharp chest pain, acute dyspnea, and cyanosis in pneumothorax and mediastinal emphysema as well as corresponding symptoms and obvious dyspnea in cardiac insufficiency and pulmonary heart diseases.

Tuberculosis Hypersensitivity Syndrome

The tuberculosis hypersensitivity syndrome includes rheumatic arthritis (Poncet syndrome), herpetic conjunctival keratitis, and erythema nodosum, whose incidence is 10–20%.

Poncet syndrome commonly occurs in young females, with symptoms of joint pain, low fever, no obvious swelling and deformity of joints, negative findings in rheumatic or rheumatoid related examinations and no therapeutic response to anti-rheumatic therapy. However, the patients with Poncet syndrome commonly show PPD skin test strongly positive or positive and favorable therapeutic response to anti-tuberculosis therapy. Further diagnostic examinations demonstrate lymph nodes TB at the hilum, mediastinum, and abdominal or pelvic cavity. Herpetic conjunctival keratitis rarely occurs, which should be considered after exclusion of viral and parasitic infections. In some patients, erythema nodosum or erythema circinatum repeatedly occurs with multiple fusible surrounding edema, which is commonly located at the surface of anterior tibial extensor or adjacent to ankles.

Systemic Symptoms

Systemic symptoms present in patients with pulmonary TB, including fatigue, night sweating, irritation, poor appetite, weight loss, changes of sexual desire, and intermittent or persistent fever after noons. Pulmonary TB in females may be accompanied by dysmenorrhea or even amenorrhea. In children, patients with pulmonary TB may present delayed development. And in the cases of pulmonary TB complicated by extrapulmonary TB, the patients may present with corresponding manifestations of the involved organs.

Signs

In the cases with pulmonary TB in a small range of involvement, no signs of TB can be detected. The signs of pulmonary TB are related to the qualitative changes and range of involvements. Along with progression of pulmonary TB, the following signs may be detected:

Superficial Lymphadenectasis

Superficial lymphadenectasis may be detected in patients with primary pulmonary TB.

Enlarged Liver and Spleen, Fundus Choroidal Nodule, and Miliary Skin Rash

In the cases of blood disseminating pulmonary TB, enlarged liver and spleen as well as fundus choroidal nodule may be detected. In the cases of pediatric pulmonary TB, miliary skin rash may be detected.

Different Signs of Secondary Pulmonary TB

Different signs can be detected at different stages of secondary pulmonary TB.

(1) In the cases of caseous pneumonia or at the large area exudation stage, signs of parenchymal lungs can be detected, including strong vocal fremitus by palpation, dullness by percussion as well as fine moist rales and bronchial breathing sound by auscultation
(2) In the cases of cavitary pulmonary TB, when the cavity is large, the following signs can be detected: bronchial breathing sound by auscultation.
(3) In the cases with complicating infection, moist rales can be auscultated.
(4) In the cases with large area of fibrotic cords opacity, there are thoracic collapse of the affected side and shift of trachea towards the affected side by observation, dullness by percussion, and diminished breathing sound by auscultation.

Tuberculous Pleurisy

(1) At the early stage or recovery stage, pleural rubs can be auscultated due to small quantity of pleural effusion.
(2) Along with increase of pleural effusion, shift of trachea towards the unaffected side, widened intercostal space of the affected side, and full chest can be observed. And dullness and flatness can be percussed. By auscultation, the breathing sounds are diminished or absent.
(3) At the advanced stage with obvious pleural thickening and adhesion, shift of trachea towards the affected side, narrowed intercostal space of the affected side, and thoracic collapse can be observed. By percussion, there is dullness. And by auscultation, diminished breathing sounds can be heard.

Tracheal and Bronchial TB

In the serious cases with atelectasis and airway constriction, shift of trachea to the affected side, narrowed intercostal space of the affected side, and thoracic collapse can be observed. By percussion, there is dullness or flatness. By auscultation, there is diminished or absent breathing sounds or fixed and localized wheezing.

1.4 Auxiliary Diagnostic Examinations

Diagnostic Imaging

Demonstrations by Chest X-ray and CT Scanning

By diagnostic imaging, pulmonary TB is demonstrated with polymorphous lesions, namely co-existence of infiltration, proliferation, caseous lesion, and fibrotic calcification. However, different types of pulmonary TB are demonstrated as their own characteristic lesions

Primary Pulmonary TB

Primary pulmonary TB is typically demonstrated as (1) TB lesion of the first infection; (2) lymph node TB; (3) lymphangitis; and (4) pleural inflammatory response around the TB lesion of the first infection, which may or may not be detected. Clinically, primary pulmonary TB manifests as intrapulmonary primary lesions of TB and intrathoracic lymphadenectasis or simple intrathoracic lymphadenectasis. In the cases of pediatric primary pulmonary TB, there may be caseous pneumonia, cavity and bronchial TB induced by bronchial lymph node fistula.

Chest X-ray demonstrates primary pulmonary TB as dumbbell shaped lesion. However, in some cases, only hilar lymphadenectasis can be detected. For further defined diagnosis or differential diagnosis, chest CT scanning may be necessary, which is capable of clearly demonstrating mediastinal lymphadenectasis and the density of the lesion.

(1) Hilar lymphadenectasis, especially lymphadenectasis at the posterior hilum, can be easily detected due to its contrast to the adjacent air-containing structures.
(2) Lymphadenectasis at the anterior hilum can only be detected by contrast CT scan due to many sections of local vascular branching. Enlarged lymph nodes commonly consist of surrounding granulation tissue and central caseous necrotic tissue. Therefore, contrast CT scan demonstrates typical ring shaped enhancement or marginal enhancement. By contrast CT scan, the lymph node metastatic lesion of lung carcinoma is commonly demonstrated as irregular enhancement or comparatively low-density area at the center. The demonstrations of contrast CT scan facilitate their differential diagnosis.

Blood Disseminating Pulmonary TB

By chest X-ray, the early stage of acute blood disseminating pulmonary TB is demonstrated as decreased transparency of both lungs and diffuse network like opacity. Along with progression of the disease, at 2 weeks after onset, chest X-ray typically demonstrates three-evens sign, namely even distribution, even size, and even density of miliary opacities in both lungs. However, in clinical practice, such typical cases are rare. And its diagnosis should be differentiated from bronchoalveolar cell carcinoma.

By chest X-ray, sub-acute or chronic blood disseminating pulmonary TB is demonstrated as diffuse lesions that commonly distribute at the upper and middle parts of both lungs with uneven size and uneven density. The lesions may be demonstrated to be fused.

In infants and young children, the miliary lesions are surrounded by obvious exudates and, therefore, demonstrated with poorly defined boundary and tendency of fusion. In pediatric cases of acute blood disseminating pulmonary TB, ground glass opacities may only be demonstrated.

In some patients with complications, such as chronic bronchitis, interstitial fibrosis, emphysema, and pleural thickening, the lung structures are changed. Therefore, the demonstrations of chest X-ray are atypical, with no above-mentioned characteristic signs. In such cases, chest CT scanning is necessary. CT scanning, especially HRCT, can clearly demonstrate miliary lesions of TB, interstitial structure (thickened or twisted lobular septum), emphysema, and old lesions. Therefore, CT scanning, especially HRCT, plays an important role in diagnosis and differential diagnosis of blood disseminating pulmonary TB.

Secondary Pulmonary TB

Secondary pulmonary TB commonly occurs at the posteroapical segment of the upper lung lobe, dorsal segment, and the posterior basal segment of the lower lung lobe. It may also occur at other lung lobe and segments. By chest X-ray, the demonstrations are diversifying, including:

(1) In the cases with slight secondary pulmonary TB, chest X-ray demonstrates mainly patchy, nodular, and cords like opacity. In some other cases, it demonstrates tuberculoma or solitary cavity.
(2) In the cases with serious secondary pulmonary TB, chest X-ray demonstrates multiple cavities, caseous pneumonia, and bronchial disseminating of the lesions.
(3) In the cases with repeated and prolonged progression of the disease, the affected lung may be destructed. Along with shrinkage of the affected lung, there are multiple fibrotic thick-wall cavities, secondary bronchial dilation, or accompanying multiple calcifications. The adjacent hilum and mediastinum are demonstrated to shift due to structural traction. The thorax is collapsed with pleural thickening and adhesion. And the other lung tissues are subject to compensatory emphysema as well as new and old lesions along bronchus.

Plain chest X-ray is the basic diagnostic imaging for the diagnosis of pulmonary TB. For further assessment and differential diagnosis, CT scanning, especially HRCT, should be performed. CT scanning demonstrations of secondary pulmonary TB include:

(1) lobular central, lobular, or lobular fused opacity;
(2) singular or scattering small round nodular opacity, commonly in size of 5–10 mm and located at the middle and lateral part of lungs;
(3) pneumonia-like opacity, commonly with air bronchogram inside;
(4) cavity opacity;
(5) swollen bronchial artery opacity, which is believed to be retention of parabronchial inflammatory secretions induced by complication of bronchial TB. CT scanning demonstrates consecutive thickening opacity from the hilum to the lung field.

Tracheal and Bronchial TB

Chest X-ray demonstrates different signs of tracheal TB from bronchial TB, which is closely related to the lesions at the lungs, pleura, and mediastinum. Chest X-ray demonstrations of tracheal and bronchial TB include:

(1) rapidly changing atelectasis and localized emphysema;
(2) unilaterally or bilaterally repeated bronchial disseminating lesions;

(3) enlarging or shrinking tension cavity or liquid-gas level in the cavity;
(4) no obvious lesion in lungs but the patients present with obvious stimulating cough or sputum smear test positive to acid-fast bacillus;
(5) multiple bronchial lesions, with narrowed, twisted, or deformed bronchial lumen but no obvious surrounding soft tissue mass opacity.

CT scanning demonstrations of tracheal and bronchial TB include:

(1) lesions commonly located at the upper, middle, and lingual lobes of both lungs;
(2) extensive lesions at the affected bronchus, with lesions disseminating along the bronchus;
(3) bronchial stenosis and obstruction as well as thickening of the bronchial wall;
(4) lesions in the atelectasis lung;
(5) low-intensity calcification at the bronchial wall or the bronchial intima;
(6) clear demonstrations of the bronchial lumen by virtual endoscopy, which are similar to demonstrations by fibrobronchoscopy.

Tuberculous Pleurisy

In patients with dry pleurisy and exudative pleurisy, if pleural effusion is less than 300 mL, posterior–anterior chest X-ray may demonstrate no abnormality. If pleural effusion is above 500 mL, the posterior–anterior chest X-ray demonstrates blunt costophrenic angle. At this time, a changed posture can be adopted for chest X-ray. If pleural effusion is in a moderate volume, posterior–anterior chest X-ray demonstrates exteriorly high and interiorly low homogeneous arch-shaped opacity with increased density in the inferior thoracic cavity and covered diaphragmatic opacity. If pleural effusion is in a large volume, the mediastinum is demonstrated with shift towards the healthy lung, and the lung field of the affected lung is demonstrated with evenly dense opacity with covered diaphragmatic opacity. In the cases with slow absorption of pleural effusion, tuberculous pleurisy is commonly complicated by pleural thickening and adhesion. And the condition may progress into pleural tuberculoma and pyothorax, which are demonstrated by chest X-ray as irregular dense opacity, encapsulated pleural effusion, pleural thickening and adhesion, shrinkage of the affected side of thorax, narrowed intercostal space, and shift of mediastinum.

The advantages of chest CT scanning include:

(1) CT scanning can detect pleural effusion in a small quantity of 150 mL.
(2) Chest CT scanning can demonstrate pleural changes, intrapulmonary lesions covered by thickened pleura, and atelectasis lung tissue compressed by pleural effusion regardless of the overlappings.
(3) Tuberculous pyothorax is commonly demonstrated as round or crescent-shaped liquid agglomeration, separation of visceral and parietal layers of pleura, and typical pleural thickening and pleural calcification of different degrees.

Assessment of the Lesions Activity

In the clinical practice, based on understandings about characteristic signs of different types of pulmonary TB, the lesions activity should be further assessed based on diagnostic imaging.

CT scanning demonstrations of active TB include:

(1) Patchy, flakes, or ground glass opacities with poorly defined boundary;
(2) Nodular opacity and small nodular micro-nodular opacity;
(3) Cavity opacity (except the purified cavity with no morphological change in long-term follow-ups);
(4) Lesions disseminating along bronchus;
(5) Thickened lobular septum and liquid bronchogram.

CT scanning demonstrations of non-active TB include:

(1) Calcification opacity;
(2) Singular or several localized fiber cords opacities with well-defined boundaries;
(3) Callosity lesions;
(4) Regular follow-ups for the purified cavity with no morphological change (in clinical practice, the lesions activity can hardly be assessed based on data of once diagnostic imaging and the assessment is commonly performed based on follow-ups.);
(5) Pleural thickening, adhesion, and calcification.

Ultrasonography

Due to strong reflection of air-containing lungs to the ultrasound with interference of thoracic bones, ultrasonography can hardly demonstrate the micro-structure in deep lungs. Therefore, it has been generally believed that ultrasonography is not suitable for the diagnosis of thoracic diseases. However, liquid containing lesions, parenchymal lesions of lungs, or atelectasis of lung in many thoracic diseases constitute an acoustic window when they contact to the thorax. The acoustic window significantly improves the penetration of acoustic beam for harvesting clear ultrasonographic images. Therefore, the application of ultrasonography in the diagnosis of tuberculous pleurisy has been appraised.

The consistence rate of B mode ultrasound in the diagnosis of pleural effusion reaches up to above 98%. B mode ultrasound has the following advantages in the diagnosis of pleural effusion:

(1) A small quantity of pleural effusion, even 10 mL, can be detected.

(2) The location and volume of pleural effusion can be defined.
(3) B-mode ultrasound guided puncture for biopsy and drainage can be performed with accurate and safe localization.
(4) By B-mode ultrasound, qualitative assessment of thoracic opacity can be performed, such as qualitative assessment of pleural thickening, parenchymal mass, free liquid, or encapsulated pleural effusion.

In the cases with pleural effusion, the visceral and parietal layers of pleura are obviously separated and the formed space is demonstrated as no-echo liquid dark area.

(1) Encapsulated pleural effusion

    Ultrasonography demonstrates localized no-echo or extremely weak-echo dark area between the visceral and parietal layers of pleura or between the visceral layers of pleura. The dark area is commonly oval in shape with its medial side protruding towards the lung. The protruding arch is enhanced during inhalation and the both ends of the dark area on the section are sharp angles.

(2) Bloody effusion

    In the liquid dark area, there is a homogeneous light spot.

(3) Purulent effusion

    In the liquid dark area, there are irregular speckles and the unevenly distributed light spots are different in size.

(4) Effusion at the base of lung

    There is obviously widened no-echo area between the base of lung and the diaphragm.

(5) Pneumohydrothorax

    Under strong gas echo, liquid level dark area or speckle like gas echo in the liquid dark area is demonstrated.

(6) Pleural adhesion

    The relative migration between the visceral and parietal layers of pleura is restricted or absent.

(7) Obvious pleural thickening

    A parenchymal dark area with low-echo light spot is demonstrated between the inferior thoracic wall and bright intrapulmonary air reflection. Its fixation with no change indicates organizing.

    Ultrasonography is non-invasive with no radiation effect. The lesions can be dynamically observed via ultrasonography, which has gained wide application in the diagnosis of thoracic and abdominal diseases.

Bacteriological Test

The three sputum specimens for bacteriological test of TB have been recommended by the WHO. The specimens are:

(1) Instant sputum that the patients expectorate after deep breath when they present.
(2) Early morning sputum that the patients expectorate after deep breath immediately when they get up in the morning.
(3) Night sputum that the patients expectorate at the night before the day the sputum specimen is sent for laboratory test.

The qualified sputum specimen should be purulent, caseous, or purulent mucous in volume of 3–5 mL.

The other clinical specimens include pleural effusion, ascites, urine, cerebrospinal fluid, gastric fluid, pus (secretion or fluid collected by drainage following puncture), pathological tissue or caseous mass, stool and throat swab as well as bronchial lavage fluid.

If the condition of patients permits, the above-mentioned specimens can be repeatedly collected for diagnosis and assessment.

The microscopic examination after sputum smear and staining recommended by the diagnostic Standards for Pulmonary Tuberculosis in China (WS288-2017) includes the Ziehl-Neelsen acid-fast staining, fluorescence staining, and microscopic examination. The isolation and culture of Mtb include solid medium culture and liquid medium culture of mycobacteria.

Microscopic Examination After Sputum Smear and Staining

The sputum smear test shows low positive rate, being only 30–50%. And the positive rates of the other specimen smear test are even lower. The sensitivity of the sputum smear test to TB is low, being 10^4–10^5 bacteria per mL.

Clinical significance of the sputum smear test is as follows:

- Sputum smear test for acid-fast bacillus is the recommended laboratory test for screening and diagnosis of TB in the developing countries. It has also been the cheapest technique for the diagnosis of TB that has gained the widest application. Sputum smear test is simple and fast that requires less complicated devices. However, non-specificity and poor sensitivity are its disadvantages in the diagnosis of TB. Acid-fastness is one of the properties of mycobacteria rather than a specific property of mycobacteria tuberculosis (Mtb). Therefore, in the regions with the prevalence of non-Mtb, the diagnosis of TB in some special populations such as patients with HIV/AIDS (susceptible to Mycobacterium avium-intracellular infection) should be differentiated from non-Mtb infection. In the clinical practice, a comprehensive analysis of the patients' condition is necessary. In the well-equipped health care institutions, culture and strain identification of mycobacteria are recommended based on the findings of sputum smear positive. After preliminary screening by sputum smear test, it has been agreed that the patients with sputum smear positive should be quarantined and treated to control the source of infection and stop the spread of Mtb.

Culture and Strain Identification of Mycobacteria

In the clinical practice, the following tests are applied for the culture and strain identification of mycobacteria. And the cultures in clinical practice are as follows.

Solid Medium Culture of Sputum for Mycobacteria

Solid medium culture of sputum for mycobacteria is also known as Lowenstein–Jensen medium culture.

Rapid Culture for Mycobacteria

(1) BACTEC MGIT 960 system for bacterial metabolites as well as the other examination by Bact/ALERT 3D, ESP II, and BACTEC 460 system is applied for rapid culture of mycobacteria.
(2) Direct microscopic observation for drug sensitivity and thin-layer agar culture are applied for rapid culture of mycobacteria.
(3) Color changing liquid medium culture is also applied for rapid culture of mycobacteria.
(4) Other rapid cultures for mycobacteria include liquid medium culture with fresh coconut milk and horse serum as the basic components, and biphasic solid medium culture.

Strain Identification

Identification of Mtb from Mycobacterium bovis as well as identification of Mtb from non-Mtb is performed based on inhibition of their growth by thiophene-2-carboxylic hydrazide (TCH) and p-nitrobenzoic acid (PNB). The final strain identification should be based on typology of their growth properties and biochemical properties, such as thermal catalyst (68 °C) stability, production of nicotinic acid, and reduction of nitrate.

Clinical Significance

Culture and strain identification for mycobacteria is the diagnostic examination of pulmonary TB with the highest specificity. Therefore, pulmonary TB can be definitively diagnosed based on it. Currently, it is believed that detection of Mtb by sputum smear test can define the diagnosis of pulmonary TB, which is the pathogenically defined diagnosis. However, culture and strain identification are more sensitive than the sputum smear test and it can be considered to be the golden standard for the diagnosis of pulmonary TB. But its disadvantages include complicated operational procedures, investments in complicated equipment, and longer period of time consumed in culture. In the clinical practice, we recommend simultaneous anti-tuberculosis medication with culture and strain identification for mycobacteria. After the culture and strain identification, the therapeutic plan is further formulated. Along with the increase of drug-resistant bacteria, drug sensitivity test is recommended to define the diagnosis.

Molecular Biology

PCR is now a common and often indispensable technique based on exponential amplification of a single copy (or more) of a DNA sequence to generate thousands to millions of more copies of that particular DNA segment. The individual steps common to most PCR methods are initialization, denaturation, annealing, and extension/elongation. The detection of Mtb based on PCR includes the following steps: extraction of Mtb DNA, PCR amplification, and detection of the amplified Mtb DNA [5].

PCR technique shows high specificity and sensitivity with simple operational procedures. In a PCR report, negative control negative indicates no contamination of the reaction system and the results are reliable. The negative control shows positive amplification, indicating re-amplification is necessary. The positive control negative indicates failed amplification. In clinical practice, the Mycobacterium tuberculosis complex can be rapidly identified from non-Mtb based on PCR of Mtb DNA and RNA segments. Compared to sputum smear test, it shows high detection rate. And compared to culture, it is more rapid. However, we should know that molecular biology positive only indicates infection of Mtb and thus cannot be basis for its definitive diagnosis. And the definitive diagnosis should be based on comprehensive analysis of the clinical symptoms, diagnostic imaging, and other laboratory tests.

Immunologic Assay

Clinical immunologic assays for the diagnosis of TB are based on disinfection-centered protective immune responses and necrosis-centered pathogenic immune responses.

Cellular Immunologic Assays for the Diagnosis of TB

Tuberculin Skin Test (TST)

Within 4–8 weeks after infection of Mtb, sensitized lymphocytes are produced in the human body. Intracutaneous local injection of Mtb antigen produces allergic reactions at the local skin, such as erythema, callosity, and blisters. Based on these findings, infection of Mtb can be diagnosed.

Seventy-two hours (48–96 h) after inoculation of Mtb antigen at local skin, skin callosity is checked for the diagnosis of Mtb infection. In the cases with no local skin reaction or the average diameter of callosity being less than

5 mm, the tuberculin skin test is considered negative. In the cases with the average diameter of callosity being more than 5 mm or with local double rings, blisters, necrosis, and lymphangitis, the tuberculin skin test is considered positive. The positive reactions are further classified into common positive, moderate positive, and strong positive. In the cases with the average diameter of callosity being more than 5 mm but less than 10 cm, the tuberculin skin test is considered common positive. In the cases with average diameter of callosity being more than 10 mm but less than 15 mm, the tuberculin skin test is considered moderate positive. In the cases with the average diameter of callosity being more than 15 mm, the tuberculin skin test is considered strong positive. In the cases with the average diameter of callosity being less than 15 mm but with double rings, blisters, necrosis, and lymphangitis, the tuberculin skin test is also considered strong positive.

The clinical significance of tuberculin skin test positive is as follows:

(1) With no inoculation of BCG vaccine and no interference of non-Mtb, Mtb infection can be diagnosed for the cases with the diameter of callosity being no less than 5 mm in PPD test.
(2) In the regions with prevailing inoculation of BCG vaccine and non-Mtb, Mtb infection can be diagnosed for the cases with the diameter of callosity being no less than 10 mm in PPD test.
(3) In the regions with prevailing inoculation of BCG vaccine and non-Mtb, the populations of HIV positive and receiving immunosuppressant for above 1 month should be diagnosed with Mtb infection in the cases with the diameter of callosity being no less than 5 mm in PPD test.
(4) Children aged under 5 years with close contacts to sputum smear-positive TB patients should be diagnosed with Mtb infection, if the average diameter of callosity is no less than 5 mm in the PPD test.
(5) The cases with the average diameter of callosity being no less than 15 mm in PPD test or with blisters, necrosis, and lymphangitis should be diagnosed as Mtb strong positive.

Generally, the tuberculin skin test negative indicates no Mtb infection or failed inoculation of BCG vaccine. However, the following PPD test false negative should be excluded in the diagnosis of Mtb infection:

(1) Expired tuberculin reagent;
(2) Operational errors in the tuberculin skin test;
(3) Prophase of allergic responses (within 4–8 weeks after infection of Mtb, sensitized lymphocytes are produced in the human body. Before the production of sensitized lymphocytes, TST test shows negative.);
(4) Compromised immunity or interfered immune responses in populations of patients with HIV/AIDS, neoplasms, sarcoidosis, serious TB, or acute infectious diseases (such as pertussis, measles, and diphtheria), the elderly, and the patients with malnutrition.

Interferon γ Release Assays (IGRAs)

The antigen used in IGRAs is the encoded protein of Mtb RD1 and RD16 instead of antigen expressed by BCG strain. Such antigen is capable of stimulating mononuclear cells in the peripheral blood to produce interferon γ. And the IGRAs commonly consumes about 12–18 h.

IGRAs show high specificity and sensitivity that consume a shorter period of time. And the patients no longer present repeatedly. In addition, Chinese people are commonly inoculated with BCG vaccine, which does not impact on the specificity and sensitivity of IGRAs. By application of IGRAs, BCG vaccination can be easily differentiated from Mtb infection. But the cost of IGRAs is high, which limits its wide application in China. It remains controversial between the CDC of the USA and the WHO about substitution of TST by IGRAs [6].

Humoral Immunologic Assays for the Diagnosis of TB

The humoral immunologic assays for the diagnosis of TB include antibody detection, antigen detection, and circulating immune complex detection. And the specimens for the immunologic assays include serum, plasma, whole blood, cerebrospinal fluid, pleural effusion, ascites, sputum, and bronchial lavage fluid.

Antibody Detection for TB

The commonly applied immunologic assays for antibody detection of TB include enzyme-linked immunosorbent assay (ELISA), dot immunochromatographic assay (DICA), dot immunofiltration assay (DIFA), protein chip, and immunoblot assay.

The patients with active TB show hyperactive humoral immune response, with elevated Mtb antibody (mainly IgG) in the serum and other body fluids. Along with anti-tuberculosis treatment, the Mtb antibody in the serum gradually decreases. The cured patients from Mtb infection and the patients with non-Mtb infection may show positive in the antibody detection of TB. However, the patients with serious TB, blood disseminating pulmonary TB, and systemic weakness may show negative in the antibody detection of TB. In addition, the antibody detection of TB plays an important role in the diagnosis of TB in postoperative patients after organ transplantation. Therefore, the diagnosis of TB based on antibody detection should be in combination of clinical manifestations.

Antigen Detection for TB

The commonly applied immunologic assays for antigen detection of TB include latex particle agglutination test (LPA), double-sandwich ELISA, dot immunochromatographic assay (DICA), and dot immunofiltration assay (DIFA).

After infection of Mtb, antigen of TB is firstly produced. And the detected antigen of TB is the direct evidence supporting the existence of Mtb, which avoids the false negative in cellular and humoral immunologic assays due to inactive immune response. Therefore, detection of antigen-specific to Mtb is valuable in early diagnosis of TB. A study has demonstrated that the sensitivity of antigen detection for TB in the cerebrospinal fluid is up to 79–100% and its specificity is 95–100%.

Detection of Circulating Immune Complex (CIC)

There are many techniques for detection of CIC. The commonly applied techniques include polyethylene glycol precipitation, ELISA, and solid phase of Clq. The detection of Mtb specific CIC is superior to detection of the antibody against Mtb in the diagnosis of active TB. However, the detection of Mtb specific antigen is superior to detection of Mtb specific CIC in the diagnosis of active TB.

In patients with active TB, the immune complexes of specific IgG obviously increase, which decrease along with improved condition. Therefore, the detection of Mtb specific CIC in the body fluids is significant in the diagnosis of active TB. In some patients with active TB, the bacteriological sputum test shows positive but serum antibody detection for Mtb shows negative due to persistent existence of Mtb or its antigen. The persistently existing Mtb or its antigen specifically binds to the produced Mtb antibody to form Mtb specific CIC.

Fibrobronchoscopy

By using fibrobronchoscopy, we can directly observe the anatomical structures, openings, lumens and mucosa of trachea, bronchus, lung lobes, lung segments and sub-segments, and even secondary segmental bronchus. And the respiratory secretions and lavage fluid can be aspirated and tissues can be harvested by using fibrobronchoscope for bacteriological, cytological, pathological, and immunological examinations. The electronic fibrobronchoscopy is even equipped with camera. Therefore, fibrobronchoscopy can be applied for data collection and storage as well as dynamic observations.

Fibrobronchoscopy can be applied for the following conditions:

(1) Long-term stimulating cough with no known reason;
(2) The patients with bacteriologically negative TB (for pathological and bacteriological evidence via secretion aspiration, brushing, tissue harvest for biopsy, and bronchial lavage fluid collection);
(3) The patients with hemoptysis or bloody sputum with no known reason;
(4) The patients with hilar mass opacity, atelectasis, or obstructive pneumonia for definitive diagnosis;
(5) The patients with respiratory secretions and foreign bodies for their elimination;
(6) The patients with tracheal lesions for treatment.

It has been reported that the Mtb positive rates of fibrobronchoscopic brushing for smear and culture are 27% and 53%, respectively, in the bacteriologically negative TB patients. And the Mtb positive rates of lavage fluid smear and culture are 20.9% and 44.3%, respectively. Due to fibrobronchoscopic irritation, the sputum tests in the consecutive 3 days after fibrobronchoscopy show increased detection rates, with sputum smear-positive rate and culture positive rate of 37% and 55.7%, respectively. By fibrobronchoscopy, the reason and source of hemoptysis can be defined.

Under a fibrobronchoscope, bronchial TB is demonstrated as follows:

(1) Slight or moderate mucosa congestion is common in patients excreting Mtb. In the cases with serious Mtb infection, mucosa edema can be observed with no luster. The cartilage rings are poorly defined or absent.
(2) In the cases of bronchial intima TB, the bronchial intima shows no luster but has erosion and ulceration. On the surface of bronchial intima, there may be caseous substances or thick moss like secretions. The mucosa and submucosal layer around the ulcerations are subject to congestion and edema, which may further progress into mucosal hypertrophy and necrosis.
(3) The tuberculous stenosis and contraction are concentric, with smooth mucosa and obvious cicatricial stenosis in funnel shape or with occlusion of bronchial opening. Commonly no infiltrations or neoplasm can be observed. Changes due to compression to lumens are rare.
(4) In the cases of bronchial lymph node fistula, there are congestion and edema around the fistular orifice at the acute stage. The old fistular orifice is demonstrated as brownish small pit.
(5) In the cases of TB, there are black patches on the bronchial intima.

Thoracoscopy and Other Endoscopic Examinations

Thoracoscopy is invasive. Therefore, its application should be strictly indicated although serious complication is rare. Clinically, thoracoscopy is classified into diagnostic and therapeutic.

Diagnostic thoracoscopy is performed to observe or harvest tissue for biopsy. It is indicated to the following conditions:

pleural effusion with no known reason, pleural mass with no known reason, diffuse lung lesions, marginal lung lesions, hemothorax, pneumothorax, diaphragmatic lesions, mediastinal lesions, and pericardial disease.

The other endoscopic examinations include mediastinoscopy and ultrasonography via esophagoscopy. By using mediastinoscopy and ultrasonography via esophagoscopy, the mediastinal structures, mediastinal masses, and enlarged lymph nodes can be directly or indirectly observed. In addition, pathological and bacteriological diagnosis can be made based on fine needle aspiration or direct biopsy.

Biopsy of Tissues from Pleura and Lungs

Based on all above examination, if the diagnosis cannot be defined, pathological examinations following the harvest of tissues from the pleura or lung can define the diagnosis. The biopsies include biopsy following intracutaneous fine needle aspiration, biopsy of lung tissue via fibrobronchoscopy, biopsy of pleura tissue via thoracoscopy, biopsy of lung tissue via thoracoscopy, biopsy of pleura, and lung tissue following laparotomy. In addition, tissues from superficial enlarged lymph nodes can also be harvested for biopsy to obtain indirect evidence for the diagnosis.

Pathology

Infection of Mtb induces cellular immune responses and type IV allergic responses, showing 3 types of basic but characteristic pathological changes.

Exudative Lesion

Exudative lesion occurs at the early stage of Mtb infection. Otherwise, it occurs in patients with compromised immunity and infection of Mtb in a large quantity with strong toxicity. It manifests as serous inflammation or serous cellulitis. And it is pathologically characterized by main components of serous fluid and fibrin as well as cellular components of lymphocytes and macrophages. Based on the detection of Mtb in the exudative lesions, the diagnosis of TB can be defined.

Proliferative Lesion

Proliferative lesion commonly occurs at the middle and advanced stages of Mtb infection. Otherwise, it occurs in patients with competent immunity, infection of Mtb in a small quantity with weak toxicity, and chronically progressing condition. The proliferative lesion mainly manifests as the formation of granuloma with cellular components of epithelioid cells and multinucleated giant cells. It had been believed that the finding of tubercular nodus, especially those with central caseous necrosis, is the basis for the diagnosis of TB. But nowadays, it is believed that the definitive diagnosis should be based on additional finding of Mtb in the lesion.

Degenerative Lesion

In the patients with compromised immunity or strong allergic responses and infection of Mtb in a large quantity with strong toxicity, the exudative lesions and proliferative lesions are subject to pathological changes that are predominantly necrosis. Under a microscope, the tubercular necrotic lesion is red stained structureless particles. By the observation of naked eyes, it resembles to cheese, which is therefore known as caseous necrosis. There may be calcification in the caseous necrosis and Mtb may be detected. Caseous necrosis is of importance in the diagnosis of TB. But the definitive diagnosis should be based on the pathogenic evidence.

The above three pathological changes are commonly concurrent with one as predominant and they are interchangeable. Although the pathological changes of TB are characteristic, it has been believed that the definitive diagnosis should be based on finding of pathogenic bacteria in the range with lesions. When Mtb is not detected by acid-fast staining, PCR should be applied to detect the DNA of Mtb.

1.5 Diagnostic Treatment

The diagnosis of bacteriologically negative TB and TB with no pathological evidence should be discussed and defined by collaborative efforts of radiologists and clinicians. For those bacteriologically negative patients whose diagnosis cannot be defined by consultations and those patients who refuse to receive invasive investigations, if indicated, diagnostic anti-infection treatment and diagnostic anti-tuberculosis treatment are recommended. Close follow-ups should be performed during diagnostic treatment to observe any changes of symptoms. Based on the observation of radiological indices after diagnostic treatment, the diagnosis can be defined in combination to the clinical manifestations and auxiliary investigations.

Diagnostic Anti-inflammation Treatment

For the cases with diagnostic imaging inconsistent to the typical demonstrations of pulmonary TB and nonexclusive pneumonia, diagnostic anti-inflammation treatment is recommended for about 2 weeks based on the condition and other indices. The anti-inflammatory drugs with anti-tuberculosis efficacy should be avoided, such as quinolones and aminoglycosides.

Diagnostic Anti-tuberculosis Treatment

For the patients whose diagnosis still cannot exclude active TB after anti-inflammation treatment, other investigations should be performed to define the diagnosis. If the patients refuse the further investigations or the hospital is poorly equipped to perform the investigations, diagnostic anti-tuberculosis treatment can be administered with informed consent from the patients or their family members. The following points should be paid close attention during the diagnostic anti-tuberculosis treatment.

Therapeutic Plan for Initially Treated Patients at the Intensive Stage of Active TB

The therapeutic plan for initially treated patients at the intensive stage of active TB is recommended for diagnostic anti-tuberculosis treatment. And the therapeutic course is commonly 1–2 months. During the diagnostic anti-tuberculosis treatment, the patients should be closely observed. If the condition permits, relative investigations should be performed to define the diagnosis.

No Improvement After Diagnostic Anti-tuberculosis Treatment

After receiving the anti-tuberculosis treatment for 3–4 weeks, if the patients remain pyrexial, secondary infection, drug fever, or infection of drug-resistant Mtb should be suspected for differentiation. In addition, extrapulmonary TB, such as cerebral TB and mesenteric lymph node TB, should be suspected for differentiation.

Deterioration

During the diagnostic anti-tuberculosis treatment, if the condition progresses or deteriorates, the following points should be paid close attention:

(1) Herxheimer-liked reaction
    When receiving chemical treatment with highly efficient bacteriocide containing isoniazid or rifampicin, some patients may present new infiltrative lesion or enlarged primary lesion, pleural effusion, and/or more and enlarged superficial/hilar mediastinal lymph nodes. In some cases, even meningitis, more or enlarged cerebral tuberculoma and pericarditis occurs.
(2) Diagnostic error or concurrence with other diseases
    During the diagnostic anti-tuberculosis treatment, if the condition progresses or deteriorates, there may be diagnostic error. Otherwise, TB may be concurrent with other diseases.
(3) Infection of other pathogenic bacteria during treatment
    During the diagnostic anti-tuberculosis treatment, if the condition progresses or deteriorates, the patients may suffer from infection of other pathogenic bacteria during the treatment.
(4) Unreasonable therapeutic protocol
    During the diagnostic anti-tuberculosis treatment, if the condition progresses or deteriorates, the patients may receive an unreasonable therapeutic protocol.
(5) Infection of non-Mtb or drug-resistant Mtb
    During the diagnostic anti-tuberculosis treatment, if the condition progresses or deteriorates, the patients may suffer from infection of non-Mtb or drug-resistant Mtb. If the condition permits, the diagnosis should be firstly defined. If the condition does not permit, diagnostic anti-tuberculosis treatment should be administered.

1.6 Non-reactive TB

Non-reactive TB is a serious type of TB, which is rarely encountered in the clinical practice. It commonly occurs in patients with seriously compromised immunity, especially cellular immunity. Clinically, it is characterized by extensively distributed lesions possibly involving all tissues and organs in human body, acute onset with chills, high fever, accompanying multiple pains of headache, chest pain, abdominal pain and bone pain as well as hepatomegaly, splenomegaly, and systemic lymphadenectasis. However, PPD skin test commonly shows negative. Therefore, the condition is known as non-reactive TB. Chest X-ray demonstrates non-reactive TB as hilar mediastinal lymphadenectasis, pleural effusion, late or atypical demonstrations of blood disseminating pulmonary TB in lungs. Pathologically, it is characterized by a large quantity of caseous miliary lesions or multiple abscess necrosis. Under a microscope, the necrotic lesions are demonstrated with a large quantity of acid-fast bacilli but less or absent characteristic proliferative inflammation (epithelioid nodule and tuberculous granuloma). There are less or no epithelioid cells, Langhans giant cells, and lymphocytes around the lesion. Its early diagnosis is challenging. And the condition progresses rapidly with high mortality rate. The definitive diagnosis is commonly made based on autopsy.

Generally speaking, the diagnosis of TB is mainly based on the clinical symptoms, chest X-ray, and sputum test for Mtb. For the cases with bacteriologically negative in the sputum test, all the above investigations including biopsy are necessary to define the diagnosis. During the diagnosis of TB, differential diagnosis is also necessary to exclude the possibility of other diseases with similar symptoms and demonstrations [7, 8].

1.7 Differential Diagnosis

For the Cases with Secondary Pulmonary TB and Infiltrative Lesion, the Disease Should be Differentiated from the Following Conditions

Bacterial Pneumonia

The patients commonly present with cough and expectoration of purulent sputum with accompanying chills, fever, and chest irritation. Physical examination demonstrates moist rales and/or signs of parenchymal changes of lung. Routine blood test commonly shows increased percentages of white blood cells and neutrophils. The symptoms can be rapidly alleviated by symptomatic anti-infection therapy. Diagnostic imaging demonstrates rapid absorption of the lesions.

Fungal Pneumonia

The patients commonly suffer from basic disease, immune disorder, or receiving medications of antibiotics and immunosuppressants for a long period of time. Laboratory G test and GM test show positive. The sputum specimen from deep inside respiratory tract with no contamination shows positive to fungal culture. And anti-fungal therapy is effective.

Pulmonary Parasitosis

The patients have a history of contacts in the disease affected region. Laboratory test shows elevated serum specific antibody. In other cases, parasite eggs can be detected in specimens of sputum or pleural effusion for diagnosis.

Pulmonary Tuberculoma Should be Differentiated from the Following Conditions

Lung Carcinoma

The patients commonly report a history of smoking or a family history of neoplasm, especially men aged above 40 years. Clinically, it manifests as chronic progressive stimulating cough with accompanying chest pain. Diagnostic imaging demonstrates lesions with spikes and lobulations but no satellite lesions. Neoplasm cells detected by cytology of sputum exfoliative cells or evidence from biopsy for pathological examination are the basis for definitive diagnosis.

Inflammatory Pseudotumor

Inflammatory pseudotumor is benign lesion of lung whose pathogenesis remains elusive. Most of the patients report a history of lung infection. Diagnostic imaging demonstrates round or oval-shaped lesion with smooth and sharp margin. Shrinkage of the lesion can be detected after anti-infection treatment.

Pulmonary Hamartoma

Pulmonary hamartoma is commonly a benign neoplasm that is caused by abnormal embryonic development of lung tissue. Diagnostic imaging demonstrates solitary round or oval-shaped lesion at peripheral lung with well-defined boundary and typical popcorn liked calcification. Nowadays, it has been agreed that it should be surgically removed at its early stage.

Pulmonary Sequestration

Pulmonary sequestration is a hereditary disease whose intrapulmonary cystic mass is composed of lung tissues supplied by abnormal systemic circulation. In the cases with no accompanying secondary infection, it is commonly asymptomatic. It commonly occurs at the basilar posterior segment of lower lung lobe. Diagnostic imaging demonstrates opacity with well-defined boundary but uneven density, possibly with lobulation and cystic dilation. The diagnosis can be defined based on arterial angiography. And if CT scanning demonstrates entry of abnormally supplying artery into the lesion of pulmonary sequestration, the diagnosis can also be defined.

Blood Disseminating Pulmonary TB Should Be Differentiated from the Following Conditions

Alveolar Cell Carcinoma

The patients present with cough, expectoration, chest distress, chest pain, shortness of breath, and hemoptysis. However, the patients present with no obvious tuberculosis poisoning symptoms. Diagnostic imaging demonstrates multiple infiltrative nodules at middle and lower lung fields of both lungs, which are different in size with uneven distribution. The diagnosis can be defined based on cytology of sputum exfoliative cells and pathological biopsy.

Pulmonary Hemosiderosis

Pulmonary hemosiderosis is the condition that the deposition of hemosiderin in the pulmonary interstitium due to pulmonary capillary bleeding causes pulmonary fibrosis. The patients commonly present with repeated cough, hemoptysis, and iron deficiency anemia. At its early stage, diagnostic imaging demonstrates extensive cloud like opacity that is different in size with uneven density. The opacity may partially fuse. After its repeated onset, diagnostic imaging demonstrates evenly distributed miliary opacity or network like opacity with fine dot at the middle and medial parts of lung fields. The sputum test shows hemosiderin particles in the macrophages, which facilitates the diagnosis. The diagnosis can be defined based on pathological biopsy.

Diffuse Interstitial Lung Disease

The manifestations of diffuse interstitial lung disease are pulmonary parenchymal diffusion and alveolar inflammation as well as interstitial fibrosis. The patients commonly present with progressive dyspnea. In the cases with a long history of illness, accompanying hypoxemia may occur. Diagnostic imaging demonstrates intrapulmonary diffuse opacity or nodular interstitial opacity, which are more common at the middle and lower lung fields as well as the medial and middle parts of lung. The diagnosis should be based on comprehensive analysis of clinical manifestations, imaging demonstrations, pulmonary ventilation, diffusion, and pathological biopsy.

Bronchial Lymph Node TB Should Be Differentiated from the Following Diseases

Lung Carcinoma

The patients commonly report a history of smoking or a family history of neoplasm, especially men aged above 40 years. Clinically, it manifests as stimulating dry cough, hemoptysis, and chest pain, commonly with no tuberculosis poisoning symptoms. Diagnostic imaging demonstrates lesions with spikes and lobulations but no satellite lesions. Neoplasm cells detected by cytology of sputum exfoliative cells or evidence from pathological biopsy are the basis for definitive diagnosis.

Lymphoma

Lymphoma is a malignancy originated from lymphoid hematopoietic system. The clinical manifestations include painless lymphadenectasis, which may involve all the tissues and organs in human body. Diagnostic imaging demonstrates unilateral or bilateral hilar lymphadenectasis. The definitive diagnosis is based on pathological biopsy of lymph nodes or involved tissues and organs.

Sarcoidosis

Sarcoidosis is a systemic non-caseous necrotic granulomatous disease with no known reason, which commonly invades lung tissue or possibly multiple organs. Diagnostic imaging demonstrates bilaterally symmetric hilar and/or mediastinal lymphadenectasis with or without intrapulmonary grid-like, nodular or flakes of opacity. The hormone therapy shows therapeutic efficacy. The diagnosis should be based on clinical symptoms and signs as well as pathological biopsy and exclusion of the other granulomatous diseases.

Pulmonary Tuberculous Cavity Should Be Differentiated from the Following Diseases

Lung Cancerous Cavity

The lung cancerous cavities are polymorphous, but commonly eccentric cavities with irregular wall and no surrounding satellite lesion. The outer wall of cavity is lobulated, commonly with short spikes. The intima of the cavity is irregular or has nodular protrusions. The vascular vessels around the cavity are rigid and thickened. And the diagnosis can be defined based on pathological evidence.

Pulmonary Cyst

Pulmonary cyst is a condition that there are gas filling or liquid and gas filling cysts of different sizes in lung caused by congenital aplasia or acquired infection of lung tissue. Diagnostic imaging demonstrates cystic lesions with smooth margin and even density but no satellite lesions. In the cases of secondary infection, there may be liquid level in the cavity. In the cases of no secondary infection, the patients are commonly asymptomatic. The lesions show no obvious change in the long-term follow-ups.

Cystic Bronchiectasis

Cystic bronchiectasis is essentially bronchiectasis, which is clinically characterized by long-term repeated chronic cough and expectoration. Diagnostic imaging demonstrates lesions commonly at the middle and lower lung fields of both lungs. The diagnosis can be made based on demonstrations of thin layer CT scanning and case history.

Tuberculous Pleurisy Should Be Differentiated from Pleural Transudate, Cancerous Effusion, and Parapneumonic Pleural Effusion

Pleural Exudate and Transudate

Pleural effusion can be further classified into pleural exudates and pleural transudates. The exudates are from diseases that invade the pleura, cause the vascular permeability to increase, or cause the pleural lymphatic return to decrease. The pleural transudates are caused by disorders of intrathoracic hydrostatic pressure and colloid osmotic pressure in normal pleural system. Tuberculous pleural effusion is actually pleural exudates. And its differentiation from transudates is based on serum lactic dehydrogenase (LDH) level and total protein level in the pleural fluid (PF) by light standards. If the indices reach one or more than one standards, the pleural fluid may be exudates:

(1) Ratio of protein in PF to serum protein is above 0.5.
(2) Ratio of LDH in PF to serum LDH is above 0.5.
(3) LDH in PF is higher than two-thirds of the upper limit in the normal range of serum LDH.

Tuberculous Pleural Effusion Should Be Differentiated from the Following Conditions

Cancerous Pleural Effusion

The patients commonly present with progressively deteriorating dyspnea, persistent chest pain, and stimulating dry cough. Otherwise, the patients present with corresponding clinical manifestations of primary lesions, possibly with accompanying cachexia. The pleural effusion is commonly a large quantity of bloody effusion. The diagnosis can be defined based on cytology of effusion and pathological biopsy of pleura. Biochemical investigations are recommended if necessary.

Parapneumonic Pleural Effusion

Parapneumonic pleural effusion is intrapulmonary infection and accompanying pleural effusion. Clinically, the patients present with symptoms and signs of corresponding intrapulmonary infection. The effusion can be rapidly absorbed after effective anti-infection treatment. The diagnosis of complex parapneumonic pleural effusion should be based on biochemical analysis and bacteriological culture [9].

Differentiation of Pulmonary TB from Non-Mtb-Induced Pneumonosis

The clinical symptoms and signs of non-Mtb-induced pneumonosis are similar to those of pulmonary TB. However, the patients with non-Mtb-induced pneumonosis commonly suffer from basic diseases, such as silicosis, bronchiectasis, and pulmonary TB, and/or compromised immunity, such as HIV/AIDS and those receiving long-term treatment of immunosuppressant. Diagnostic imaging demonstrates inflammation lesion and singular/multiple thin-wall cavities that commonly involve the anterior and apical segments of upper lung lobes, but the spherical nodular lesion, fibrous callosity, and pleural exudates are comparatively rare.

Pulmonary TB should be differentiated from non-Mtb-induced pneumonosis based on the following points.

Etiology

Based on acid-fast staining positive in the sputum smear test, Mtb infection and non-Mtb infection cannot be differentiated. The bacterial strain identification following bacteria culture should be performed for differentiation.

Pathology

The histopathological changes of Mtb infection and non-Mtb infection are similar. However, histologically, non-Mtb infection is more commonly demonstrated with epithelioid granuloma, no obvious caseous necrosis, and commonly glass like collagen fibrous hyperplasia.

Clinical Therapeutic Efficacy

Non-Mtb infection cannot be improved by anti-tuberculosis treatment due to drug resistance to anti-tuberculosis drugs by most non-Mtb. So far, there are no effective chemical treatment and standardized protocol for non-Mtb infection of lung. Therefore, combined use of anti-tuberculosis drugs with other antibiotics is recommended for the treatment of non-Mtb infection of lung. The combination of 3–5 drugs is appropriate. Generally, after negative conversion of acid-fast bacilli in the cases of non-Mtb infection, the treatment needs to be continued for 18–24 months or at least 12 months, which is obviously different from treatment for TB.

1.8 Ways of Recording

Incubated Infection of TB

The sequence of recording: diagnosis, investigations, and the reports of the ordered investigations. For the PPD test, the values from measurement should be recorded as follows: transverse diameter (mm) × diameter (mm). And findings of blisters and double rings should be recorded. For the interferon γ release assay, the values should be recorded. For example, a patient with incubated infection of TB, PPD test 15 × 18 mm, and double rings.

Active TB

Active Pulmonary TB

The sequence of recording: the type of pulmonary TB, location, results of bacteriological test, drug sensitivity test to anti-tuberculosis drugs, and history of treatment

Example 1: acute blood disseminating pulmonary TB, both lungs, smear (−), culture (−), initially treated.

Example 2: secondary pulmonary TB, bilateral upper and middle lungs, smear (−), culture (+), isoniazid resistant, re-treated.

Active Extrapulmonary TB

The sequence of recording: location of extrapulmonary TB, bacteriological test (specimen specified), drug sensitivity test to anti-tuberculosis drugs, history of treatment.

Example 3: Tuberculous meningitis, CSF smear (−), culture (+), sensitive, initially treated.

Example 4: TB at the left hip joint, joint fluid smear (−), culture (−), initially treated.

Non-active TB

The sequence of recording: location of TB lesion, demonstrations of diagnostic imaging.

Example 5: non-active TB, right upper lung, calcification (solitary)

2 Treatment and Prevention

TB is a common disease with high incidence that seriously threatens human health. And most of the cases are pulmonary TB.

In the fight against TB, the therapies for TB and its preventive measure have been explored to reduce, control, and finally end it. The whole-course DOTS and the whole-course management under the five principles of early, regular, whole-course, appropriate dose, and combined medication are keys in successful treatment of TB.

According to *the Standard for Classification of Tuberculosis in China* (WS196-2017), TB is classified into latent infection of Mtb, active TB (including pulmonary TB and extrapulmonary TB), and non-active TB (including non-active extrapulmonary TB and non-active pulmonary TB).

Patients with active pulmonary TB are the main source of infection. The progression of active pulmonary TB decreases the life quality of the patients and increases the social burden. Therefore, the patients with active pulmonary TB are the key population for TB control. In some cases, the latent infection of Mtb develops into active pulmonary TB. And it is necessary for some patients with latent infection of Mtb to receive prophylactic anti-tuberculosis treatment.

Anti-tuberculosis treatment is mainly a standardized chemical treatment. But due to complex complications of TB, simple chemical treatment can hardly achieve favorable outcome. Therefore, in the clinical practice, collapse therapy, surgical treatment, interventional therapy, immunotherapy, nutritional support, and traditional Chinese medicine have been tried to treat TB. In addition, individualized therapeutic protocol has also been tried for more favorable therapeutic outcomes.

2.1 Principles of the Chemical Treatment for Active Pulmonary TB

TB is a serious pulmonary infectious disease that seriously threatens human health and life security. According to the Law of P. R. China on the Control of Infectious Diseases, pulmonary TB is categorized into class B infectious disease. And the DOTS strategy is focused on detecting and curing patients with sputum smear positive for acid-fast bacilli and/or culture positive for mycobacteria, especially the initially treated patients with sputum smear positive. The detection and treatment of such patients are intended to control the source of infection and stop the spread of TB. And the key for successful chemical treatment of active pulmonary TB is the management of the patients with TB. The patients should receive standardized DOTS or at least DOTS during the intensive stage of active TB.

The principles of chemical treatment for pulmonary TB are early treatment, appropriate dosage, regular treatment, combined medication, and whole-course treatment. The whole therapeutic protocol is composed of two stages, namely the intensive stage treatment and the continuation stage treatment. The formulation of the principles is based on the following underlying mechanisms of pulmonary TB:

Early treatment:

(1) In the early stage of pulmonary TB, there is a large quantity of Mtb in the lesion. At this stage, their metabolism and production is active and they are sensitive to anti-tuberculosis drugs. The combined medication should be administered at this stage to rapidly kill the Mtb.
(2) In the early stage of pulmonary TB, the alveolar wall is subject to congestion and edema. And there are infiltration and exudation of inflammatory cells. In and around the lesion, the lung tissue is well supplied with favorable permeability of the drugs. And an effective blood concentration of drugs can be reached for absorption of the lesion.
(3) In the early stage of pulmonary TB, the responsive hyperplasia of macrophages is active. And the proliferating and active macrophages can engulf the Mtb, which plays a collaborative role with the anti-tuberculosis drugs for favorable tissue repair and recovery.

Based on the above three points, the chemical treatment for pulmonary TB should be administered as early as possible.

Regular Treatment

Regular intake of anti-tuberculosis drugs can keep the blood concentration of drugs relatively stable to kill Mtb. Irregular intake of drugs makes the blood concentration of drugs unstable. At a low blood concentration, Mtb cannot be killed and inactivated. Contrarily, drug resistance by Mtb can be induced to negatively impact on the recent therapeutic efficacy and to cause relapse of the disease. The drug resistance by Mtb causes the treatment more challenging. Studies have demonstrated that patients receiving whole-course regular medication show a cure rate of 96%. And if the regular medication reduces by 10%, the cure rate decreases to 40%. Therefore, regular standardized medication is the key for successful treatment of TB and for prevention of secondary drug resistance by Mtb.

Whole Course

After 2–3 weeks medication of anti-tuberculosis drugs, most of the sensitive Mtb are killed and the symptoms are correspondingly improved. However, Mtb non-sensitive to drugs, intracellular Mtb, and persistently existing Mtb are still alive. Only persistent medication can finally kill all of the pathogenic Mtb to prevent relapse of the disease. Therefore, whole-course medication guarantees favorable therapeutic efficacy.

Appropriate Dosage

Patients with pulmonary TB are generally weak or suffer from concurrent diseases. In formulating the therapeutic protocol, appropriate dosage of anti-tuberculosis drugs should be administered. Insufficient dosage may cause failed treatment or induce drug resistance of Mtb, while overdose induces more adverse reactions that the patients cannot tolerate. Therefore, appropriate dosage of anti-tuberculosis should be administered based on the age, body weight, and reference table for dosage of anti-tuberculosis drugs.

Combined Medication

In the lesions of TB, there are different metabolic flora of Mtb, which show different sensitivity to anti-tuberculosis drugs. The combined medication is the combined use of different drugs with different mechanisms of killing Mtb. Based on the combined medication, therefore, different metabolic flora of Mtb can be killed and inactivated to prevent drug resistance and improve the therapeutic efficacy. In addition, naturally drug-resistant Mtb may exist, and the combined medication can kill the correspondingly sensitive Mtb via cross bactericidal action. The reproduction of drug-resistant Mtb is thus restricted and occurrence of secondary drug-resistant TB is avoided. In currently formulated therapeutic protocol of combined medication, the anti-tuberculosis drugs play collaborative roles to improve the therapeutic efficacy.

Based on the drug resistance, active pulmonary TB can be classified into non-drug-resistant pulmonary TB and drug-resistant pulmonary TB. Different types of TB should be treated by different therapeutic protocols.

Standardized Regular Chemical Treatment

Dosage and Medication Route of Commonly Applied First-Line Anti-tuberculosis Drugs

Isoniazid Tablet

(1) Route of administration

Isoniazid tablet should be taken orally, once a day recommended. For the cases with serious condition, isoniazid injection is recommended to substitute tablets.

(2) Dosage

For adults, daily oral intake in a dose of 5 mg/kg body weight should be administered and the total daily dose should not exceed 0.3 g. For the patients with serious condition, obesity or blood disseminating pulmonary TB, the dose can be appropriately increased. Based on the weekly 2–3 times oral intake, the daily dose should be 15 mg/kg body weight and the maximal daily dose should be within 0.9 g.

For children, daily oral intake in a dose of 10–20 mg/kg body weight should be administered and the total daily dose should not exceed 0.3 g. For the patients with serious condition, obesity, blood disseminating pulmonary TB, or tubercular meningitis, the dose can be appropriately increased. The daily dose can reach as high as 30 mg/kg body weight and the total daily dose should not exceed 0.5 g.

(3) Contraindications

Isoniazid is contraindicated to patients with serious abnormal liver functions, epilepsy, and psychiatric disorders.

Rifampicin Capsule

(1) Route of administration

Rifampicin capsule should be taken orally, once a day before meal recommended. For the patients with serious condition, rifampicin injection should be administered instead of capsule.

(2) Dosage

For adults, the daily dosage should be 0.45–0.6 g and the total daily dosage should not exceed 1.2 g. For the patients receiving 2–3 times oral intake a week, the daily dosage should be 0.6 g and the total daily dosage should not exceed 1.2 g. For the patients who are elderly or with weak condition, the daily dosage should be 10 g/kg body weight and the total daily dosage should not exceed 0.6 g.

For children, rifampicin should be orally intake every day. And the daily dosage should be 10–20 mg/kg body weight and the total daily dosage should not exceed 0.6 g.

(3) Contraindication

Rifampicin is contraindicated to the patients who are allergic to it or who are allergic to rifomycins, patients with serious liver function insufficiency, patients with biliary obstruction, and women within 3 months pregnancy.

Rifapentine Capsules

(1) Route of administration

Rifapentine capsule should be taken orally, once a day before meal recommended.

(2) Dosage

For adults, oral intake of 1–2 times a week and 0.6 g for each time should be administered. For the patients with a body weight of less than 55 kg, the dosage should be appropriately decreased.

(3) Contraindication

Rifapentine is contraindicated to the patients who are allergic to it or allergic to rifomycins, the patients with serious liver function insufficiency, biliary obstruction, or women within 3 months pregnancy.

Pyrazinamide Tablet

(1) Route of administration

Pyrazinamide tablet should be taken orally, once a day recommended.

(2) Dosage

For adults, daily oral intake of 15–30 mg/kg body weight should be administered, and the total daily dosage should not exceed 2 g. Weekly oral intake for three times can also be administered with daily dosage of 50–70 mg/kg body weight and a total daily dosage not exceeding 3 g. Weekly oral intake of two times is another way of administration with a daily dosage of 50–70 mg/kg body weight and a total daily dosage not exceeding 4 g.

(3) Contraindication

No experiment so far has been conducted for its contraindications and there is no reference for it.

Ethambutol Hydrochloride Tablet or Capsule

(1) Route of administration

Ethambutol hydrochloride tablet or capsule should be orally taken, once a day recommended.

(2) Dosage

For adults, the daily intake should be administered with 15 mg/kg body weight and the total daily dosage should be within 0.75–1.0 g. For weekly oral intake of three times, the daily dosage should be 20–30 mg/kg body weight and the total daily dosage should not exceed 2.5 g. For weekly oral intake of two times, the daily dosage should be 50 mg/kg body weight and the total daily dosage should not exceed 1.5 g. For re-treated patients with serious pulmonary TB at the intensive stage, the dosage should be based on 25 mg/kg body weight and the total daily dosage should not exceed 1.5 g.

The children aged under 13 years, ethambutol hydrochloride tablet or capsule should be avoided. And for children aged above 13 years, the route of administration and the dosage should refer to those of adults.

(3) Contraindication

No experiment so far has been conducted for its contraindications and there is no reference for it.

Streptomycin Injection

(1) Route of administration

Streptomycin injection should be administered via intramuscular injection.

(2) Dosage

Streptomycin injection can be injected twice a day, with injection of 0.5 g every 12 h. Otherwise, streptomycin injection can be injected once a day, with injection of 0.75 g. For the elderly patients, daily injection for once is recommended in a dose of 0.5–0.75 g. Interval injection can also be administered for 2–3 times a week in a dose of 1 g each time.

(3) Contraindication

Streptomycin injection is contraindicated to the patients who are allergic to it or allergic to aminoglycosides. Skin test is recommended before administration, when the batch is changed or after retrieval of the medication for more than 48–72 h. Only the patients with skin test negative can receive the medication [10].

Ethamidoprazine and Rifampicin Tablet

(1) Route of administration

Ethamidoprazine and rifampicin tablet should be taken orally, once a day recommended.

(2) Dosage

A tablet of the high dose ethamidoprazine and rifampicin tablet contains 150 mg rifampicin, 75 mg isoniazid, 400 mg pyrazinamide, and 275 mg ethambutol hydrochloride. The patients with a body weight of 30–37 kg should once oral intake of two tablets a day. The patients with a body weight of 38–54 kg should oral intake once of three tablets a day. The patients with a body weight of 55–70 kg should oral intake once of four tablets a day. The patients with a body weight of above 71 kg should oral intake once of five tablets a day. And the patients with a body weight of under 30 kg, ethamidoprazine and rifampicin tablet is not recommended.

A tablet of the low dose ethamidoprazine and rifampicin tablet contains 75 mg rifampicin, 37.5 mg isoniazid, 200 mg pyrazinamide, and 137.5 mg ethambutol hydrochloride. The patients with a body weight of 30–37 kg should oral intake once of four tablets a day. The patients with a body weight of 38–54 kg should oral intake once of six tablets a day. The patients with a body weight of 55–70 kg should oral intake once of eight tablets a day. And the patients with a body weight of above 71 kg should oral intake once of ten tablets a day. Medication of ethamidoprazine and rifampicin tablet for the patients with a body weight of under 30 kg is not recommended.

(3) Contraindication

Medication of the tablet is not recommended to the patients who are allergic to any component or pharmaceutical adjuvant of the tablet. The tablet is contraindicated to the patients with serious liver function insufficiency, serious kidney function insufficiency, biliary obstruction, women within 3 months pregnancy, epilepsy, psychiatric disorders, gout, diabetes complicated by fundus change, or porphyria. And it should not be combined use with protease inhibitor and voriconazole.

Rifampicin and Isoniazid Tablet

(1) Route of administration

Rifampicin and isoniazid tablet should be taken orally and once a day is recommended.

(2) Dosage

A tablet of rifampicin and isoniazid tablet contains 300 mg rifampicin and 150 mg isoniazid. The patients with a body weight of above 50 kg should oral intake once of two tablets a day. The patients with a body weight of under 50 kg should take appropriately decreased dose of rifampicin and isoniazid tablet or take the tablets of bulk package.

(3) Contraindication

The tablet is contraindicated to the patients who are allergic to it, women within 3 months pregnancy, with serious liver function insufficiency, biliary obstruction, epilepsy, or psychiatric disorders.

Chemical Treatment Protocol for Initially Treated Patients with Secondary Pulmonary TB

The chemical treatment protocol is recommended for the initially treated patients with bacteriologically positive or negative TB plus any one of the following conditions:

(1) The patient has never received anti-tuberculosis drugs for treatment of TB;
(2) The patient ever received anti-tuberculosis drugs for treatment of TB but the treatment was not regular and lasted for less than 1 month;
(3) The patient is receiving initial regular anti-tuberculosis drugs for treatment of TB but the therapeutic course has not been completed.

The recommended chemical treatment protocol is as follows:

2FDC-HRZE/4FDC-HR

During the intensive stage of TB, combined use of 4 drugs is administered for 2 months. And during the intensive stage of TB, the ethamidoprazine and rifampicin tablets are administered for oral intake once a day that lasts for 60 days.

During the continuation stage of TB, combined use of two drugs is administered for 4 months. And during the continuation stage of TB, rifampin and isoniazid capsule is administered for once a day that lasts for 120 days.

2HRZE/4HR

During the intensive stage of TB, combined use of 4 drugs, isoniazid, rifampicin, pyrazinamide, and ethambutol, is administered for 2 months. The drugs should be taken orally once a day that lasts for 60 days.

During the continuation stage of TB, combined use of two drugs, isoniazid and rifampicin, is administered. The drugs should be taken orally once a day that lasts for 120 days.

$2H_3R_3Z_3E_3/4H_3R_3$

During the intensive stage of TB, combined use of four drugs, isoniazid, rifampicin, pyrazinamide, and ethambutol, is administered for 2 months. The drugs should be taken orally once every other day, or three times a week which is rarely applied, for 30 times of intake within 60 days.

During the continuation stage of TB, combined use of two drugs, isoniazid and rifampicin, is administered. The drugs should be taken orally once every other day, or three times a week which is rarely applied, for 60 times of intake within 120 days.

3FDC-HRZE/4FDC-HR or 3HRZE/4HR or $3H_3R_3Z_3E_3/4H_3R_3$

During the standardized anti-tuberculosis treatment, if the initially treated patients with bacteriologically positive TB show acid-fast bacilli positive in the sputum smear test after 2 months treatment, the present treatment protocol is applied.

Notes:

(1) For convenient medication and favorable compliance of medication, FDC complex preparations are recommended.
(2) When the management of DOT strategy cannot be well implemented, interval therapy should be possibly avoided to reduce the chances of multidrug resistance.
(3) Administration of ethambutol in children should be avoided.
(4) For the patients with a history of close contacts to TB, strain identification and drug sensitivity tests are recommended for correct selection of drugs. If the patients report a definitive history of contacts to the patients with DR-TB, the drug sensitivity test of the infection source (patients with DR-TB) should be referred to and the treatment protocol of DR-TB should be applied.
(5) In the initially treated patients with bacteriologically negative TB, any bacteriologically positive during the treatment indicates failed treatment. In the initially treated patients with bacteriologically positive TB, any bacteriologically positive after 5 months standardized treatment indicates failed initial treatment. For the patients with failed initial treatment, sputum culture and drug sensitivity test should be supplemented. The treatment protocol should be formulated based on the drug sensitivity test. If the strain identification and drug sensitivity test show non-drug-resistant Mtb, the treatment protocol for re-treated patients should be adopted.

Chemical Treatment Protocol for Re-treated Patients with Secondary Pulmonary TB

The chemical treatment protocol for re-treated patients with secondary pulmonary TB should be administered to re-treated patients with bacteriologically positive or negative TB plus one of the following conditions:

(1) The patients received anti-tuberculosis treatment for TB, but the treatment was irregular or the therapeutic course lasted for at least 1 month.
(2) The patients never received anti-tuberculosis medication for TB.

(3) The initial treatment failed and DR-TB has been excluded.
(4) The patients suffer from relapse of TB and DR-TB has been excluded.

2FDC-HRZES/6FDC-HRE

During the intensive stage of TB, combined use of five drugs is administered for 2 months and complex preparation of ethamidoprazine and rifampicin tablets should be administered orally once a day during the intensive stage of TB. Intramuscular injection of streptomycin should simultaneously be administered once a day for 60 days.

During the continuation stage of TB, combined use of three drugs is administered for 6 months. Rifampin and isoniazid capsules and ethambutol tablets or capsules are administered once a day for 180 days.

3FDC-HRZE/6FDC-HRE

During the intensive stage of TB, combined use of four drugs is administered for 3 months. The complex preparation of ethamidoprazine and rifampicin tablets is administered once a day for 90 days.

During the continuation stage of TB, combined use of three drugs is administered for 6 months. Rifampin and isoniazid capsules and ethambutol tablets or capsules are administered once a day for 180 days.

2HRZES/6HRE

During the intensive stage of TB, combined use of five drugs, isoniazid, rifampicin, pyrazinamide, and ethambutol, is administered for 2 months. The drugs should be taken orally once a day. Meanwhile, intramuscular injection of streptomycin should simultaneously be administered once a day for 60 days.

During the continuation stage of TB, combined use of 3 drugs, isoniazid, rifampicin, and ethambutol, is administered once a day for 180 days.

3HRZE/6HRE

During the intensive stage of TB, combined use of four drugs, isoniazid, rifampicin, pyrazinamide, and ethambutol, is administered for 3 months. The drugs should be taken orally once a day for 180 days.

During the continuation stage of TB, combined use of three drugs, isoniazid, rifampicin, and ethambutol, is administered once a day for 180 days.

$2H_3R_3Z_3E_3S_3/6H_3R_3E_3$

During the intensive stage of TB, combined use of five drugs is administered. Oral intake of isoniazid, rifampicin, pyrazinamide, and ethambutol is administered every other day. Meanwhile, intramuscular injection of streptomycin should simultaneously be administered once every other day for 60 days.

During the continuation stage of TB, combined use of three drugs, isoniazid, rifampicin, and ethambutol, is administered once every other day for 180 days.

$3H_3R_3Z_3E_3/6H_3R_3E_3$

During the intensive stage of TB, combined use of four drugs is administered. Oral intake of isoniazid, rifampicin, pyrazinamide, and ethambutol is administered every other day for 90 days.

During the continuation stage of TB, combined use of three drugs, isoniazid, rifampicin, and ethambutol, is administered once every other day for 180 days.

Notes:

(1) For the re-treated patients with smear-positive TB, if sputum smear test still shows positive to acid-fast bacilli after 2 months treatment, the treatment for the intensive stage of TB should be prolonged for 1 month and the treatment for the continuation stage of TB should remain the same. The correspondingly changed treatment protocol is as follows: 3FDC-HRZES/6FDC-HRE, 4FDC-HRZE/6FCD-HRE, 3HRZES/6HRE, 4HRZE/6HRE, $3H_3R_3Z_3E_3S_3/6H_3R_3E_3$, and $4H_3R_3Z_3E_3/6H_3R_3E_3$.
(2) For the re-treated patients receiving regular treatment, bacteriological positive after 5 months treatment or after the completion of therapeutic course indicates failed re-treatment.
(3) Before re-treatment of any reason, sputum culture for mycobacteria, strain identification, and drug sensitivity tests should be performed before the re-treatment to define DR-TB and the infected strain. Based on these tests, a reasonable treatment protocol can be formulated. For the patients with no drug resistance, sufficient dosage of medication should be administered.
(4) For the re-treated patients with bacteriologically negative TB, the diagnosis should be cautiously made.

Recommended Chemical Treatment for Tuberculous Pleurisy (Interpretation of the Protocol Should Refer to the Above Texts)

(1) 2FDC-HRZE/10FDC-HRE
(2) 2HRZE/10HRE
(3) $2H_3R_3Z_3E_3/10H_3R_3E_3$

Note: Due to different degrees of tuberculous pleurisy, the therapeutic course can be accordingly shortened or prolonged. But the whole therapeutic course should be at least 9 months.

Tracheal and Bronchial TB

(1) 2FDC-HRZE/10FDC-HRE
(2) 2HRZE/10HRE

(3) $2H_3R_3Z_3E_3/10H_3R_3E_3$

Note: At the intensive stage of TB, medication should be administered along with aerosol treatment or interventional fibrobronchoscopy. The therapeutic course can be appropriately prolonged according to the condition of the patients. The drug for aerosol inhalation is recommended to be one of the administered anti-tuberculosis drugs.

Primary Pulmonary TB

For adult patients with primary pulmonary TB, the treatment protocol should refer to that of secondary pulmonary TB, but individualized treatment protocol is recommended based on the specific condition of the patients.

For pediatric patients with primary pulmonary TB, the medication of ethambutol should be extracted from the treatment protocol. And a reasonable treatment protocol should be formulated based on the specific condition of the patients.

Blood Disseminating Pulmonary TB

The condition of blood disseminating pulmonary TB is complex and the pathogenic bacteria tends to invade extra-pulmonary tissues and organs. Overall investigations are recommended before treatment. The condition of the patients should be well understood for individualized treatment protocol. Within the range of safe medication dosage, the maximal dosage is recommended.

Treatment Interrupted or Returned to Patients (Tables 4.1 and 4.2)

Table 4.1 Diagnosis and treatment of initial active TB patients

Treatment duration	Interruption duration	Need sputum smear test	Sputum smear test result	Regimen
Unlimited	<2 week	No	No	Continue with original regimen
<1 month	2–8 week	No	No	Start initial treatment
>1 month	2–8 week	Yes	Smear negative	Continue with original regimen
1–2 month	2–8 week	Yes	Smear positive	Add 1-month intensive phase to original regimen
>2 month	2–8 week	Yes	Smear positive	Start smear-positive re-treatment regimen

Table 4.2 Diagnosis and treatment of re-treatment TB patients

Treatment duration	Interruption duration	Need sputum smear test	Sputum smear test result	Regimen
Unlimited	<2 week	No	No	Continue with re-treatment regimen and finish the intensive phase
<1 month	2–8 week	No	No	Continue with re-treatment regimen and finish the intensive phase
>1 month	2–8 week	Yes	Smear negative	Add 1-month intensive phase to original regimen
1–2 month	2–8 week	Yes	Smear positive	Reformulate the re-treatment regimen
>2 month	2–8 week	Yes	Smear positive	Reformulate the re-treatment regimen

Corticosteroid Therapy

Treatment of TB with corticosteroid therapy has remained controversial. The mechanism of the therapy for TB is as follows:

(1) Its anti-inflammatory effects;
(2) Its immunosuppressive effects;
(3) Its anti-toxic effects;
(4) Its anti-shock effects;
(5) Its anti-fibrotic effects;
(6) Favorable bactericidal effects due to its stimulation on metabolism of Mtb.

The indications of corticosteroid therapy are as follows:

(1) Blood disseminating pulmonary TB;
(2) Tuberculous polyserositis;
(3) Caseous pneumonia;
(4) Tuberculous allergy syndrome;
(5) Tuberculosis complicated by intractable hemoptysis;
(6) Tuberculosis complicated by pulmonary heart disease, respiratory failure, and/or pulmonary encephalopathy.
(7) Serious allergic reactions induced by anti-tuberculosis drugs;
(8) Tuberculosis and other diseases that should be treated by corticosteroid.

In treating TB, corticosteroid therapy has no absolute contraindications. And the following conditions are the relative contraindications of corticosteroid therapy in the treatment of TB:

(1) Tuberculosis complicated by active peptic ulceration and postoperation of intestinal anastomosis;

(2) Pulmonary TB complicated by serious hypertension, atherosclerosis, and/or heart failure;
(3) TB of pregnancy;
(4) Diabetes complicated by TB;
(5) HIV/AIDS complicated by TB;
(6) Psychiatric disorders.

In the clinical practice, the mechanisms, indications, and contraindications of corticosteroid therapy should be well understood by the clinicians. And flexible administrations of corticosteroid therapy according to the condition of the patients are recommended. However, corticosteroid therapy may induce multiple complications. Without concurrent medication of sensitive and effective anti-tuberculosis drugs, corticosteroid therapy may deteriorate the condition or induce other overlapping conditions with TB. Therefore, the administration of corticosteroid therapy should not exceed 1 month.

2.2 Prophylactic anti-tuberculosis treatment

Populations that Should Receive Prophylactic Anti-tuberculosis Treatment

According to the guideline for the management of patients with latent infection of Mtb by the WHO and the clinical experience for TB control in China, the populations that should receive prophylactic anti-tuberculosis treatment include: (1) patients with HIV/AIDS, (2) children aged under 5 years who have a history of close contacts to patients with active pulmonary TB; and (3) primary and secondary school students who have a history of close contacts to patients with active pulmonary TB.

Mechanisms of Prophylactic Anti-tuberculosis Treatment

(1) The administration of one or multiple anti-tuberculosis drugs can reduce the quantity of infected Mtb in human body and thus reduce the chance of its pathogenicity.
(2) During the prophylactic anti-tuberculosis treatment, new cases of Mtb infection can be effectively avoided.

Procedures of Prophylactic Anti-tuberculosis Treatment

The prophylactic anti-tuberculosis treatment is for populations with latent infection of Mtb. Therefore, the populations that should receive prophylactic anti-tuberculosis treatment should be appropriately selected. And after exclusion of populations who are contraindicated, the therapeutic protocol is formulated.

Selection of Populations that Should Receive Prophylactic Anti-tuberculosis Treatment

Currently, the following populations should receive prophylactic anti-tuberculosis treatment after exclusion of patients with active pulmonary TB.

Children Aged 1–5 Years Who have a History of Close Contact to Patients with Sputum Smear-Positive TB

(1) Screening of suspected symptoms of TB

The symptoms of cough and expectoration for above 2 weeks, bloody sputum, or hemoptysis are suspected symptoms of pulmonary TB. In children with pulmonary TB, the development may be delayed. The children aged 1–5 years who have a history of close contact to patients with sputum smear-positive TB but show negative in the screening of suspected symptoms should receive prophylactic anti-tuberculosis treatment.

(2) Tuberculin test and other investigations for TB

The individuals showing positive in the screening of suspected symptoms should receive sputum tuberculin test and other investigations for TB, such as sputum test for Mtb and chest X-ray. If active pulmonary TB is excluded, prophylactic anti-tuberculosis treatment should be administered.

Primary and Secondary School Students with Tuberculin Test Strong Positive

(1) Screening of suspected symptoms of TB

The primary and secondary school students who have a history of close contact to patients with sputum smear-positive TB but show negative in the screening of suspected symptoms should receive prophylactic anti-tuberculosis treatment.

(2) Investigations for TB

The individuals showing positive in the screening of suspected symptoms should receive sputum tuberculin test and chest X-ray. If active pulmonary TB is excluded, prophylactic anti-tuberculosis treatment should be administered.

Patients with HIV/AIDS

(1) Screening of suspected symptoms of TB

In the follow-ups for or newly detected patients with HIV/AIDS, suspected symptoms of TB should be screened with questionnaires or necessary physical examinations for TB should be performed.

(2) Investigations for TB

In the follow-ups for or newly detected patients with HIV/AIDS, the sputum tuberculin test and chest X-ray for TB should be performed at least once a year. If active pulmonary TB is excluded, prophylactic anti-tuberculosis treatment should be administered.

Populations Contraindicated to Anti-tuberculosis Drugs

Populations that should receive prophylactic anti-tuberculosis treatment should be assessed before medication.

Case History

The population that should receive prophylactic anti-tuberculosis treatment should be asked in detail about their past history, medication history, allergy history, history of contact to patients with TB, and history of contact to patients with drug-resistant TB.

Investigations

Routine blood test, liver function test, and kidney function test should be performed to exclude contraindications to anti-tuberculosis drugs.

Selection of Anti-tuberculosis Drugs

Based on the results of investigations and case history, appropriate anti-tuberculosis drugs should be selected for prophylactic anti-tuberculosis treatment.

Individuals Inappropriate for Prophylactic Anti-tuberculosis Treatment

Individuals with one of the following conditions should not receive the prophylactic anti-tuberculosis treatment.

(1) Patients who are receiving treatment for active viral hepatitis or with accompanying hyperlipidemia (abnormal liver function);
(2) Individuals with allergic constitution or individuals in allergic period;
(3) Patients with epilepsy or psychiatric disorder or patients who are receiving anti-psychiatric drugs;
(4) Patients with deficiencies of platelets ($<50 \times 10^9$/L) and/or leukocytes ($<3000 \times 10^9$/L);
(5) Patients with known poor compliance before medication;
(6) Patients with PPD test strongly positive and have finished therapeutic course of anti-tuberculosis treatment for TB within past 3 years.

Treatment Protocol

Isoniazid

For adults, 300 mg/day for 6–9 months is recommended for prophylactic anti-tuberculosis treatment.

For children, 10–15 mg/kg body weight per day for 6–9 months is recommended and the total daily dosage should not exceed 300 mg.

Isoniazid Plus Rifampicin

For adults, 300 mg isoniazid per day and 450–600 mg rifampicin per day for 3 months are recommended for prophylactic anti-tuberculosis treatment.

For children, isoniazid of 10–15 mg/kg body weight per day and rifampicin of 10 mg/kg body weight per day for 3 months are recommended for prophylactic anti-tuberculosis treatment. The total daily dosage of isoniazid should not exceed 300 mg and the total daily dosage of rifampicin should not exceed 450 mg.

Notes:

(1) The protocol is indicated to high-risk populations of any age group.
(2) The protocol is indicated to individuals with or possibly with a history of close contact to patients with isoniazid or rifampicin resistant TB.

Isoniazid Plus Rifapentine

For adults with a body weight above 50 kg, isoniazid of 600 mg each time and twice per week is recommended for prophylactic anti-tuberculosis treatment. And for adults with a body weight less than 50 kg, isoniazid of 500 mg each time and twice a week is recommended. For children, isoniazid of less than 300 mg each time (10–15 mg/kg body weight) and twice a week is recommended.

For adults with a body weight above 50 kg, rifapentine of 600 mg each time and twice a week with isoniazid is recommended for prophylactic anti-tuberculosis treatment. And for adults with a body weight less than 50 kg, rifapentine of 450 mg each time and twice a week with isoniazid is recommended. For children aged above 5 years, rifapentine of 10–20 mg/kg body weight each time that less than 450 mg each time and twice a week with isoniazid is recommended. The therapeutic course is 3 months.

Note: The protocol is mainly for adults because there is no recommendation on the dosage of rifapentine for children. And the above recommended dosage can be referred to in the clinical practice.

Others

A study has demonstrated that administration of isoniazid and rifapentine once a week for 12 times (3 months) has the same effect as the above protocol, which still needs more evidence supporting its application.

2.3 Collapse Treatment

The currently applied collapse treatments for TB include artificial pneumoperitoneum (APP), artificial pneumothorax, and thoracic cavity tamponade. And its indications should be well known by clinical physicians for treatment of TB.

The indications of artificial pneumoperitoneum include:

(1) Extensive lesions in unilateral or bilateral lungs and/or cavity or suspected cavity, sputum bacteriologically positive, unconditional drug sensitivity test, and no improvement after 3 months treatment;

(2) Extensive lesions in unilateral or bilateral lungs and/or cavity or suspected cavity, persistent Mtb positive in the sputum test, and resistance to anti-tuberculosis drugs;
(3) Pulmonary TB complicated by massive hemoptysis, and failed hemostasis by other treatments;
(4) Re-treated patients with cavity or suspected cavity in unilateral or bilateral lungs;
(5) Cavity in the lower lung lobe that is predicted to be incurable by anti-tuberculosis drugs.

Artificial pneumothorax is indicated for the following conditions:

(1) TB lesions at unilateral upper lung and/or cavity or suspected cavity, sputum Mtb positive, unconditional drug sensitivity test, and no improvement after 3 months treatment;
(2) TB lesions at unilateral upper lung and/or cavity or suspected cavity, sputum Mtb positive, and resistance to anti-tuberculosis drugs;
(3) TB lesions at unilateral upper lung that is complicated by massive hemoptysis and failed hemostasis by other treatments;
(4) Re-treated patients with cavity or suspected cavity at unilateral upper lung.

Thoracic cavity tamponade for TB is indicated for the following patients:

(1) Patients with chronic fibro-cavitary pulmonary TB whose cavity is located at the apex or upper part of lung and the range with lesions not exceeding the 6th or the 7th posterior rib;
(2) Patients with pulmonary TB and repeated hemoptysis that is ineffectively treated by internal medicine and may induce suffocation and death.
(3) Patients with drug-resistant pulmonary TB who have lung function insufficiency, poor systemic condition and intolerance to surgeries, artificial pneumoperitoneum, and artificial pneumothorax.

2.4 Surgical Treatment for Pulmonary TB

Currently, it has been believed that patients with pulmonary TB should firstly receive chemical treatment. And surgical treatment is an alternative to the necessary chemical treatment for pulmonary TB. Surgical treatment for pulmonary TB is indicated to the following conditions:

(1) No improvement by standardized chemical treatment;
(2) Disclosure of cavity in initially treated and re-treated patients after standardized treatment protocols for 9–12 months, and persistent or intermittent bacteriologically positive in the sputum test, especially the patients with DR-TB;
(3) Lung destruction of one lobe or one lung;
(4) Cavity and secondary aspergilloma;
(5) Thick-wall cavity that resistant to multiple anti-tuberculosis drugs;
(6) Pulmonary TB complicated by pyothorax and/or pneumothorax;
(7) Tuberculous pyothorax;
(8) Bronchial pleural fistula;
(9) Tuberculoma;
(10) Localized large caseous lesion;
(11) Repeated infection or repeated intractable hemoptysis induced by tuberculous bronchiectasis;
(12) Bronchiostenosis induced by endobronchial TB.

The surgical treatment is contraindicated to the following conditions:

(1) Poor systemic condition or cardiopulmonary compensatory dysfunction that the patients are intolerant to the surgery;
(2) Acute progression of TB or emergence of new infiltrative lesion at other body parts during treatment;
(3) The elderly patients who should receive function tests of major organs before the surgery to predict their tolerance to the surgery;
(4) Poor pulmonary compensatory function predicted before the surgery;
(5) Complication of extrapulmonary TB and its deterioration despite of systemic anti-tuberculosis treatment.

According to different conditions of the patients, the adoptable surgical approaches include: segmentectomy, lobectomy, total pneumonectomy, wedge-shaped excision of lung, video-assisted thoracoscopic surgery, and mediastinoscopy. In addition, pleura dissection for tuberculous pyothorax, thoracic reconstruction, pleuropulmonary resection, and muscle flap filling with vascular pedicle can also be performed.

2.5 Interventional Treatment

Currently, the commonly applied interventional treatments include fibrobronchoscopic intervention, percutaneous lung puncture for drug injection, and implant of tracheal stent.

Fibrobronchoscopic Intervention

The anti-tuberculosis drugs can be directly administered into the lesion of bronchial TB via fibrobronchoscopy. Otherwise, the anti-tuberculosis drugs can be directly injected into the cavity of pulmonary TB via guidance of fibrobronchoscopy.

Based on the fibrobronchoscopy assisted approach, pulmonary TB and bronchial TB can be treated. Local administration of anti-tuberculosis drugs via fibrobronchoscope has been widely applied in the clinical practice. However, the following points should be paid close attention during its application:

(1) Based on the systemic condition of the patients, reasonable therapeutic plan should be formulated for systemic treatment. Local injection of anti-tuberculosis drugs via fibrobronchoscopy only plays adjuvant role. The combination of systemic treatment and fibrobronchoscope guided injection should be applied for better therapeutic efficacy.
(2) Fibrobronchoscopic intervention shows unfavorable therapeutic efficacy for multiple cavities, fibrous thick-wall cavity, and lung destruction. In the clinical practice, its indications should be well known by the clinicians for its application.
(3) For patients with poor systemic condition or new cases of hemoptysis and severe cough, fibrobronchoscopic intervention should be avoided.
(4) Close attention should be paid on sterile operation to avoid or reduce the chances of infections.

Percutaneous Lung Puncture for Drug Injection

Percutaneous lung puncture for drug injection is commonly applied for patients with cavitary pulmonary TB. It has been believed that the approach facilitates local hyperplasia of granulation tissue and promotes purification of the cavity.

Percutaneous lung puncture for drug injection is guided by chest X-ray or CT scan. The effective anti-tuberculosis drugs, commonly isoniazid and amikacin, are injected into the cavity to directly kill the Mtb in the cavity. In addition, repeated puncture can weaken the barrier of cavity wall and the drug can also erode the cavity wall, both of which promote to soften the caseous lesion. The necrosis tissue thus sheds off and is discharged.

The precautions of percutaneous lung puncture for drug injection include the following:

- The patients should try to hold their breath during drug injection. To prevent severe cough during drug injection, a small quantity of lidocaine (0.5–1 ml) can be firstly injected into the cavity. And drug injection should be performed after the puncture needle is confirmed in the cavity. After drug injection, the filling of drug in the cavity should be confirmed. And the patients should be closely observed for occurrence of pneumothorax.

Implant of Tracheal Stent

Implantation of tracheal stent is mainly applied for tuberculous bronchiostenosis. Based on the staging and grading of tracheal and bronchial stenosis as well as the systemic condition of the patients, microwave therapy, laser therapy, cryotherapy, high-frequency electric surgical knife, balloon dilation, and implantation of airway stent can be selected. When implantation of tracheal stent is chosen, the following points should be paid close attention.

Time for Implantation

Implantation of tracheal stent is applicable for soft tuber wall type of bronchial TB and cicatricial stage of endotracheal TB during which dyspnea may be induced by tracheal stenosis. During the early stage of bronchial TB such as the ulceration and necrosis stage and proliferation stage, stenosis may relapse after implantation of tracheal stent. Therefore, implantation of tracheal stent is not applicable for early stage bronchial TB.

Condition of the Trachea

(1) For patients with tracheal stenosis with accompanying major bronchial stenosis or bilateral major bronchial stenosis, implantation of tracheal stent may induce local congestion, edema, bleeding, and obstruction of trachea by necrotic tissues that may further cause suffocation. Therefore, implantation of tracheal stent should be cautious for such patients and corresponding preventive measures should be formulated.
(2) Intact distal bronchial lumen of the stenotic area is the pre-condition of tracheal stent implantation.

Notes: Tracheal hemostasis via bronchoscope should be performed if strictly indicated. Especially when the approach is selected via fibrobronchoscope or electronic bronchoscope, rapid suction of blood may fail to cause suffocation in patients with large quantity of hemoptysis. Therefore, bronchial arterial embolism, suction of blood via tracheal intubation, or rigid bronchoscopic intervention should be appropriately selected based on the general condition of the patients.

2.6 Immunotherapy

Currently, it is believed that the occurrence of pulmonary TB is closely related to the immunity of organisms. Clinically, application of immunosuppressants in the treatment of pulmonary TB has achieved success, especially in patients with compromised immunity. The commonly applied immunosuppressants are as follows.

Cytokines

The cytokines in the immunotherapy for pulmonary TB include IL-2, IL-12, INF-γ, INF-α, TNF-α inhibitor, rhu-GM-CSF, and TGF-β.

Biologicals and Other Immunosuppressants

The biological and other immunosuppressants include Mycobacterium vaccae vaccine, Mycobacterium phlei vaccine, BCG-polysaccharide nucleic acid, transfer factor, thymic peptide, and thymopentin.

Anti-tuberculosis Vaccines

The anti-tuberculosis vaccines include DNA vaccine, subunit vaccine, and recombinant BCG vaccine.

Immunotherapy is indicated to TB with accompanying compromised immunity, serious pulmonary TB, extensive drug-resistant TB, multidrug-resistant TB, non-reactive TB, and TB with accompanying immunodeficiency. Vaccines are capable for enhancing the immune responses of organisms. At the different pathophysiological stages, the same vaccine may aggravate the pathological lesions and induce immunologically protective responses. Therefore, the time for immunotherapy should be appropriately chosen. The combination of standardized chemical treatment and appropriate anti-tuberculosis vaccination can enhance the immunity of the patients, which, in response, inhibits the reactivation of Mtb and improves the therapeutic efficacy.

However, it has been believed that the treatment of TB should be predominantly based on chemical treatment, and immunotherapy plays only an adjuvant role.

2.7 Nutritional Support

TB is an infectious disease that is related to malnutrition. TB commonly occurs in the malnutritional population after infection of Mtb. And the patients with TB show further deteriorating malnutrition. After infection of Mtb by health populations, multiple factors contribute to the onset of TB. The important factors include immunity of the infected population as well as the quantity and toxicity of infected Mtb. Currently, it has been believed that in population with competent immunity and infection of a small quantity of weakly toxic Mtb, the infected Mtb remains in a state of dormancy and the infection is latent. Otherwise, the infection of Mtb induces occurrence and progression of TB. And the immunity is largely related to the nutritional state of the hosts.

About 90% patients with TB suffer from malnutrition. The pyrexial response after infection of Mtb may induce gastrointestinal dysfunction, poor appetite, decreased intake of nutrients, glucose metabolism disorder, increased catabolism, and decreased anabolism. Therefore, the adipose deposits in human body decrease and the loss of protein increases. The patients with pulmonary TB are characterized by consumption and body weight loss.

Pulmonary TB is a chronic disease, with prolonged illness course. The longer its illness course is, the worse the nutritional state of the patients is, especially seriously ill patients and the re-treated patients with pulmonary TB. On the contrary, the patients with malnutrition show low level of protein, which further weakens the capability of self-repair. And the lesion progresses and the illness course is prolonged. Based on the mechanism, it is recommended that the protein level and the cellular immunity of the patients should be monitored in the clinical practice. The therapeutic plan should be appropriate and nutritional support should be enhanced for the patients.

Currently, during the anti-tuberculosis treatment, diet of four highs is recommended for the patients. The four highs include high calorie, high protein, high vitamins, and high dietary fiber with water. And the key point is supplementation of high calorie and high protein.

High Calorie

Pulmonary TB is a chronic consuming disease and the patients consume more calorie than healthy population. Sufficient supplementation of calorie can reduce the catabolism of the protein and improve the negative nitrogen balance. Nowadays, fat milk and glucose as well as their reasonable composition are recommended for the patients with pulmonary TB. Excessive supplementation of glucose adds burden to the lungs and liver. 30–40 kcal/day/kg body weight with a total daily supplementation of 2000–2400 kcal is recommended for the patients with pulmonary TB. And the daily supplementation of calories for critically ill patients and the patients working in intensive labor should be formulated according to their actual needs.

High Protein

The patients with pulmonary TB show increased catabolism and thus are susceptible to negative nitrogen balance. Therefore, active supplementation of protein, especially branched chain amino acids and the other necessary amino acids, can decrease the breakdown of the protein, which facilitates healing of the lesions. The recommended supplementation of protein is 1.2–1.5 g protein per day per kg body weight with a total daily intake of 80–100 g. And the daily supplementation of protein for critically ill patients and the patients working in intensive labor should be formulated according to their actual needs. High-quality protein is recommended, such as meat, eggs, milk, and aquatic products.

High Vitamins

Supplements of vitamins, calcium, and iron are also necessary for patients with pulmonary TB. Such supplements can improve the appetite of the patients and promote the absorption of nutritional substances. Therefore, their immunity can be improved to promote healing.

High Dietary Fiber and Water

Dietary fiber and water can regulate the intestinal functions to maintain smooth bowel movements and to prevent absorption of toxins. Therefore, the acid-base balance can be maintained. The recommended foods with high dietary fiber and water include fresh vegetables, fruits, and roughly processed grains.

Nutritional support plays a supplementary role in the treatment of TB. For slightly ill patients, reasonable food intake and improved eating habit are recommended to improve the nutritional state of the patients.

2.8 Traditional Chinese Medicine

In Chinese medicine, pulmonary TB is categorized into lung phthisis, which is an infectious chronic consuming disease of lungs due to weak right qi external infection of pathogens. It is characterized by flush, night sweat, fatigue, cough, expectoration, hemoptysis, and gradual emaciation. And the principles of treatment include killing the pathogens and nourishing asthenia. In the *Orthodox Tradition of Medicine* (yī xué zhèng zhuàn), it was proposed that phthisis should be treated by killing the pathogens and nourishing the right qi.

In traditional Chinese medicine, differential pattern of the syndrome is important. And some scholars differentiate it based on its pathological properties of yin, yang, qi, and blood deficits. Some other scholars in traditional Chinese medicine typed it based on the diseased location of lung, spleen, and kidney. And the other scholars in traditional Chinese medicine typed it based on the severity of the disease. Currently, its typing has been based on pathological properties in combination with location.

The commonly applied formulae for TB include:

(1) For patients with lung yin deficit, yin should be nourished, lungs moisturized, and pathogens killed. The recommended formula is Yuehua pills with modifications.
(2) For patients with fire excess from yin deficiency, yin should be nourished and pathogenic fire reduced. The recommended formula is Baihe Gujin decoction and Qinjiu Biejia powder with modifications.
(3) For patients with qi yin consumption, qi and yin should be tonified. And the recommended formula is Baozhen decoction and Shenling Baizhu power with modifications.
(4) For patients with both deficiencies of yin and yang, yin should be nourished and yang tonified. The recommended formula is Butian Dazao pills with modifications.

In treating pulmonary TB, traditional Chinese medicine has limitations. And it should play an adjuvant role in the treatment.

3 Therapeutic Surveillance

Pulmonary TB is a chronic respiratory infectious disease whose treatment lasts for a comparatively long period of time. Different changes may occur during the treatment and the toxic and side effects of anti-tuberculosis drugs are commonly reported. Therefore, the therapeutic surveillance during the treatment is especially important for patients with pulmonary TB. With no effective therapeutic surveillance, the patients may experience irregular medication, deterioration of the condition, persistent or intermittent excretion of Mtb, and many other adverse effects on the patients themselves and the society. The therapeutic surveillance is thus an important procedure to reduce drugs withdrawal, secure the safety of the patients, increase the cure rate, and control the spread of the disease. The therapeutic surveillance of anti-tuberculosis treatment includes the following three aspects: patient surveillance, therapeutic efficacy assessment, and management of the toxic and side effects.

3.1 Patient Surveillance

The patient surveillance mainly includes the record of treatment and the surveillance on the compliance to medication.

Records of Treatment

A complete record on the treatment is a necessary part of therapeutic surveillance and the information about treatment should be recorded throughout the whole process of treatment. The records of treatment include the following:

Case Record

Case record shows various data about the patients, including the diagnosis, treatment, and follow-ups. The basic data includes chief complaint, present history, past history, personal history, marital and delivery history, family history, physical examination, auxiliary investigations (such as diagnostic imaging and laboratory tests), the diagnosis, treatment protocol and medication, treatment course, and summary of treatment.

Data of the Diagnostic Imaging

The data of the diagnostic imaging mainly includes the images harvested from chest X-ray, CT scanning (MRI, PET, and radionuclide for special cases), and B-mode ultrasound.

Various Registry Books

The various registry books include the initial presentation registry book, the laboratory registry book, and other registry books.

Table 4.3 Symptom and sign scale for tuberculosis

Symptoms/sign	Grading criteria and scoring			
	Degree 0 (0 credit)	Degree 1 (1 credit)	Degree 2 (2 credit)	Degree 3 (3 credit)
Cough	No	Intermittent cough during daytime/not affect daily life	Between 1–3 degree	Cough frequently
Cough phlegm	Daily phlegm <20 mL	Daily phlegm at 20–50 mL	Daily phlegm at 50–100 mL	Daily phlegm >100 mL
Hemoptysis	No	Hemoptysis <50 mL each time	Hemoptysis at 50–200 mL each time	Hemoptysis at 200–500 mL or above each time
Chest pain	No	Dull pain, 2–3 times a day	Continuous and severe pain that could affect sleep, >3 times a day	Severe pain that affects routine activity
Dyspnea	No	Dyspnea in rest. When there is increased movement, no need for oxygen absorption	Restless in quiet which can only be improved by intermittent oxygen absorption	In addition to Degree 2, there is cyanosis, pale, cardiac failure, or coma which cannot be alleviated by oxygen absorption
Debilitation	No	Mild	Moderate	Severe
Weight lose	No	Mild	Moderate	Severe
Fever	No	<38 °C	38–40 °C	>40 °C

Electronic Information System

The electronic information system includes the data from the electronic DOTS system and APP-based video-assisted DOTS system.

Surveillance on the Compliance of Patients

The treatment of pulmonary TB lasts for a long period of time with many difficulties. Currently, DOT is recommended by the WHO for favorable compliance of the patients due to its effectiveness and flexibility. If the patients cannot get to the place for directly observed treatment, sending the anti-tuberculosis drugs to the patients' home for directly observed treatment, DOT via electronic on-line system, and APP-based video-assisted DOT can be the alternatives for directly observed treatment.

3.2 Therapeutic Efficacy Assessment

The therapeutic efficacy assessment includes the therapeutic efficacy assessment for individual patient and the therapeutic efficacy assessment for cohort of patients.

Therapeutic Efficacy Assessment for Individual Patient

The following indices are applied to assess the therapeutic efficacy of the treatment for individual patient: symptoms and signs, bacteriological test, diagnostic imaging, and laboratory test. Among the indices, the bacteriological test and diagnostic imaging are the most important.

Symptoms and Signs

Symptoms and signs are the simplest indices demonstrating the therapeutic efficacy. The improved or absence of symptoms as well as changes of breathing rales indicate favorable therapeutic efficacy. However, the assessment is subjective rather than objective. Clinically, different scales are applied to quantitatively assess the changes of symptoms and signs (Table 4.3).

Bacteriological Indices

Bacteriological indices are one of the most important indices in assessment of the therapeutic efficacy. The indices include sputum smear test, sputum culture, and molecular biology. And the sputum smear test is the most widely applied indices in assessing the therapeutic efficacy. But due to its low positive rate, the sputum culture for detection of Mtb has gained wider application, especially during the treatment of DR-TB. Therefore, if the conditions permit or it is necessary for the patients, sputum culture for Mtb detection and strain identification can be performed to assess the therapeutic efficacy.

Initially Treated Patients with Pulmonary TB

For the initially treated patients with pulmonary TB, a night sputum specimen, a morning sputum specimen, and a randomly selected sputum specimen should be collected before the treatment is administered for the sputum smear test to define the diagnosis of sputum smear positive or negative. If standardized treatment is administered, a night sputum specimen and a morning sputum specimen should be collected after 2 months treatment, 5 months treatment, and 6 months treatment (or after the therapeutic course is completed) for sputum smear test.

Re-treated Patients with Pulmonary TB

For the re-treated patients with pulmonary TB, a night sputum specimen, a morning sputum specimen, and a randomly selected sputum specimen should be collected before the treatment is administered for the sputum smear test to define the diagnosis of sputum smear positive or negative. If standardized treatment is administered, sputum specimens are collected at different time points due to different treatment protocols:

(1) If the patients receive 8 months treatment (including 2 months intensive treatment and 6 months continuation treatment), a night sputum specimen and a morning sputum specimen should be collected after 2 months treatment, 5 months treatment, and 8 months treatment for sputum smear test.
(2) If the patients receive 9 months treatment (including 3 months intensive treatment and 6 months continuation treatment), a night sputum specimen and a morning sputum specimen should be collected after 2 months treatment, 3 months treatment, 5 months treatment, and 9 months treatment for sputum smear test.

Patients with Sputum Smear-Positive TB

After 2 months treatment, if the sputum smear test shows positive, another sputum smear test should be performed again after 3 months treatment.

Initially Treated Patients with Sputum Smear-Negative TB

After 2 months of treatment, if the sputum smear test converses to positive, the initial treatment is preliminarily assessed to be failed and re-treatment protocol should be implemented. Meanwhile, strain identification and drug sensitivity test should be performed.

Definitively Diagnosed and Registered TB Patients with Sputum Smear Negative

If the patients fail to receive standardized anti-tuberculosis treatment, bacteriological test of sputum should be performed at 2 and 6 months after the definitive diagnosis and registry.

Diagnostic Imaging

The diagnostic imaging includes chest X-ray, CT scanning, and B-mode ultrasound, and chest X-ray is the most widely applied. In the Guideline for Prevention and Treatment of Tuberculosis in China, it has been stipulated that chest X-ray should be performed before and after the anti-tuberculosis treatment. And for some patients, such as those with serious or deteriorating condition, chest X-ray should be more frequently performed. Chest CT scanning is superior to chest X-ray in demonstrating changes of lesion, which can also be applied for therapeutic efficacy assessment.

Note: For pediatric patients aged under 5 years, chest X-ray should be ordered with caution.

Laboratory Test

The laboratory tests include erythrocyte sedimentation rate (ESR) and C reactive protein (see the Chap. 1.1 concerning the diagnosis of pulmonary TB for details).

Therapeutic Efficacy Assessment for Cohort Patients

Therapeutic efficacy assessment for cohort patients is cohort analysis of the treatment and prognosis in patients who begin their treatment during a certain period of time. The cohort analysis shows the relationship between the treatment time and its efficacy. And cohort analysis of the therapeutic efficacy can be applied to assess the quality of TB control within a country or a region.

3.3 Detection and Management of the Toxic and Side Effects

Currently, adverse reactions of anti-tuberculosis drugs occur in about 12–20% of the patients in China and they are the important reason for the patients to discontinue the treatment. Therefore, timely detection and management of the adverse reactions facilitate to improve the compliance of the patients and thus to improve the cure rate. The adverse reactions of anti-tuberculosis drugs are shown in Table 4.4.

Table 4.4 Main adverse effects of common anti-TB drugs

Drugs	Common adverse effects	Rare adverse effects
Isoniazid	Hepatotoxicity, peripheral neuritis	Convulsions, pellagra, arthralgia, agranulocytosis, lupoid reaction, rash, acute psychosis
Rifampicin	Hepatotoxicity, gastrointestinal reaction, allergy	Acute respiratory failure, stroke, thrombopenia, rash, influenza syndrome, pseudomembranous colitis, pseudoadrenal crisis, osteomalacia, hemolytic anemia
Pyrazinamide	Hepatotoxicity, gastrointestinal reaction, gouty arthritis	Rash, sideroblastic anemia
Ethambutol	Visual disturbance, visual field contraction	Rash, arthralgia, peripheral neuropathy
Streptomycin	Hearing disturbance, dizziness, allergy	Rash, renal dysfunction
Rifapentine	Hepatotoxicity, gastrointestinal reaction, allergy	Acute respiratory failure, stroke, thrombopenia, rash, influenza syndrome, pseudomembranous colitis, osteomalacia, hemolytic anemia

In formulating the treatment protocol, the common adverse effects of the anti-tuberculosis drugs should be considered. In combination with the history of allergy and the past medical history of hepatic and/or renal diseases, the anti-tuberculosis drugs should be selected with caution. Before taking the drugs, the patients should be informed about the possible adverse effects of the drugs. Once occurred, the adverse effects should be reported to the physician immediately. In the following medications, the adverse effects of the drugs can be reported via the following ways.

Surveillance of the Symptoms and Signs Due to Adverse Effects of the Drugs

The adverse effects of the drugs present as certain symptoms and signs. Therefore, the patients should be educated about the related symptoms. The physicians should seriously and carefully analyze the complaints of the patients. And the physical examination should be performed carefully. The detection and management of adverse effects are vitally important.

(1) Nausea, vomiting, or jaundice are commonly related to impairments of the liver.
(2) Depression and irritation are commonly related to psychiatric disorder.
(3) Skin itch and rash are commonly caused by allergy to drugs.
(4) Muscular soreness and joint swelling are possibly caused by uratic arthritis.

In the clinical practice, the adverse effects of the anti-tuberculosis drugs are diverse, which should be carefully differentiated by the physicians.

Surveillance of Vital Organs

Monitoring the function of vital organs is the main way to detect adverse effects of anti-tuberculosis drugs.

The commonly applied indices include body weight, routine blood and urine tests, liver and kidney function tests, vision, and hearing assessments. The indices of liver and kidney function tests include levels of aspartate transaminase (AST), alanine aminotransferase (ALT), bilirubin, blood urea nitrogen, and serum creatinine.

Generally, the baseline data of these indices should be collected before treatment, which are then compared to the dynamic data collected during treatment. Once the levels change, adverse effects should be considered and appropriately managed.

The duration of surveillance and selection of the indices show great regional and institutional variance due to the absence of unified standards. It has been generally believed that the high-risk populations (such as patients with basic hepatic and/or renal disease) affected by adverse effects during the intensive treatment should be more frequently monitored, for example, once per 2–4 weeks. For some patients, the frequency should be further increased. For instance, for patients diagnosed with hepatic and/or renal disease, the surveillance of the liver and/or kidney function should be performed once a week or even several times a week. In the clinical practice, the frequency should be chosen by the physicians based on the fact analysis (Table 4.5).

Investigations Before the Treatment

The investigations before the treatment include the sputum smear test, chest X-ray or CT scan, routine blood test, routine urine test, the liver function test, and electrocardiography for baseline data collection. If necessary, electrolytes, vision, visual field, and hearing are examined and tested.

Investigations During the Treatment

During the treatment, the liver function test, the kidney function test, routine blood test, routine urine test, diagnostic imaging of chest, and electrocardiography should be regularly performed for surveillance. And investigations related to specific signs and symptoms should be performed. For instance, for patients with symptoms of

Table 4.5 Common monitoring projects and suggested frequency

	Time and frequency		
Check projects	Before treatment	During treatment	After treatment
Urine-RT/blood-RT	√	Check after 2-week treatment and keep once-a-month frequency	√
Liver and kidney function	√	Check after 2-week treatment and keep once-a-month frequency	√
		Increase frequency if results are abnormal	
Electrolyte	√	Patients using capreomycin keep once-a-month frequency	√
		Increase frequency if results are abnormal	
Hearing and eyesight	√	Check after 2- to 4-week treatment and keep once-a-month or once-2-month frequency	√
Chest X-ray	√	Check after 4-week treatment and keep once-2-month or once-3-month frequency	√
Cardiogram	√	Patients using fluoroquinolones keep once-a-month or once-2-month frequency	√

nausea, vomiting, aversion to oil, and hepatalgia, the liver function test should be re-examined.

Individualized Investigations

In the clinical practice, the conditions of the patients are diverse. Therefore, the indices and frequency of investigations cannot be standardized. The indices and frequency of investigations should be based on the basic constitution of the patients, the treatment protocol, and the therapeutic responses of the patients [11–24].

4 Prognostic Assessment

The therapeutic efficacy of tuberculotherapy is assessed mainly by bacteriological indices. However, due to the limitations of the bacteriological assessment, the combination of bacteriology with diagnostic imaging is recommended. If necessary, the clinical manifestations and laboratory tests results should be referred to assess the prognosis.

4.1 Indices for Therapeutic Assessment

Cure

For patients with the sputum smear test positive and/or sputum culture for mycobacteria positive before the treatment, two consecutive sputum bacteriology tests at 1 month before completion of the therapeutic course and when the therapeutic course is completed should be performed. If both negative, the patients are cured.

Completed Treatment

(1) For patients with the sputum smear test negative and/or sputum culture for mycobacteria negative before the treatment, the sputum bacteriology test should be performed when the therapeutic course is completed. If negative or the test is not performed, the patients complete the treatment.
(2) For patients with the sputum smear test positive and/or sputum culture for mycobacteria positive before the treatment, the last sputum bacteriology test before the therapeutic course is completed shows negative. But the sputum test is not performed when the therapeutic course is completed. Such patients complete the treatment.

Failed Treatment

(1) For patients with the sputum smear test negative and/or sputum culture for mycobacteria negative before the treatment, the sputum bacteriology test shows positive when the intensive treatment is completed. The treatment is considered failed.
(2) For patients with the sputum smear tests positive and/or sputum culture for mycobacteria positive before the treatment, the sputum bacteriology test still shows positive after at least 5 months treatment. The treatment is considered failed.
(3) If patients with TB suffer from MDR-TB during the treatment, no matter positive or negative in the sputum smear test, the treatment is considered failed.

Death

During the treatment, if death occurs. Whatever the reason is, the prognosis is assessed as death. The causes of death include death from TB and death from other reasons.

(1) Death from TB
    Death may be caused by progression of TB or complications of TB.
(2) Death from other reasons
    Death may also be caused by other reasons than TB.

Transferred

If the patients are transferred to other health-care institutions, the prognosis should be assessed as transferred.

Loss

For patients who are receiving treatment, if the treatment is discontinued for at least 2 months due to any reason, the prognosis should be assessed as loss.

For patients who have been transferred to other health-care institutions, if no information about the patients can be harvested for consecutive 2 months, the prognosis should be assessed as loss.

Successful Treatment

Successful treatment means that the patients have completed the treatment and are cured.

4.2 Indices of Sputum Bacteriology Test and Diagnostic Imaging

Sputum Bacteriology Test

The commonly applied sputum bacteriology tests include the sputum smear test and sputum culture for mycobacteria. For the patients with no sputum, throat swab is recommended. Before the sputum specimen is collected, the mouth should be rinsed with clear water and attempts should be made to collect the sputum from deep lung tissue.

Standards

Negative: no findings of Mtb in the sputum bacteriology test.

Positive: findings of Mtb in the sputum bacteriology test.

Conversion to negative: the sputum bacteriology test negative for consecutive 2 months. The sputum bacteriology test should be performed three times a month. And the results from the two tests are referred for judgment.

Return to positive: the sputum bacteriology test positive for consecutive 2 months after persistent sputum bacteriology test negative.

Indices

Conversion to negative after intensive treatment

Conversion to negative after the therapeutic course is completed

Sputum bacteriology test 2 years after the treatment

Indices of Chest X-ray or CT Scan

Obvious Absorption of Lesion

The area of lesion absorption is no less than one half of primary lesion. For patients with cavity, the shrinkage of cavity diameter is no less than one half of primary cavity.

Absorption of Lesion

Compared to the size before the treatment, the lesion is smaller. But the area of absorption is less than one half of the primary lesion. For patients with cavity, the cavity is smaller but the shrinkage of the cavity diameter is less than one half of the primary cavity.

No Change of Lesion

The size of lesion or cavity is demonstrated with no obvious change.

Deterioration of Lesion

After the treatment, the lesion is enlarged or there are new or disseminated lesions at other parts of human body. For patients with cavity, the cavity diameter is longer than the primary cavity.

Indices of B-mode Ultrasound

For patients with tuberculous pleurisy, after the therapeutic course is completed, B-mode ultrasound demonstrates no pleural effusion or a small quantity of encapsulated pleural effusion. And by dynamic observation, the quantity of encapsulated pleural effusion is demonstrated with no increase or decrease. Such patients are considered cured.

4.3 Indices of Fibrobronchoscopy

For patients with tracheal or bronchial TB, if the therapeutic course is completed, the therapeutic efficacy is assessed by the sputum bacteriology test, diagnostic imaging of chest, and fibrobronchoscopy. When the patients with tracheal or bronchial TB are cured, fibrobronchoscopy demonstrates no congestion, edema, ulceration, and necrosis. However, fibrobronchoscopy may demonstrate scar tissue and the resultant luminal stenosis of the trachea. Due to great individual difference, the severity of scar tissue and the resultant luminal stenosis of the trachea cannot be assessed via unified standards [25, 26].

References

1. Ma Y, Zhu LZ, Pan YX, et al. Tuberculosis. Beijing: People's Medical Publishing House; 2006. p. 152–91.
2. Tang SJ, Gao W, et al. Clinical tuberculosis. Beijing: People's Medical Publishing House; 2011. p. 8–167.
3. Bureau of Disease Control & Department of Medical Administration, the Health Ministry of China. Center for Disease Control of China. Technical guideline for tuberculosis control planning in China (2008). Beijing: Peking Union Medical College Press; 2009. p. 20–8.
4. Ge JB, Xu YJ, et al. Internal medicine. 8th ed. Beijing: People's Medical Publishing House; 2013. p. 61–75.
5. Chen XY, Wang HP, Jin YS, et al. Detection of mycobacterium tuberculosis DNA by Taqman polymerase chain reaction and its clinical application. Chin J Tuberc Respir. 2000;23(5):284–8.
6. Xie L, Ma Y, Gao WW, et al. Interferon gamma release of mononuclear cells in peripheral blood after antigen stimulation: its clinical application in the diagnosis of mycobacterium tuberculosis infection. Chin J Tuberc Respir. 2005;28:545–9.
7. Arend SM, Andersen P, van Meijgaarden KE, et al. Detection of active tuberculosis infection by T cell responses to early-secreted antigenic target 6-kDa protein and culture filtrate protein 10. J Infect Dis. 2000;181(5):1850–4.
8. Ewer K, Deeks J, Alvarez L, et al. Comparison of T-cell-based assay with tuberculin skin test for diagnosis of Mycobacterium tuberculosis infection in a school tuberculosis outbreak. Lancet. 2003;361(9364):1168–73.
9. Spieler P. The cytologic diagnosis of tuberculosis in pleural effusions. Acta Cytol. 1979;23(5):347–9.
10. Ozekinci T, Ozbek E, Celik Y. Comparison of tuberculin skin test and a specific T-cell-based test, T-Spot. TB, for the diagnosis of latent tuberculosis infection. J Int Med Res. 2007;35(5):696–703.
11. Ma Y, Zhu LZ, Pan YX, et al. Tuberculosis. Beijing: People's Medical Publishing House; 2006. p. 507–93.
12. Tang SJ, Gao W, et al. Clinical tuberculosis. Beijing: People's Medical Publishing House; 2011. p. 167–333.
13. Bureau of Disease Control & Department of Medical Administration, Ministry of Health; CDC of China. Technical guideline for tuberculosis control planning in China (2008). Beijing: Peking Union Medical College Press; 2009. p. 40–59.
14. Li L, Li Q, Xu SF, Gao WW, et al. Treatment of tuberculosis. Beijing: People's Medical Publishing House; 2014. p. 16–242.
15. Chinese Medical Society. Clinical guideline for diagnosis and treatment of tuberculosis. Beijing: People's Medical Publishing House; 2005. p. 106–9.
16. Lin Y, Harries AD. Tuberculosis infection control measures in diabetes clinics in China: a rapid assessment of 10 hospitals. Trop Med Int Health. 2015;20(9):1196–200.
17. Rezakovic S, Pastar Z, Kostovic K. Cutaneous adverse drug reactions caused by antituberculosis drugs. Inflamm Allergy-Drug Targets. 2014;13(4):241–8.

18. Arslan K, Kanbur M, Karabacak MZ, et al. Genotoxic effects of some antituberculosis drugs and mixtures in rats. Drug Res. 2014;65:219–22.
19. Gumbo T, Lenaerts AJ, et al. Nonclinical models for antituberculosis drug development: a landscape analysis. J Infect Dis. 2015;211(suppl 3):s83–95.
20. Ma Y, Zhu LZ, Pan YX, et al. Tuberculosis. Beijing: People's Medical Publishing House; 2006. p. 556–72.
21. Bureau of Disease Control and Department of Medical Administration, Ministry of Health. Center for Disease Control of China. Technical guideline for tuberculosis control planning in China (issued in 2008). Beijing: Peking Union Medical College Press; 2009. p. 54–9.
22. Li L, Li Q, Xu SF, Gao WW, et al. Treatment of tuberculosis. Beijing: People's Medical Publishing House; 2014. p. 167–72.
23. Pageaux JF, Duperray B, Dubois M, Pacheco H, Pacheco Y, Brun J, Perrin-Fayolle M, Kofman J. Hepatic function monitoring during tuberculotherapy (author's transl). Therapie. 1979;34(4):505–13.
24. Quenard F, Fournier PE, Drancourt M, Brouqui P. Role of second-line injectable antituberculosis drugs in the treatment of MDR/XDR tuberculosis. Int J Antimicrob Agents. 2017;50(2): 252–4.
25. Li L, Li Q, et al. Treatment of tuberculosis. Beijing: People's Medical Publishing House; 2014. p. 167–72.
26. Chinese Medical Society. Clinical guideline for diagnosis and treatment of tuberculosis. Beijing: People's Medical Publishing House; 2005. p. 84–7.

Management of Migrating Population with Tuberculosis

5

Sheng-yuan Liu, Li-juan Wu, Xu-jun Guo, Juan He, Yi-ting Luo, and Wei-guo Tan

1 Management of Migrants with Tuberculosis

It has been proposed by the WHO to end TB in the year of 2035, which means that the incidence of TB across the world should decrease to 100 per million by the end of 2035. The goal proposed by the WHO indicates that the global incidence of TB should be at a low level and attempts should be made by the countries with a low incidence of TB to further decrease the incidence of TB. TB should be preliminarily eliminated (10 per million), followed by gradual elimination (1 per million). The realization of the great goals is necessarily based on scientific breakthroughs and consistent international and national TB control. Along with the increasing mobility of populations around the world, the treatment and prevention of TB in migrants will definitely be the key work in countries with low and high incidence of TB.

Currently, there are 1 billion migrants and the problems concerning migrants are the commonality in countries around the world. But the background culture of migrants is diverse. In the way of migrating, various environmental conditions greatly impact on their physiological and mental status. And they fail to be secured with the social welfare in the immigrating countries. Some of them are more susceptible to infection of Mtb. The healthy migrants develop TB due to multiple factors. And the interaction of these factors increases risks of Mtb infection and TB in the migrants and causes unfavorable therapeutic outcome. Therefore, migrants are the important population in TB control. The management of migrants with TB is vitally important in the realization of goal proposed by the WHO, end TB in 2035.

S.-y. Liu (✉) · L.-j. Wu · X.-j. Guo · J. He
Shenzhen Nanshan Center for Chronic Disease Control, Shenzhen, Guangdong, China

Y.-t. Luo
Shenzhen Center for Chronic Disease Control, Shenzhen, Guangdong, China

W.-g. Tan
Department of Tuberculosis, The Shenzhen Center for Chronic Disease Control, Shenzhen, Guangdong, China

1.1 Migrants and Health

Definition of Migrant [1]

In 1922, it was firstly proposed in the Fourth Session of the International Labour Conference that unified standards should be formulated to define international migrants due to involvement of different countries. It was recommended by the conference that the participating countries should negotiate to clearly define the basic concepts concerning international migrants, such as emigration and immigration. In 1953, it was proposed by the Department of Economic and Social Affairs Statistic Division of the UN that the statistics of international migrants should be standardized, including the definition of permanent non-local residents (citizen and non-citizen). The international migrants herein were defined with two categories, non-local residents living in a country for above 1 year, and local residents of long-term emigration including those living in another country for above 1 year (including residence with citizenship and residence with no citizenship). It was the first proposal by the UN that one of the standards for international migrants is living in another country for above 1 year.

In 1976, the above standards and definitions were revisited by the Department of Economic and Social Affairs Statistic Division of the UN. In the new standards and definitions, the international migrants include intension of long-term residence in another country, living in another country for above 1 year, and continuing residence in that country. The international migrants also include those with intension of long-term residence in another country but living in that country for less than 1 year, and those living in another country for above 1 year but not presently living in that country. Due to complex standard and definition stipulated in 1976 with no operability, the standards and definitions were revisited by the Department of Economic and Social Affairs Statistic Division of the UN in 1997. And in 1998, the

W.-y. Yu et al. (eds.), *Tuberculosis Control in Migrating Population*, https://doi.org/10.1007/978-981-32-9763-0_5

Recommendations on Statistics of International Migration was announced. Although the experts in the international society have been in disagreement about the standards and definitions, the standards proposed in the Recommendations on Statistics of International Migration have been applied for national statistics of international migrants.

In the Recommendations, the international migrants are defined as all the people who live in another country. But the populations with temporary change of the living country, such as travelers for leisure, holiday, business, health-care service, and religious pilgrimage are excluded.

As the supplements to the above basic definition, the international migrants are classified into long-term migrants and short-term migrants in the Recommendations. The long-term migrants are those living in another country for at least 1 year and the country they are living in is their new residence country. The short-term migrants refer to those living in another country for at least 3 months but less than 1 year. However, travelers for leisure, holiday, visiting friends and relatives, business, health-care service, and religious pilgrimage should not be categorized into the short-term migrants.

Migrants and TB

Migrants are those living in another country. The comprehensive effects of push and pull cause migration of population. The push means migration of population due to their fears to persecution or natural disasters, while the pull means migration of population for better socioeconomic status. Therefore, there have been migrants with diverse intensions [2, 3]. However, no matter what the intension is, all the migrants leave their primary residence country for a new residence in another country, who suffer from losses of the primary family as well as social and emotional supports. And they need to adapt to the new customs, laws, and regulations in a socially, culturally, and economically new environment [4].

In the year 2015, there were 1 billion migrants in the world, equivalent to one migrant in every seven individuals, with 244 million cross the national boundaries [5]. Half of the migrants are females, and nearly 70% migrants live in high-income countries. More than 150 international migrants are migrating workers, with about 21 million victims of forced labor (including one-third of underaged labor) [6]. According to statistics, there are 50 million migrants with unconventional or undocumented migration [7].

Migration across geographic regions or nations affects the behaviors seeking health-care and pursuing health, which finally impact the health of migrants [8]. TB is a major public health issue. In 2015, the WHO announced 30 countries with high TB burden [9]. And TB is a consequence of interacting sociocultural factors with biomedical factors [10]. Migration itself affects the epidemic of TB, especially in the countries with low incidence of TB. In addition, migrants are exposed to risks of Mtb infection, onset of TB and DR-TB due to poorly conditioned living and working environment, unsecured health-care service, and discrimination. However, due to variance in gender, age, and legal status, some migrants are more vulnerable to TB [11]. And insufficient knowledge about the causes, symptoms, spreading routes, and treatment of TB, migrants behave inadequately in seeking health [12].

For migrants with sufficient knowledge about the symptoms of TB, their legal status in the residence countries is one of the factors influencing their therapeutic outcome of TB [13]. For migrants with undocumented migration, they are afraid of seeking health-care service because they are trying their best to avoid being detected by the police and being deported on conviction [14]. Without documentations of identity or residence, many migrants seek health-care service in private clinics for sense of security [15].

TB is commonly related to sense of humiliation. Due to exaggeration and misunderstandings about TB, migrants are believed to increase the risk of TB spread in the community. Based on such knowledge, the migrants in the countries with low incidence of TB may suffer from sense of humiliation [16]. When the migrants with TB seek health-care service, the attitude of health-care staff affects the compliance and outcomes of the treatment [17]. Unfriendly health-care service, such as xenophobic health-care staff, no health-care interpreter, and no social worker, negatively impacts the outcome of treatment in migrants with TB [18].

The living environment after migration is related to the risk of Mtb infection and TB onset. For migrants living in overcrowded place, seeking asylum in cities, living in the reception center or residence center, poor ventilation, and insufficient food may increase their susceptibility to TB [19]. Poor conditions at the workplace, no opportunity to seek health-care service, and insufficient awareness of health-care insurance cause unfavorable or delayed behaviors seeking health-care service, which further result in low detection rate of TB, delayed diagnosis of TB, and poor compliance for treatment [20].

If no free-in-charge policy for treatment of TB in migrants is adopted and implemented, migrants with TB may sustain catastrophic economic burden due to direct or indirect expenses on anti-tuberculosis treatment. Otherwise, they may face additional risks, such as decreased budget on health-care service for non-citizens due to economic crisis [21]. Even though the anti-tuberculosis treatment is free-in-charge, the allowances for auxiliary investigations and well-nourished foods may be terminated [22].

1.2 Overview on TB in Migrants

Populations tend to migrate from countries with high incidence of TB to countries with low incidence of TB [23]. Most migration is forced by violence and poverty. When the migrating population arrives in another country, their health and life are poorly secured [23]. Therefore, latent infection of TB and active TB are more likely to be detected in migrants. The risk of active TB in migrants is far higher than that in local residents [24]. And the migrants with active TB include those with progression from latent infection into active TB and new occurrence of TB in immigrated countries.

It has been estimated that migrants with TB account for 35–70% of all cases of TB in countries with low incidence of TB. And most migrants with TB suffer from re-activated Mtb infection in the immigrated countries following latent infection of TB in the emigrated countries. And the high-risk period of re-activation may as long as 10 years [25]. In addition, undocumented migrants account for 5–10% of all the migrants with TB. In the USA, the cases of DR-TB in migrants are the three times as many as those in local residents, which are 1.2% and 0.4%, respectively [26]. Although the conclusions of some studies are in disagreement, it has been generally believed that screening and treatment of migrants with latent Mtb infection or active TB are sociologically healthy with economic benefits, especially in young migrants from countries with high TB burden.

Recent epidemiological data from Italy indicated that the reported incidence rate of TB is 5.8 per 0.1 million, with 62.6% born in another country [27]. Although the cases of TB in local residents of Italy have been decreasing in the past decade, the incidence of TB in migrants has remained stable during the same period of time. The report incidence rates of TB in local residents of the Netherlands and immigrants born in another country show significant difference, being 1.5 per 0.1 million and 33.8 per 0.1 million, respectively. In the reported cases of TB in Norway, 92.9% is from immigrants born in another country, and the percentage is one of the highest in European countries reported by the WHO [28]. The incidence of TB in Britain ranks the second in the west European countries, being 10 per 0.1 million in 2015 and 69.1% from immigrants born in another country (most from countries with high TB burden) [29]. In 2016, the incidence of TB slightly increased in the USA, with the total cases being 9551, and the incidence remained at 3.2 per 0.1 million. In the past 23 years, the incidence of TB failed to be decreased and the cases in immigrants born in another country accounted for 66.2% [30].

According to a report by the Department of Economic and Social Affairs Statistic Division of the UN, Chinese mainland has not been a country of immigration. In 2000, 2005, and 2010, the immigrants amounted to 0.508 million, 0.59 million, and 0.686 million, respectively (mainly from developing countries). It has been estimated by the UN that foreigners living in Chinese mainland amounted to 0.8485 million in 2013, with an average annual increase of 3.9% in the recent decade. And the increase was higher than the average annual increase of 3.0% during 1990–2000. According to the data from the 6th census of population in Chinese mainland in 2000, foreigners living in Chinese mainland ranked from the highest number to the lowest number are Korean, American, Japanese, Burmese, Vietnamese, Canadian, French, Indian, German, and Australian. Except Indian, the other nine countries have a lower incidence of TB than Chinese mainland.

Along with the proposal of One Belt One Road, the trans-regional commercial connections are strengthened, which further impacts on the international migration in China, Asia, Africa, and countries related to One Belt One Road. Meanwhile, cross border investment, trade, and businesses cause upward migration of populations along the industrial service chain. Therefore, being affected by One Belt One Road, immigration into China will be increased.

China is still one of the 30 countries with high TB burden in the world with annual new cases amounting up to about 0.9 million, which ranks the second in the world. Along with the increase of immigrants into China, the currently implemented management of patients with TB is challenged. The measures for first national gate-keeping from TB, measures against influx of TB into China, and surveillance of TB after its influx deserve focused attention and scientific research.

1.3 Surveillance and Management of Migrants with TB

TB Control Strategy Adapted to Migrants

Consistent countermeasures are necessary to control the scale of migrants, their risk of infecting TB, and their difficulties seeking health-care service. The United Nations agenda for sustainable development is established on the principles that promote the realization of the goals. The principles include no one left behind, definitive goal concerning health (including whole population coverage concerning health and end epidemic of TB in 2030), safe and orderly migration (emphasis on the relationship between health and migration to promote sustainable development) [31]. The end TB strategy proposed by the WHO is based on end epidemic of TB and understandings about epidemic of TB. It especially emphasizes coverage of health-care service and social protection for the uncovered populations, including migrants and other vulnerable and marginal populations [32]. In the global stop TB strategy, more attention should be paid on the key populations, including migrants and migrating population at high risk of TB, populations receiving limited health-care service, and populations possibly missed coverage of health-care service [33]. Another key guideline is a framework of end TB strategy on the background of low incidence, including focused attention on migrants [34].

Management of TB in Migrants

Health Examination Before Migration to Prevent International Spread of TB

In the recent guideline for TB control issued in 2013 by the WHO, screening of active TB has been confirmed to be appropriate and effective as a component of TB control. The guideline provided a clear blueprint to identify the screening population based on the morbidity of active TB in baseline population and its development. Although no specific examination has been recommended by the guideline, it emphasized the necessity of optimizing the cost-effectiveness ratio in screening of active TB [35]. At the same time, there has been no unified and migrants specific screening for patients with latent Mtb infection across the world. In 2015, the first guideline for diagnosis and management of latent tuberculosis infection (LTBI) was issued by the WHO. In the guideline, the limitations of currently applied interferon-γ release assays (IGRAS) and tuberculin skin test (TST) were pointed out [36]. Therefore, the currently traceable evidence has been the nation-level experience, especially data from countries with low incidence of TB. The experience is applied to screen the migrants from countries with moderate and heavy TB burden.

In many countries, screening of infectious diseases has been performed in all immigrants, targeting mainly on TB based on historical background, political reason, and fears to infectious diseases in local residents [37]. The simplest way to select high-risk populations of TB and latent TB infection in migrants is to refer the incidence of TB in their original country reported by the WHO. Meanwhile, the uncertainty of reported data by some countries or regions with poorly performed health-care system is considered. Evidence has demonstrated that in Germany and the Netherlands, such screening is time-saving and financially economic, with optimal effectiveness.

According to the guideline by the CDC of the USA, the screening of TB in immigrants includes case history, physical examination, and chest X-ray (chest CT scan if necessary). If necessary, immunological assays for antigen of Mtb including IGRAS and TST as well as sputum bacteriology test can be performed.

(1) For applicants aged above 15 years

For applicants aged above 15 years, the screening includes case history, physical examination, and chest X-ray. If the chest X-ray indicates TB and patients are symptomatic of TB or HIV positive, the applicants should provide three sputum specimens for microscopy following acid-fast staining as well as Mtb culture and strain identification at least the level of Mtb complex.

(2) For applicants aged 2–14 years who come from countries with an estimated incidence of TB by the WHO being above 20 per 0.1 million

For applicants aged 2–14 years who come from countries with an estimated incidence of TB by the WHO being above 20 per 0.1 million, TST or IGRA should be performed. If TST $\geq$10 mm or IGRA positive or the applicants are symptomatic of TB or are HIV positive, chest X-ray should be performed. If the applicants are aged under 10 years, posterior–anterior or anterior–posterior and lateral chest X-rays should be performed. If the applicants are aged above 10 years, posterior–anterior chest X-ray should be performed. If chest X-ray indicates TB and the applicants are symptomatic of TB or are HIV positive, the applicants should provide three sputum specimens for microscopy following acid-fast staining as well as Mtb culture and strain identification at least the level of Mtb complex.

(3) For applicants aged under 2 years who come from countries with an estimated incidence of TB by the WHO being above 20 per 0.1 million

For applicants aged under 2 years who come from countries with an estimated incidence of TB by the WHO being above 20 per 0.1 million, physical examination is necessary. The case history should be provided by the parents or responsible adults who know the related information about the children. Those applicants with signs and symptoms of TB or with HIV infection should receive TST, IGRA, and chest X-ray (anterior–posterior chest X-ray or posterior–anterior chest X-ray and lateral chest X-ray). Three sputum specimens should be provided for microscopy following acid-fast staining as well as Mtb culture and strain identification at least the level of Mtb complex.

(4) For applicants aged under 15 years who come from countries with an estimated incidence of TB by the WHO being lower than 20 per 0.1 million

For applicants aged under 15 years who come from countries with an estimated incidence of TB by the WHO being lower than 20 per 0.1 million, physical examination is necessary. The case history should be provided by the parents or responsible adults who know the related information about the children. Those applicants with signs and symptoms of TB or with HIV infection should receive TST or IGRA and chest X-ray. For children aged under 10 years, anterior–posterior or posterior–anterior and lateral chest X-rays should be performed. For children above 10 years, posterior–anterior chest X-ray should be performed. In addition, three sputum specimens should be provided for microscopy following acid-fast staining as well as Mtb culture and strain identification at least the level of Mtb complex.

In Canada, for applicants for long-term residence or short-term residence of more than 6 months, the screening of TB includes case history, physical examination, and chest X-ray. If chest X-ray indicates abnormality, sputum smear test and sputum Mtb culture are performed. For applicants who are defined with active TB, residence is approved after the treatment. The officially identified high-risk populations of TB (with documented history of TB or abnormality by chest X-ray) receive regular surveillance of TB after immigrated. For population with latent TB infection, there have been no routinely performed screening and treatment before and after migration.

Some studies from countries with low incidence of TB have demonstrated that screening of LTBI in applicants from countries with high incidence of TB shows optimal cost-effectiveness ratio. However, the best threshold for screening remains undefined. In addition, more studies are needed to optimize the nursing cascade after screening of LTBI. If the therapeutic outcome after screening of LTBI is unfavorable, the value of LTBI screening is undermined. In some countries, screening of LTBI has been implemented and in some other countries, screening of LTBI is planned to be implemented. For instance, pilot work for LTBI screening has been conducted in different populations of immigrants in the Netherlands to assess the feasibility of LTBI screening before their immigration.

Management of TB in the Major Immigrant Countries

In the USA, TB Net has been developed by a non-profit organization, which is one of the components of its health-care network. It is an innovative bridge pattern for management of TB cases, which is intended to treat TB in geographically, linguistically, and culturally diverse migrants. The TB Net is intended to provide national and international nursing for patients who need persistent health-care service. If necessary, the management of TB patients, transfer of medical records, continuing health-care service, and other supports are provided via the TB Net [38]. Initiated in 1996, the TB Net has been integrated into the health-care network since 2010 and is intended to focus on migrants with TB. It is now a comprehensive project which provides health-care service for migrants with any health problems. By January 1st, 2016, TB Net had provided health-care service for 1737 migrants living in the USA and flowing between the USA and other 111 countries. In the past decade, the TB Net shows a completion rate of above 84%, which is close to the completion rate of 87% in non-flowing population in the USA.

TB Net shows an extremely optimal cost-effectiveness ratio in treating and curing LTBI in immigrants in the USA. [39]. The working staffs at the TB Net communicate with patients all over the world, government officials and clinicians. The clinicians from the federal law enforcement agencies, health-care centers, local or state health management branches, or other health-care institutions submit the data about patients to the TB Net. The TB Net assistants, namely the patient administrators, approve and register the cases and directly contact with the patients. The project is then introduced to the patient with the language chosen by the patient. After the informed consent is obtained from the patient, the medical and personal information about the patient is then publicized. In addition, the assistant may seek more information about the traveling plan of the patient. For international migrants with TB, the TB Net assistant contacts to the TB control agency in the immigrated country to determine the local clinic at the next destination. The case record is then transferred and the TB Net assistant keeps contact to the patient to make sure the communication between the patient and the local clinic. Lastly, the TB Net assistant keeps contacts with the patient and the new health-care institution to trace the compliance of the patient. When the treatment is finished, the TB Net assistant sends the complete case record to the registry health-care institution and all the involved health-care institutions. The chief medical officer in the TB net approves the case record and confirms the completion of treatment.

Papua New Guinea is a country with the highest TB burden in the Pacific Ocean Area. It has been estimated that the incidence of TB is up to 432 per 0.1 million. And the cases of DR-TB and MDR-TB have been increasing year by year. In Australia that is less than 5 km away from Papua New Guinea, the incidence of TB is less than 6 per 0.1 million [40]. Therefore, the incidence of DR-TB in Australia can be greatly attributed to the cases in Papua New Guinea. In addition to treating immigrant patients in Australia, health-care officials from Australia negotiated with those from Papua New Guinea in 2011 for construction of infrastructural facilities such as laboratories and health-care institutions. The strategy is intended to improve diagnosis and treatment of TB in Papua New Guinea, including construction of quarantine wards. And the international communication between health-care staffs of the two countries is also improved to trace and transfer patients.

A 5-year action planning (2015–2020) was formulated in Britain to solve the problem of TB. In addition to screening before entry, LTBI screening was proposed for immigrants from countries with incidence of TB above 150 per 0.1 million and flowing population into Britain in the past 5 years and the screening threshold remains undefined. In addition, the health care administrations and clinicians from other countries who treat TB keep in contact to ensure the continuity of the treatment. If the contact is discontinued, they seek help from the WHO.

In Norway, the immigrants excluded from TB by screening are transferred to local health-care centers for follow-ups. All the immigrants in Norway can receive systemic anti-tuberculosis treatment. If the immigrant patients go back to their original country or migrate into another country, the local health-care administrations keep contact with the counterpart in the destination country and the WHO acts as liaison.

About 20 patients with TB travel to the Netherlands for anti-tuberculosis treatment each year. Most of them choose to continue their treatment after communicating with clinician. And some patients resume their treatment there. By the Migrant Law, the undocumented patients with TB can stay in the Netherlands during the treatment. And their housing, health insurance, and living expense are included. The regulation is applied to about 10–20 patients with TB (2–3% of all the cases) each year.

1.4 Problems in Management of TB in Migrants

Chest X-ray is the first-line management for screening of TB in clinical practice. But it is not the sensitive and specific way for screen of TB [41] and it fails to screen LTBI, while LTBI constitutes the main source of TB in immigrant countries.

The management of immigrants itself shows limitations. In different countries, the applications of immigration are dealt with at different time, which usually lasts for several months or even longer. There is a long time interval from the health examination of applicants to their arrival in the immigrating countries. During the time interval, infection of TB or re-activation of LTBI increases the cases of active TB in the migrants.

In addition, only specific international travelers are compulsory to health examination. In many countries, only applicants for permanent residence are compulsory to screening of TB. In some countries, travelers for long-term stay are compulsory to medical assessment, while the short-term visitors usually do not receive screening. Actually, the amount of short-term visitors is far more than the migrants. The undocumented migrants (including illegal immigrants and individuals who stay after deportation) usually do not receive screening unless there are specific screening program targeting on such populations and accessible health-care facilities [18].

Some immigrants are afraid of being deported and thus try to avoid health-care service. Therefore, no refusal for or deportation during the anti-tuberculosis treatment is important to secure the completion of treatment. For effectiveness of the screening, the diagnosis and treatment of TB should be free-in-charge. No risk of deportation is also a precondition for completion of the treatment.

In some countries, supporting health-care policies targeting on migrants have been issued. But the migrants are still facing difficulties, such as misconceptions and poor performance of the migrants' administrators [42]. Therefore, migrants with TB are a population who needs scientific management with national and international political commitments. We still need a long period of time to end TB. Joint efforts are necessary from countries, regional institutions, departments of the UN, non-official social organizations, migrants' communities, and donators.

2 Management of Trans-regional Patients with TB

2.1 Background

Migrating population remains to be undefined in the world. Generally, migrating population is a group of people migrating from one region to another to work and live. In China, migrating population refers to the group of people who leave their permanent registered residence and live at another place. The migrating population is defined by the National Bureau of Statistics in China as population with separated actual residence from permanent registered residence and the separation within one city should be excluded [43]. Internationally, the migrating population is defined as internally migrating population. Along with rapid economic development in China, the migrating population has been increasingly larger. They leave their permanent registered residence for higher salary and better life. In 2017, the migrating population amounted up to 245 million [44].

It has been a long history that the migrating population attracts focused attention in TB control. In China, the morbidity of TB is higher in low-income population of western rural areas [45]. And the migrating population flows from rural areas to urban areas, from economically underdeveloped region to the economically well-developed region, and from the middle-west to the east coastal region of China. Epidemiologically, the migrating population flows from the regions with high incidence of TB to the regions with low incidence of TB, with resultant input epidemic of TB [46]. The migrating population is characterized by poor awareness about health, overcrowded housing, and malnutrition. Therefore, they are exposed to higher risks of TB than local residents [47, 48]. Due to the low income, they rarely seek health-care service when they feel sick. Instead, they tend to restrain themselves or neglect the illness. Otherwise, they buy drugs in drug stores by themselves or present to the illegal health-care clinics. The resultant delayed diagnosis of TB causes its serious and persistent spread [49]. Even though they present to health-care institutions with specialty in TB, due to the duration of treatment for at least 6–8 months, they are likely to interrupt the treatment due to various personal reasons that are commonly related to flow. The failed treatment further causes secondary drug-resistant TB [47, 49, 50]. These factors repeatedly contributed to a vicious cycle. And the migrating population is the seriously affected population of TB.

Therefore, it is mandatory to establish a mechanism of chain treatment in trans-regional flowing population. That is to say, when patient flows from one region to another, the TB control agencies in the two regions can sufficiently cooperate to ensure the continuation of the treatment. Meanwhile, the information about the diagnosis and treatment can be timely exchanged and feedback. Based on such a mechanism, the registry, reporting, treatment, and management of patients with TB can be interconnected with no interruption. The detection rate and cure rate of TB can thus be improved in the migrating population. A mechanism of trans-regional cooperation for detection, diagnosis, treatment, and information sharing of patients with TB is a new approach in TB control.

In 2006, trans-regional management was firstly proposed in the 5th round global funding program for TB control in China. And the Technical Procedures for Trans-regional Management of Patients with Tuberculosis was formulated in the Implementation Planning for TB Control in migrating Population [51]. The pilot work for trans-regional management of patients with TB was then conducted in 127 counties and districts in China. The trans-regional management of patients with TB is intended to connect the TB control agencies in two different regions for completion of treating patients with TB. Based on the pilot work, a notice on the Procedures for Trans-regional Management of Patients with Tuberculosis was issued by the CDC of China in 2009 [52] to promote its wider application. In the same year, the trans-regional management module was established in the TB Management Information System. Based on these works, trans-regional management of patients with TB has been applied nationwide (except in Hong Kong, Macao, and Taiwan).

Currently, the mechanism for trans-regional management of patients with TB around the world has not established. But such a mechanism has been attempted in some countries. China, as a country with high TB burden and high percentage of migrating population, the trans-regional management of patients with TB is one of the effective measures for TB control in China [53].

2.2 Technical Strategy and Working Procedure

In the trans-regional management of patients with TB, the migrating population is defined as the population who has lived in the city for above 3 months or population who has no permanent registered residence in the city but expects to live in the city for above 3 months. The travelers for tourism, visiting friends and relatives, and participating in the military army are excluded. And the population flowing within one city is not categorized into the migrating population [54]. The trans-regional patients with TB are defined as flow of registered patients with TB from one county or district into another county or district during the treatment that they cannot receive treatment and management in the primarily registered TB control agency [52]. Along with the implementation of trans-regional management, the subjects of the trans-regional management are not limited to the migrating population. The local residents who migrate into other county or district have also been integrated into the trans-regional management. However, the trans-regional management still targets mainly on the migrating population.

According to the Technical Procedures for Trans-regional Management of Patients with Tuberculosis in China [52], the county-level and district-level TB control agencies are responsible for management of patients with TB who are referred in and referred out. The management of patients with TB who are referred out includes referral-out of the patient, providing information of the patient to the referral-in TB control agency, trace of the patient during the whole treatment, and information maintenance in the Management Information System. And the referral-out of the patient includes informing the patient about the procedures in trans-regional management, reporting the registry data in the Management Information System, and prescribing anti-tuberculosis drugs during transfer. If the patient has left and cannot be contacted with, the referral-in agency should be input into the Management Information System as his/her permanent registered residence. If there is no feedback from the agency at the permanent registered residence within 3 weeks, the information should be reported to the superior TB control agency for assistance (Fig. 5.1). The management of referral-in patients includes follow-ups of the referral-in patients, providing anti-tuberculosis drugs, managing the treatment, and feedback the information to the referral-out agency (Fig. 5.2). In the Technical Procedures for Management of Trans-regional Patients with Tuberculosis in China, it has been stipulated that the primary treatment protocol should be continued for patients with no interruption of treatment and the patients with interruption of treatment for less than 2 months. For patients with interruption of treatment for no less than 2 months, the patients should be re-registered into the registry book in the referral-in agency and managed according to the Technical Guideline for TB Control Planning in China. Meanwhile, it has also be stipulated that the cost in diagnosis and treatment of TB should be paid by the TB control funding in the referral-out region before the patient is referred out, and the cost should be paid by the TB control funding in the referral-in region after the patient is transferred in.

Therefore, the trans-regional management of patients with TB includes 4 key points. They are information feedback from the referral-in agency to the referral-out agency, arrival in the referral-in agency, management by the referral-in agency, and completion of treatment in the referral-in agency (Fig. 5.3). The corresponding indices include information feedback rate, arrival rate, management rate, and treatment completion rate. These indices show the quality of trans-regional management of patients with TB.

2.3 Problems During Implementation and Strategies

Since the pilot work conducted in 2008, the trans-regional management of patients with TB has been gradually matured.

The implementation of trans-regional management and its effectiveness have been in disequilibrium due to variant

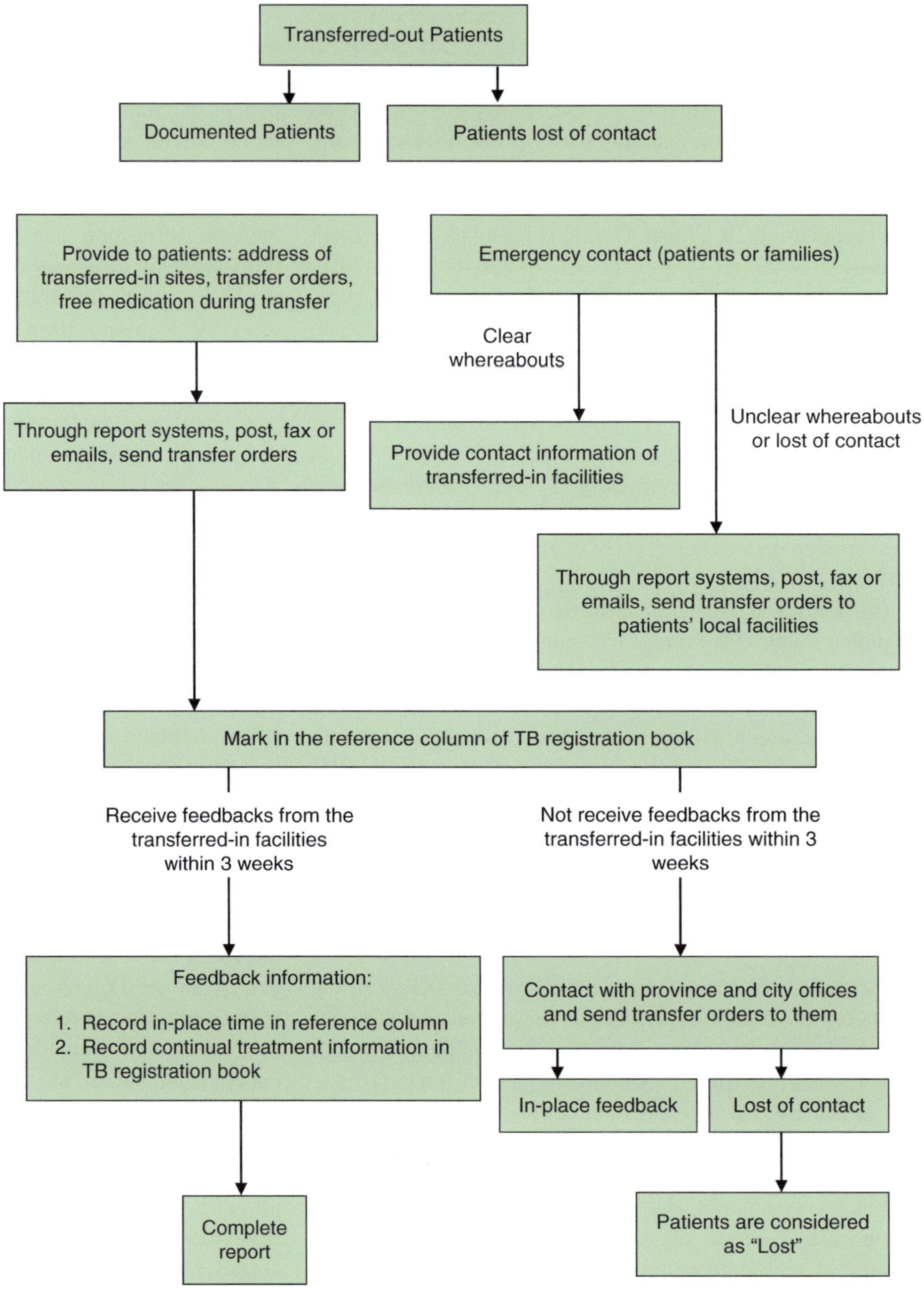

Fig. 5.1 Patients management process in transferred-out TB prevention facilities

percentage and amount of the migrating population in different regions and differently developed TB control [53, 55]. Especially at the early stage of its implementation, the information feedback rate, the arrival rate, management rate, and treatment completion rate remained low due to small amount of migrating population in some regions, insufficient experience and awareness about trans-regional management, insufficient funding, and unstable trans-regional corporation. For instance, from January to June in 2009, the arrival rate in referral-out patients from Shenzhen was 72.1%, the management rate in referral-in patients was 38.0%, and the treatment completion rate in the managed trans-regional patients was 66.7% [56]. From July to December in 2009, the arrival rate in referral-out patients from Panyu district of Guangzhou was only 21.62% and the average feedback time from the referral-in agency was 58 days [55]. During the whole year of 2009, the arrival rate of referral-out patients from Fujian province was 61.9% and the average feedback time from the referral-in agency was 42 days [57]. During the years 2009–2012, the treatment completion rate in trans-regional

Fig. 5.2 Patients management process in transferred-in TB prevention facilities

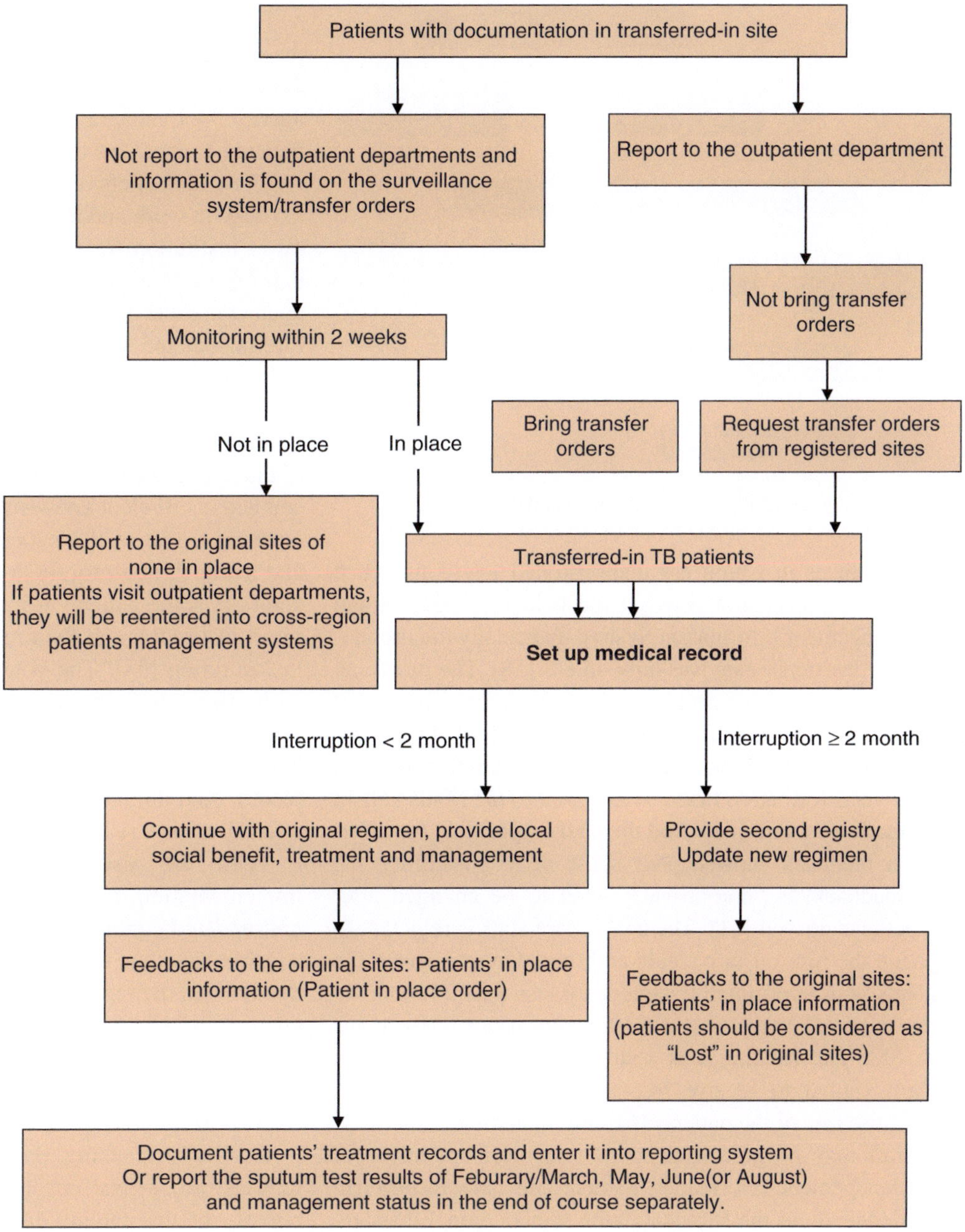

managed patients was 43.24% and the patient loss rate was 35.14% [47].

The factors influencing the quality of trans-regional management are as follows.

Before referral-out, the referral-out agency plays a basic role in the trans-regional management of the patients. The common problems include incomplete information or mistake information about the contact number of the referral-out patients, which may result in loss of the patients [58]. The health education about the procedures of trans-regional management and importance of regular medication is not conducted before the referral-out [59–61]. The trace of patients with interrupted treatment by the referral-out agency is neglected and the patients are referred out without observation of the technical procedure [62]. The referral-out is not timely or the reporting of referral-out information is delayed [56].

After referral-out, the referral-in agency plays a decisive role in the trans-regional management of the patients [63]. The problems include no information feedback, untimely information feedback, incomplete information feedback, and inconsistent information feedback about the referral-in patients in the Management Information System. A survey on trans-regional management of patients with TB in Shenzhen has demonstrated that the complete information feedback from the referral-in agency was 66.7% [56]. And another survey on the trans-regional management of the patients in

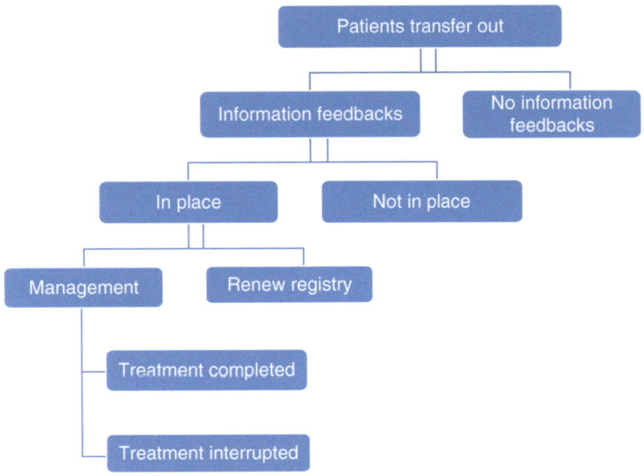

Fig. 5.3 Cross-regional patients' management flow

four provinces in China has demonstrated low consistence rate of the information between the field investigation and the Management Information System. Especially the prognosis, the consistence rate was only 45.6% [58]. The physician failed to inquire the case history and the referral-in patient was mistaken as the initially present patient [64]. The working procedures in referral-in agency were problematic and the arrival information failed to feedback to the Management Information System [61]. And the staff responsible for information feedback showed poor sense of responsibility, the first feedback as "non-arrival" failed to be changed after the patients arrived [61]. The health-care staff is reluctant to manage the referral-in patients and they may re-register the patients with interrupted treatment for less than 2 months in order to complete the task of treating smear-positive patients [58, 65]. The funding was insufficient and the referral-in patients failed to receive free-in-charge treatment, which may cause loss of the patients [61, 66]. In addition, the working staff may be unfamiliar to the technical operations of the Management Information System and have insufficient knowledge about the stipulations on trans-regional management. And the referral-in patients failed to receive attention by the referral-in institution [66].

The common problems in both referral-out and referral-in agencies include non-standardized technical procedures in trans-regional management [58], insufficient training for clinic physicians, and staff operating the Management Information System [58]. The referral-out and referral-in patients were not timely followed up and the communication between the referral-out and referral-in agencies was not sufficient [59]. Generally, the trans-regional management in the areas with global funding is more standardized than that in the areas with no global funding [53, 67]. And the trans-regional management in the economically well-developed regions is more standardized than that in the economically underdeveloped regions [68–70].

Patient is also one of the important factors influencing the quality of trans-regional management [67]. A study has demonstrated that the reasons for non-arrival in the referral-in agency for treatment included: (1) economic reason that the patients cannot pay for the cost of diagnosis and treatment (70.8%), (2) beliefs that the disease has been cured (54.2%), (3) busy in work and inconvenient transportation to the referral-in institution for treatment (37.5%), and (4) no faith in the referral-in agency (16.7%). Some patients changed their contact number after referral-out and lost their contact to both referral-out and referral-in agencies [61]. Some patients presented to the health-care institution that was not responsible to reporting in the Management Information System [61]. Further analysis indicated that some patients were unaware of the importance of standardized treatment and management and had insufficient knowledge about the trans-regional management. Most of the patients were insufficiently educated and it was difficult for them to find the referral-in agency. In addition, some patients were afraid of payment in the referral-in institution and then refused to present in the referral-in institution [58]. The potential reason also includes fears to discrimination after being known as patient with TB [61]. The factors influencing the arrival of patients in the referral-in agency include completeness of the contact number in the record. And duration of treatment for above 1 month before referral-out is a risk factor of patient loss [71].

There are also some other reasons that affect the implementation of trans-regional management, such as non-updated contact number of the institutions [58], unreasonable function settings in the Management Information System that the reported data cannot be updated or occasionally occurring system breakdown during operations [61, 62]. The quality of trans-regional management was only assessed in the referral-out agencies instead of both referral-out and referral-in agencies [67].

Generally speaking, due to the above-mentioned variant reasons, low arrival rate in the referral-in agencies and re-registry of the patients by the referral-in agencies against the regulation are the two main problems in trans-regional management. Consequently, the health-care resources are wasted, the patients have heavy economic burden, the incidence of adverse reactions increase, the treatment fails or drug resistance develops, and the risk of TB spread increases. In addition, the malpractice causes national data distortion, which may further negative affect the formulation of policies [61, 65].

Along with further implementation of trans-regional management, multiple interventional measures have been conducted in many TB control agencies. The indices of information feedback rate, patient arrival rate, and management rate have been increasing year by year. For instance, via health education for trans-regional transfer in the Guangzhou Thoracic Disease Hospital, the informed rate about TB and compliance behaviors have been significantly improved. In Nanshan district of Shenzhen, health education about the initial presentation targeting on the trans-regional management has been reinforced [72]. After that, a series of studies have been conducted and multiple interventional measures have been implemented. The interventional measures include: (1) management by specific staff and regular assessment of the management performance; (2) health education at the initially presented patients; (3) telephone communication during the whole process of trans-regional management; (4) close communication with the referral-in agency via multiple routes; (5) incentives for management in the referral-in agencies; and (6) intervention of superior agency to collaborate. After comprehensive application of multiple interventional measures, the information feedback rate, the patient arrival rate, the management rate, and treatment completion rate have increased from 87.36%, 51.72%, 2.30%, and 2.30% in 2007 to 100.00%, 90.74%, 83.33%, and 81.40% in 2013, respectively [62]. Targeting on non-arrival in the referral-in agency after referral-out, a survey was conducted via telephone interviews to the non-arrival patients and the referral-in agencies. The survey has demonstrated that there was mistake information feedback from the referral-in agency. Targeting on the problem, the collected data about patients was then increased and real-time bidirectional confirmation of patient arrival was conducted. In addition, the mistake feedback information was corrected in the referral-in agency. The patient arrival rate then increased from 62.47% to 82.62%. And the experience deserves wider application in TB control agencies in other regions [61].

Other scholars have also proposed many advice and measures for trans-regional management. Targeting on the management of referral-out, health education, sufficient and frequent communications with patient, timely reporting of referral-out in the Management Information System, and correctly informing the patient about the address and contact number of the referral-in agency, prescribing necessary anti-tuberculosis drugs have been advised [58]. It was also recommended that the referral-out agency should be in close contact with the referral-in agency for information feedback and continuing management [56], which is a key procedure in the trans-regional management. Targeting on the management of referral-in, the health-care staffs in the referral-in agencies should improve their sense of responsibility and commission [59]. And the arrival of patients in the referral-in agency should be timely recorded in the Management Information System and the patients should be followed up [56, 63]. The health administrations should reinforce the organization and their leadership to define the responsibilities of the institution and working staffs in the trans-regional management. The performance of institutions and working staffs should be regularly assessed. And in the professional health-care institutions, the working staffs should be sufficiently guided and trained [58].

3 Management of Homeless Population

3.1 Overview

TB is closely related to poverty. And homeless population is susceptible to TB due to malnutrition and compromised immunity induced by their economic difficulty and homelessness. In countries with low incidence of TB in North America, west Europe, and west Pacific area, high morbidity of TB in homeless population has attracted focused attention from the governments and social organizations. In the early twentieth century, the relationship between homelessness and TB was better known. Homeless population refers to the population who is constantly on the move or lives at the sanctuary, house of detention, or other poorly equipped place due to low socioeconomic status. In the year 2009, at the Conference of European Statisticians, a homeless individual was defined as an individual who has no residence and lives at the street or an individual who has no permanent residence and constantly changes his/her lodging place [73].

Multiple international reports [74–77] have demonstrated that the percentage of homeless individuals in outbreak of TB has been increasing. In high-income countries with low incidence of TB, homeless population accounts for a large proportion. In 2017, the surveillance report issued by the CDC of the USA (https://www.cdc.gov/tb/statistics/reports/2016/default.htm) indicated that the new cases of TB had generally decreased during 1993–2016, but the number of decrease in homeless population had been small. Due to drug abuse, HIV/AIDS, and poor aggregation environment, homeless population has been exposed to high risk of TB. Meanwhile, the places of homeless population aggregation have been unfixed, which promotes the spread of TB. However, homeless population commonly fails to receive insufficient health-care service for early diagnosis of TB. And the public health-care service is rarely harvested by this population. Before their diagnosis of TB and standardized treatment, there may be a prolonged period of time, which causes challenges for TB control in this population. In addition, the accessibility of health insurance and social security has been limited in this population. The social security mechanism for homeless population is far less enough to cover their expenses on clinic consultation, hospitalization, diagnostic examinations, and transportation.

3.2 Data About Homeless Population

Since early twentieth century, statistics of homeless population has been conducted by national and local governments or social organizations. Surveys have been commonly conducted by the governments to collect data of homeless population from aid agencies. In other countries and regions, hundreds and thousands of volunteers have been called together for field statistics at the streets and under the bridges to test the accuracy of the data. However, due to limitations of environment and conditions, the actual size of homeless population is far larger than the released data [78].

The size of homeless population is closely related to the economic development of the country or region. And the definition of homeless population shows national and regional variance. Therefore, comparison can hardly be performed with one set of standards. Generally speaking, in developed countries with more humanitarian assistance, homeless population accounts for a comparatively smaller proportion of the whole national population. According to a survey report by scholars from Yale University in the USA in 2017, the homeless population in the world estimated to be 150 million (https://yaleglobal.yale.edu/content/cities-grow-worldwide-so-do-numbers-homeless, https://en.wikipedia.org/wiki/List_of_countries_by_homeless_population#cite_note-49). According to another survey report by the Department of Housing and Urban Development in the USA in 2017, the homeless population in the USA is as large as about 0.55 million, accounting for 0.17% of the whole population of the USA [79]. And survey data about China released in 2012 indicated that the homeless population was as large as about 2.58 million, accounting for 0.18% of the whole population of China [80]. According to the census of population in India in 2011, there was at least 78 million homeless population, including 18 million street children (https://homelessworldcup.org/homelessness-statistics/). The countries and regions with comparatively smaller size of homeless population include Korea (0.022% in 2016) (http://www.mohw.go.kr/react/al/sal0301vw.jsp?PAR_MENU_ID=04&MENU_ID=0403&CONT_SEQ=342148&page=1) and Chinese Hong Kong (0.02% in 2014) [81].

Homeless population is economically poor and they are susceptible to climate, violence, and conflicts. According to the United Nations work report by the general secretary (https://www.un.org/annualreport/zh-hans/), the newly registered homeless population has enlarged totally by 30.60 million in 143 countries and regions in 2017, including 18.80 million due to natural disasters. Meanwhile, the homeless population due to conflicts has reached 40 million by the end of 2017. The new homeless population needs humanitarian assistance under effective collaboration.

Because the survival environment of homeless population has been insufficiently monitored by the governments and non-profit organizations, a high percentage of homeless population is subject to unnatural death. And most of homeless people suffer from substance abuse and psychiatric disorders. A study in the Netherlands in 2018 indicated that the most common cause of death in homeless population is unnatural death, and infectious diseases are one of the main reasons affecting the variance of death rate [82, 83]. A study in Spain targeting on the hospitalized homeless population ($n = 163$) has demonstrated that the average age of hospitalized homeless population is 48 years and 76.5% of them are males. In addition, 83.7% of them suffer from psychiatric disorders and 77.6% of them are believed with overdose of drugs [83].

3.3 Prevalence of TB in Homeless Population

Due to the economic dilemma and high mobility, the health-care service for early diagnosis of TB can hardly be available for homeless population. After the diagnosis of TB, the treatment and management can hardly be implemented, which may further deteriorate the epidemic of TB. If patients with sputum smear-positive TB are transferred to other sanctuaries or detention centers, the patients themselves become mobile source of infection. According to results of international surveys, the morbidity of active TB in the homeless population is higher than that in the local residents. When active TB is detected in the homeless population, the disease has commonly developed into the advanced stage with high incidence of DR-TB. In low-income but densely populated countries, the infection rate of latent TB is also high.

A report by the WHO has indicated that the incidence of TB in homeless population in industrialized countries is far higher than that in common population. A survey about epidemic of TB in the USA in 2017 ($n = 457$) has demonstrated that there are 204 cases of TB who are homeless before the definitive diagnosis during 2009–2015, accounting for 45% of the study subjects. Compared to the data from 2002 to 2008, the homeless patients are doubled [75]. Another survey conducted in the USA indicated that there are 16 thousand homeless in 0.27 million patients with TB and the homeless patients account for 6.1% of all the patients with TB [84]. A study in London in 2016 by ADDIN EN. CITE [85] has demonstrated that 550 patients with TB have a history of homelessness in 12,908,000 patients with TB, and the patients with a history of homelessness account for 4.3%. In addition, in 231 homeless individuals, 134 show sputum smear positive, accounting for 58% of the homeless individuals, and the positive rate is far higher than the common population [86, 87]. The percentage of homeless population remains low in China. A survey in Beijing in 2017 targeting on patients with psychiatric disorders and TB ($n = 251$) has demonstrated that the homeless subjects account for 38.6%, suggesting that homelessness may be one important factor for occurrence of psychiatric disorders in patients with TB [88]. All of the surveys suggest that homeless population is important in TB control. And essential health-care service and welfare housing are necessary to cover the homeless population for TB control.

Due to the special social attributes of homeless population, the treatment and management after the diagnosis of TB is more complex than those in common populations. And the incidence of complications in homeless patients with TB is higher than that in the common populations. But the cure rate remains low, with poor prognosis. A survey in Portuguesa in 2017 has demonstrated that the incidence of TB in homeless population is 122 per 0.1 million, which is approximately five times as high as that in non-homeless population. In addition, the possibility of HIV infection in homeless patients with TB is about 3 times as high as that in common population. But the cure rate of TB in homeless patients is 60.4%, which is lower than 81.3% in non-homeless patients [76]. The possible reasons influencing completion of therapeutic course and healing include age, intravenous drug use (IDU), and HIV/AIDS. In addition, the average life expectancy in homeless population is low but the number of deaths from TB is high. A retrospective analysis on 615 homeless individuals [87] has demonstrated that the average life expectancy of homeless individuals is 17.5 years lower than that in common population but the mortality is higher than that in the common population. In addition, the most common cause of death in homeless individuals is cardiovascular diseases (33.8%) and death occurs in a comparatively high proportion of the subjects due to TB (2.15%).

In recent years, latent TB infection has been one of the focuses in TB control in high-income countries. Latent TB infection (LTBI) is defined as a condition which the human body shows persistent immune responses to stimulation of Mtb with no clinical manifestations of active TB [89]. It has been estimated by the WHO that one-third of the global population suffers from Mtb infection. And the infection rate of latent TB is higher in countries with more frequent flow of populations. In addition, the infection rate of latent TB is higher in population born in another country than in local residents [89]. A survey in London in 2018 targeting on homeless population (n = 491) has demonstrated that the infection rate of latent TB in homeless population is 16.5% and in populations born in another country is 28.0%, which is far higher than 9.5% in local residents. The homeless population with a history of imprisonment is believed to be more susceptible to TB [90]. The homeless immigrants are believed to be more susceptible to latent TB infection. In a globalized world, TB can widely spread along with international traveling and commerce, which presents challenges to TB control in nationally and internationally flowing populations. Via national collaboration and international cooperation, latent TB infection in homeless population can be treated and managed, which terminates the onset and spread of TB from its sources.

3.4 Intervention of TB in Homeless Population

Several international surveys have demonstrated that the early diagnosis of TB can hardly be performed in homeless population. And smoking, alcoholism, and imprisonment are closely related to the high morbidity, unfavorable compliance, and poor prognosis of TB in homeless population. In hospitalized patients with TB, the emergency admission rate, drugs retrieval rate, death rate, and admission rate to ICU in homeless individuals are higher than common population. To prevent homeless patients with TB acting as mobile source of infection, active and effective treatment are necessary for homeless patients with TB from hospitals to communities. Meanwhile, the detection of homeless patients with TB should be paid close attention. And screening of and health education about TB should be well performed in homeless population. With these as the background, a working framework was formulated by the WHO and the European Respiratory Society (ERS) to eradicate TB in countries with low incidence of TB. In the framework, priority actions were performed for homeless population and other vulnerable populations [73].

Screening of TB in Sanctuary and Refuge

Detection of patients with TB is the most effective strategy in TB control. In many regions, the misdiagnosed patients with TB constitute high TB burden, especially in homeless population. In recent years, screening of TB in homeless population has been performed in some countries [91–95]. In the year 2000, health education about TB was widely performed in houses of detention, night sanctuaries, and daytime retention centers with aggregations of homeless population in London. Screening of TB was performed in about 2000 homeless individuals living in the houses of detention in London. Once TB was suspected, a case manager was responsible to contact with him/her and arrange his/her presentation in thoracic clinics. And negotiation was then made between the house of retention and local thoracic clinic for referral as soon as possible. If necessary, the suspected cases could be transferred to the local clinic on the day of screening [96]. In Switzerland, the immigrants seeking shelter there received screening of TB but it has not been conducted in homeless population [95]. In 2017, spatial analysis was conducted targeting on outbreak of TB in Fulton County, Georgia in 2008. The analysis has demonstrated that the geographic distribution of homeless population and patients with DR-TB largely overlaps [97]. Spatial analysis with multiple addresses can more rapidly capture the geographic information about homeless population and other high-risk populations. Combined with traditional epidemiological analysis, the spatial analysis based on geographic information can provide data for more significant interventional measures in future TB control.

Since early 1990s of the twentieth century, active screening has been gradually conducted on key populations in TB control programs in China. Health examinations have been conducted in supervision places, such as prisons, watchhouses, detention houses, re-education centers, compulsory isolated drug-quitting centers, and compulsory health-care institutions and in special populations, such as homeless population for early detection of infection source. Along with rapid economic development, health-care service has been possibly available for screening of TB in homeless population based on national and regional prevalence of TB, capability of the health-care system, and availability of the resources.

In addition, in regions with outbreak of TB in homeless population, screening of TB has been conducted in the aid institutions as soon as possible. In 2002–2003, there are outbreaks of TB in several sanctuaries in Washington, DC [98]. The screening and follow-ups to individuals with contact to patients in the sanctuaries have demonstrated that 48 cases are related to the outbreak in 313 definitively diagnosed cases. The outbreaks in sanctuaries and other aid institutions reflect the vulnerability of homeless population, suggesting necessity the role of government in preserving a strong TB control planning. Based on understandings about the homeless population in regions with TB epidemic, a systemic screening of TB can be scientifically formulated for better precaution of TB epidemic.

Concerning the mode and way of screening, past studies have been conducted for feasibility of chest X-ray and GeneXpert from perspectives of resource demands and benefits. And a comprehensive mathematical model of spread-dynamics and health-economy has been established to provide suitable and feasible screening of TB for homeless population. Chest X-ray is characterized by rapidity, convenience, and favorable compliance. Mobile chest X-ray for screening of TB facilitates to expand the coverage of screening and to improve the early diagnosis rate of TB. Thus, it has optimal cost-effectiveness ratio in homeless population who has only limited access to insufficient health-care service. In addition to GeneXpert screening and sputum smear test after active referral, TB can be early detected in homeless population. In this way, spread of TB in homeless population can be terminated and the health of this population can be benefited.

Incentives for Screening of Latent TB Infection in Homeless Population

The high morbidity of TB in homeless population has been believed to be related to high infection rate of latent TB. To prevent outbreak of TB in homeless population, in addition to establishment of a complete surveillance system, screening and treatment of latent TB infection should be performed in homeless population and other high-risk populations. The screening of latent TB infection is a nonprofit screening for homeless population with undefined diagnosis of TB. And latent TB infection can be identified by tuberculin skin test or interferon γ release assay. To eradicate TB, management of homeless patients with latent TB infection is vitally important. In North America, Western Europe, and west Pacific area, management of latent TB infection has been paid close attention in countries with low incidence of TB.

Spread of Mtb is more common in homeless population than in non-homeless population. Occasional contact may induce spread of Mtb in homeless population and the common population. A molecular epidemiological survey conducted in Japan in 2006 ($n = 152$) indicated that the genotypic clustering rate in homeless population significantly increases (aOR = 2.72, 95%CI = 1.42–5.20, $P = 0.002$). The result suggested that the preventive measures such as screening of latent TB infection for homeless population may be effective. A study on social support conducted in Russia in 2007 indicated that homelessness is a factor associated with unfavorable compliance in new cases of TB and the social support from the health-care institutions specialized in TB decreases the risk of unfavorable compliance [99]. Survival is commonly the first consideration in homeless population. Incentives for their active participation in screening of latent TB infection facilitate to improve the compliance in newly detected cases of TB.

Due to limitation in funding, investment is commonly put into diagnosis and treatment of active TB by the health administrations in various countries and regions. But the screening of latent TB infection in homeless population is commonly less attended. Based on the practice in Seattle of the USA, coverage of health allowance has been extended to most homeless population. In addition, an incentive-based DOT program has been conducted in the government-funded community clinics. With combined therapy of isoniazid and rifapentine, oral intake once a week, the primary therapeutic course of 9 months has been shortened to 12 weeks [100]. A randomized controlled trial has demonstrated that the completion rate is increased with increased early cost but shortened therapeutic course. Due to economical dilemma, constant change of lodging place, and restriction to alcohol during medication, the completion rate of treatment remains low in homeless population. Shortened treatment, therefore, can effectively control the epidemic of TB in homeless population, which facilitates to achieve the goal of end TB. Latent TB infection cannot prioritize in allocation of health-care resources. But screening and treatment of latent TB infection contribute greatly to effective TB control. Therefore, incentive treatment of latent TB infection in homeless population deserves exploration in countries with wide coverage of basic public health-care service.

Health Education About TB in Homeless Population in Aid Institutions

Homeless population tends to seek health-care service out of the sanctuaries, detention centers, and other aid institutions due to the social background of such institutions. That is why the diagnosis, treatment, and care of TB in homeless population are so difficult. The discrimination towards TB is the main barrier for homeless population to seek health-care service, which also affects their compliance to treatment. In addition, the primary health-care staffs commonly have insufficient knowledge about TB. The deficiency of professional health-care service is another important reason for delayed diagnosis and treatment of TB in homeless population.

Firstly, attempts should be made to eliminate the misunderstandings about communicability of TB by the government and social organizations to decrease discrimination towards TB. Government-guided health education about TB control should be extensively and regularly performed for primary health-care staffs, community residents, and vulnerable populations living in aid institutions. In the health education for TB control, coughing manners and respiratory health should be emphasized to increase the awareness rate of TB control. A case survey targeting on the homeless population conducted in the USA in 2017 ($n = 10$) indicated that people commonly acquire knowledge about HIV/AIDS and drug abuse in communities, but no knowledge about TB can be acquired in communities. Based on the finding, we know that health education about HIV/AIDS and drug abuse should be strengthened in communities. Meanwhile, systematic health education about TB should be extensively performed in community residents including homeless population.

Secondly, training of health-care staffs in aid institutions should be performed to increase the compliance to treatment. In addition to health-care staffs in the health-care institutions specialized in TB, the health-care staffs in aid constitutions should also know about the standardized procedures concerning screening, referral, diagnosis, and treatment of TB. Via close communication between the two types of institutions, the screening of TB and health education of TB control can be promoted. Matching budget should be planned for health-care staffs responsible to TB control for systemic implementations of the national TB control planning. Based on sufficient funding, care and prevention of TB can be extended to other institutions other than health-care system and administrations.

Lastly, comprehensive nursing should be performed for TB and HIV/AIDS to further implement the care strategy for patients with TB. According to the 2018 global health report on TB issued by the WHO, the cases of TB are estimated to be 10 million across the world in 2017, with 0.92 million of TB and HIV/AIDS (9%). In addition, the death cases from TB are estimated to be 1.57 million, including 0.3 million deaths from TB and HIV/AIDS. Most of the deaths occur in Africa and South-east Asia. Although comprehensive control of TB and HIV/AIDS has been proposed in the working framework to end TB by the WHO and collaboration between drug providers and health-care institutions for TB is recommended, the studies assessing comprehensive nursing for TB and HIV/AIDS are limited. An integrative health-care service for TB and HIV/AIDS indicated that concurrent anti-tuberculosis treatment and anti-retroviral therapy can decrease the mortality. Therefore, understanding about HIV/AIDS in patients with TB is vitally important. But in the European Union/the European Economic Area, only 65% of the patients with TB know about their infection of HIV/AIDS. The data is 88.5% in the USA and unpublicized in Australia and Canada. In countries and regions with high TB burden, health-care for TB and HIV/AIDS should be extended into maternal health service and preventive measures for mother-to-infant transmission of HIV/AIDS.

Government-Guided Environment Control in Aid Institutions

In TB control, actions of governments are necessary to integrate aid institutions into the national surveillance program for TB control. Effective environment control can help decrease the vulnerability to and risk of TB in homeless population. Generally, aggregation outbreak of TB may be induced in homeless population living in the aid institutions due to poor housing conditions and ineffective environment control in the aid institutions. Therefore, environment control measures should be adopted at the high-risk areas in aid institutions to decrease the risk of TB spread. Targeting on the spreading route of TB via droplets in the air, the environment control is intended to decrease the concentration of droplets in the air. The applied environment control measures in health-care institutions for disease control include natural ventilation, mechanical ventilation, and sterilization.

Firstly, from the economic perspective, natural ventilation is applicable in aid constitutions with no cases of TB but with potential risk of infection. At the specific area in aid institutions, to open the window and doors for favorable ventilation can decrease the concentration of droplets in the air for TB control.

Secondly, natural ventilation is not enough for environment control in aid institutions with cases of active TB. From the perspective of TB control, mechanical ventilation should be adopted for environment control. Mechanical ventilation is intended to strengthen the ventilation by using exhaust fan, negative pressure, and other external force. Considering its complexity and high cost, natural ventilation should be the first choice. If necessary, mechanical ventilation can be applied via seeking assistance from local health-care institutions.

Lastly, for aid institutions previously with cases of TB, sterilization is also an important way to protect homeless population from TB. When patient with TB stays at the aid institution, the things they used should be regularly sterilized. When patient with TB leaves the aid institution, the living place as well as the tables and chairs should be cleaned and sterilized. In addition, the garbage, face mask, gloves, and other medical wastes should be dealt according to the standards.

3.5 Prospects

Poverty is one of the main determinant factors of TB. Due to instant change of lodging places and malnutrition induced by poverty, the homeless population is commonly exposed to risk of TB. Studies have demonstrated that morbidity of TB and infection rate of latent TB in homeless population are higher than common population. To achieve the goal of globally end TB, screening of TB is necessary for homeless population and the population should be encouraged to participate in screening of latent TB infection. Meanwhile, health education about TB control should be performed in homeless population and health-care staffs in aid institutions. And environment control measures should be adopted in aid institutions. Alleviation of poverty and extended coverage of social welfare would greatly facilitate TB control in homeless population.

In the future 20 years, coverage of health-care service to whole population would be a major challenge. Homeless population is one of the risk and vulnerable populations of TB spread and is a major difficulty in full coverage of health-care service. To globally end TB in homeless population, health and social policies are necessary to gradually improve the social security system and extend the coverage of TB control measures. Meanwhile, all the service providers, social organizations, and communities should well collaborate. And new technologies for TB control should be developed. We expect all countries and regions participate in the management of homeless population to achieve the goal of globally end TB.

4 Health Promotion in Migrating Patients with TB

4.1 Definition of Health Promotion and Evolution of Health Promotion in Migrating Population

On November 21st, 1986, the first International Conference on Health Promotion was held by the WHO in Ottawa, Canada. The concept of health promotion was firstly proposed. Health promotion is defined in the Ottawa Charter as the process of enabling people to increase control over, and to improve, their health. It is a strategy to collaborate human being and its environment and defines personal and social responsibilities for health [101]. And the five components of health promotion have been defined as public policies promoting health, health-supporting environment, communities capable of promoting health, personal skills on health promotion and direction of health-care service [101, 102].

Broadly, health promotion refers to strategies promoting health of populations which are guided, planned, and collaborated by national government based on social development and social medicine. Based on a narrow sense, health promotion is a basic work and strategy in public health which is guided by health-care professionals. Since 1987, health promotion has been persistently advanced in China, which, however, has remained within its narrow sense of definition. Nowadays, more and more scholars believe that, in addition to clinical medicine and public health, social and cultural factors related to health should be paid close attention to develop a systemic health promotion strategy for the whole population. It has been advocated that health should be integrated into all the policies. And the integration indicates the development of health promotion in its broad sense [102].

A large migrating population is a determinant factor in social development of China. It has been defined as adults at the child bearing age those who leave their permanent registered residence and live at another place for work or personal life [103]. In the fifth nationwide census of population in 2000, the migrating population has reached about 140 million, accounting for 11.6% of the whole population in Chinese mainland. In recent decade, policies, science and technologies, social economy, and social development have greatly changed. In the sixth nationwide census of population in 2010, the migrating population has sharply increased to as large as 221 million, accounting for 16.33% of the whole population in Chinese mainland [103]. Because the migrating population is characterized by low levels of education and income, the coverage of health-care service in migrating population has always been challenging [103]. Since 1985, health promotion policies targeting on the migrating population have been formulated and issued. Based on the social needs at different stages of social development, the policies targeting on the migrating population in China have been gradually advanced [104].

In 1985–2003, family planning oriented health promotion was implemented in migrating population. The family planning in migrating population was jointly managed by the governments of the permanent registered residence and the present residence. In 2003–2010, health promotion in migrating population was comprehensively managed. And the focus was paid on the control of infectious diseases, occupational health, social security, and health-care service.

Since 2010, health promotion in migrating population has developed from management oriented to service-oriented based on their actual needs [104].

4.2 Targeting Populations in TB Control for Health Promotion of Migrating Population

TB control for health promotion is intended to improve detection rate of TB, quality of DOTS, and cure rate of TB as well as to decrease the incidence of TB based on the strategies of health education, behaviors change, policy-making, and environment control [105].

Due to different needs and functions of different populations in TB control, strategies on TB control for health promotion should be implemented targeting on different populations. The targeting populations include government officials, health-care professionals, patients with TB, individuals with close contact to patient with TB, general public, and special population.

Government Officials

Government officials are responsible for formulating and implementing health promotion policies. And they play decisive role in policy making and financial funding for TB control in migrating population. Health promotion strategies targeting on government officials include appointments with government officials for fact-to-face report about TB control, invitation for their participation in social activities for TB control, and providence of sufficient data and information to them [105, 106].

The government officials need to know about the threats and epidemic of TB as well as its negative impacts on social and economical developments. And they also need to know the shortages of financial funding, health-care institutions, human resources, and social participations in TB control. Based on such knowledge about TB control, a systemic mechanism can be established with leadership and sufficient financial funding for TB control.

Health-Care Professionals

The health-care professionals are the frontier staffs working for diagnosis, treatment, and management of patients with TB. They should be equipped with accurate knowledge about clinical management and preventive measures of TB. Based on the knowledge, they can effectively communicate with patients and their family members (individuals with close contacts to patient) for health education about TB control. The strategies for health promotion of health-care professionals include regular training, seminar, and providing brochures about TB control.

The health-care professionals for TB control need to know about advanced technologies on diagnosis, treatment, prevention, and management of TB. And they also need national guidelines for TB control for effective and standardized clinical practice.

Patients with TB

Knowledge about treatment and control of TB can eliminate the psychological barriers in patients with TB. Based on the knowledge, the compliance to treatment can be improved. The strategies of health promotion targeting on the patients with TB include oral health education about TB control for patients and their family members, providing brochures about TB control, playing videos about TB control, and psychological counseling for patients.

The patients need to raise their awareness of self-protection and other protection. If the patients live at overcrowded place, they should know that a well-ventilated and hygienic lodging place is necessary. The patients also need to know that they should not speak loudly, cough, and sneeze to the surrounding individuals. In addition, the patients need to know about free-in-charge treatment for TB and health insurance system for critical diseases. And they need to know that cure of TB is possible with regular treatment and its infectivity can be eliminated immediately after cure [106].

Individuals with Close Contacts to Patient with TB

The strategies of health promotion for individuals with close contacts to patient with TB are mainly intended to raise their awareness about self-protection. Specifically, when in accompany with patient suffering from TB for treatment, individuals with close contacts should know that sputum smear-positive TB is communicable and the individuals with close contacts can be infected. Once suspected symptoms are detected, the individuals with close contacts need to know that they should present to hospitals or health-care institutions with TB clinic as soon as possible. And they also need to know that TB is curable and the patients should be empathized instead of being discriminated [106].

Common Population

Health education to common population about the threats and symptoms of TB, health-care institutions with TB clinics and national policies for TB control can raise their awareness about TB. And the strategies for health promotion of common population are conducted during aggregation of population and in the area with aggregation of population [107]. The strategies include providing brochures, putting up posters, radio broadcasting, and field health education in community health-care centers and communities.

The common population needs to know about the threats and symptoms of TB, presentation to the health-care institutions with TB clinic when the symptoms present, and free-in-charge treatment for patients with TB. And the common population also needs to know that when an individual with suspected symptoms of TB is unwilling to present for treatment, they should attempt to persuade him/her to present for diagnosis and treatment [106].

Special Population

The strategies for health promotion in special population should be targeted on the characteristics of the population [108]. Targeting students, health promotion before and after epidemic of TB is equally important. Health promotion is intended to raise the awareness rate of TB control in students, parents, and working staffs in schools, which further improves their health-promoting behaviors [109]. The strategies of health promotion targeting on students include providing brochures that are understandable by students, such as cartoons and caricatures. Health education can also be conducted via class meeting, campus radio broadcasting, and blackboard newspaper. The health education about TB can also be integrated into related curriculum. Health education of parents via students can also further spread the knowledge into the families and communities.

The students need to know about the suspected symptoms and transmission routes of TB as well as the appropriate behaviors during epidemic of TB. They also need to know that fears and discriminations towards TB and patients with TB are unnecessary. And the strategies of health promotion targeting on high-risk populations with compromised immunity, such as patients with HIV/AIDS or diabetes, and the elderly include face-to-face talks in clinical encounters, and health education in families. They need to know about the threats and clinical manifestations of TB as well as preventive measures against TB [110].

4.3 Effects Assessment on Health Promotion of TB Control in Migrating Population

Briefly, the effects of health promotion are assessed via comparison. The actual consequence is compared to the project planning and expected goals. Assessment facilitates to summarize and analyze the reasons for successes and failures, based on which the next strategies can be optimized. If the strategies of health promotion about TB are assessed as excellent, more extensive social influence can be obtained. Meanwhile, more support and cooperation can be obtained from the targeted populations and communities. The assessment should be composed of three parts, namely how to perform the assessment, what to be assessed, and indices of assessment.

How to Perform the Assessment

Direction Comparison to the Expected Goal of the Project

At the time point of project completion, the awareness of the targeted population about TB control is collected and analyzed. Its consistency with the expected goal of the project can then be assessed.

Comparison in the Same Population Before and After the Project

No control group is defined. Before and after the project, sampling from the targeted population for questionnaire survey with the same procedures can be performed. The comparison with no control group is applicable for projects with short duration and limited funding.

Comparison Before and After the Project with Control Group

The indices are compared in project covered area and project non-covered area after the project is completed. If the control group and the intervention group are basically the same, the changes of indices are believed to be the effects of the project.

3.2 What to be assessed

Changes of Knowledge, Beliefs, Attitudes, and Values in Targeted Population

The knowledge is mainly awareness of the targeted population about the core information of TB control. Beliefs, attitudes, and values indicate the basic attitude of the targeted population towards TB and patients with TB, such as care for patients with TB, curability of TB, and inappropriate discrimination towards patients with TB.

Changes of Policy, Environment, and Service Technology

Changes of policy, environment, and service technology include policy on collaborative efforts for TB control, free-in-charge treatment of MDR-TB, and establishment of health-care institutions with TB clinic.

Changes of Behaviors in Targeted Population

The changes of behaviors in targeted population are the key marks indicating the success of the project. The appropriate behaviors include timely presentation to hospital if suspected symptoms are detected, persistence to TB treatment, and no alienation and discrimination towards patients with TB.

Realization of the Health Goal

Realization of health goal is one of the indices indicating the success of health promotion. However, the improved health should not be wholly attributed to the project of health promotion. The realization of the health goal is mainly assessed by incidence and cure rate of TB.

Indices of Assessment

Awareness Rate

Average awareness = total awareness score of the subjects/total number of the subjects

Awareness rate of certain knowledge = number of subjects with the certain knowledge/total number of the subjects × 100%

Total awareness rate of knowledge about health = total number of correct answers in all subjects/total number of subjects × number of questions

Belief Holding Rate

Belief holding rate = number of subjects hold a certain belief/total number of subjects × 100%

Behavior Change Rate

Timely presentation rate of suspected cases = number of timely presentations/number of suspected cases × 100%

References

1. Li MH. Definition and categorization of international migrants and migration in China. Overseas Chin History Stud. 2009;2:1–10.
2. Schoorl J, Heering L, Esveldt I, et al. Push and pull factors of international migration: a comparative report, 2000.
3. Van Hear, Nicholas And Brubaker, Rebecca And Bessa, et al. Managing mobility for human development: the growing salience of mixed migration; 2009.
4. Bhugra D. Migration, distress and cultural identity. Br Yearbook Int Law. 2004;69:129–41.
5. International Organization for Migration. 2015 global migration trends: IOM's Global Migration Data Analysis Centre. 2016.
6. International Labour Organization. ILO global estimates on migrant workers. Geneva: ILO; 2015.
7. United Nations Office on Drugs and Crime. The globalization of crime: a transnational organized crime threat assessment. New York: UN; 2010.
8. Gushulak BD, MacPherson DW. The basic principles of migration health: population mobility and gaps in disease prevalence. Emerg Themes Epidemiol. 2006;3:3.
9. World Health Organization. Use of high burden country lists for TB by WHO in the post-2015 era. 2016; WHO/HTM/TB/2015.29. Geneva: WHO; 2015. http://www.who.int/tb/Publications/global_report/high_tb_burdencountrylists2016-2020.pdf?ua¼1. Accessed March 2017.
10. Lienhardt C. From exposure to disease: the role of environmental factors in susceptibility to and development of tuberculosis. Epidemiol Rev. 2001;23(2):288–301.
11. Malmusi D, Borrell C, Benach J. Migration-related health inequalities: showing the complex interactions between gender, social class and place of origin. Soc Sci Med. 2010;71(9):1610–9.
12. Abarca Tomás B, Pell C, Bueno Cavanillas A, et al. Tuberculosis in migrant populations. A systematic review of the qualitative literature. PLoS ONE. 2013;8(12):1–12.
13. Heldal E, Kuyvenhoven JV, Wares F, et al. Diagnosis and treatment of tuberculosis in undocumented migrants in low- or intermediate-incidence countries. Int J Tuberc Lung Dis. 2008;12(8):878–88.
14. Berk ML, Schur CL. The effect of fear on access to care among undocumented Latino immigrants. J Immigr Health. 2001;3(3):151–6.
15. Mili D. Migration and healthcare: access to healthcare services by migrants settled in Shivaji Nagar Slum of Mumbai, India. Health. 2011;2:82–5.
16. Kamper-Jorgensen Z, Andersen AB, Kok-Jensen A, et al. Migrant tuberculosis: the extent of transmission in a low burden country. BMC Infect Dis. 2012;12:60.
17. de Vries G, Gerritsen RF, van Burg JL, et al. Tuberculosis among asylum-seekers in the Netherlands: a descriptive study among the two largest groups of asylum-seekers. Ned Tijdschr Geneeskd. 2016;160:D51.
18. Cain KP, Mac KW, Castro KG, et al. No man is an island: reducing diagnostic delays in undocumented foreign-born persons is needed to decrease the risk of tuberculosis transmission. Clin Infect Dis. 2008;47(10):1284–6.
19. Diana L, Schneider D, Mark N, et al. Tuberculosis control among people in US immigration and customs enforcement custody. Am J Prev Med. 2007;33(1):9–14.
20. Tschirhart N, Nosten F, Foster AM. Access to free or low-costtuberculosis treatment for migrants and refugees along the Thailand-Myanmar border in Tak province, Thailand. Int J Equity Health. 2016;15:100.
21. Kimbrough W, Saliba V, Dahab M, et al. The burden of tuberculosis in crisis-affected populations: a systematic review. Lancet Infect Dis. 2012;12(12):950–65.
22. Eisenberg JR, Lidji M, Gelfer E, et al. Same but different: tuberculosis treatment and care among migrants from different countries of origin in Israel. Lung. 2014;192(6):863–7.
23. International Organization for Migration (IOM). Global migration trends; 2015. Available from https://publications.iom.int/system/files/global/migration/trends/2015/factsheet.pdf. Accessed 5 Oct 2017.
24. Aldridge RW, Zenner D, White PJ, et al. Prevalence of and risk factors for active tuberculosis in migrants screened before entry to the UK: a population-based cross-sectional study. Lancet Infect Dis. 2016;16(8):962–70.
25. Dasgupta K, Menzies D. Cost-effectiveness of tuberculosis control strategies among immigrants and refugees. Eur Respir J. 2005;25(6):1107–16.
26. Schmit KM, Wansaula Z, Pratt R, et al. Tuberculosis---United States. MMWR Morb Mortal Wkly Rep. 2016;66(11):289–94.
27. European Centre for Disease prevention and Control (ECDC)/WHO Regional Office for Europe tuberculosis surveillance and monitoring in Europe, 2015. Stockholm: ECDC. 2015.
28. Lonnroth K, Mor Z, Erkens C, et al. Tuberculosis in migrants in low-incidence countries: epidemiology and intervention entry points. Int J Tuberc Lung Dis. 2017;21(6):624–37.
29. European Centre for Disease Prevention and Control/WHO Regional Office for Europe. Tuberculosis surveillance and monitoring in Europe 2016. 2016.
30. Salinas JL, Mindra G, Haddad MB, et al. Leveling of tuberculosis incidence - United States, 2013-2015. MMWR Morb Mortal Wkly Rep. 2016;65(11):273–8.
31. Tulloch O, Machingura F, Melamed C. Health, migration and the 2030 agenda for sustainable development. Bern: Swiss Agency for Development and Cooperation; 2016.
32. Uplekar M, Weil D, Lonnroth K. WHO's new end TB strategy. Lancet. 2015;385:1799–801.
33. World Health Organization. Global strategy and targets for tuberculosis prevention, care and control after 2015. WHA67/2014/REC/1(WHA67.1). Geneva: WHO; 2014.
34. Lonnroth K, Migliori GB, Abubakar I, et al. Towards tuberculosis elimination: an action framework for low incidence countries. Eur Res. 2015;45:928–52.
35. World Health Organization. Systematic screening for active tuberculosis: principles and recommendations. WHO/HTM/TB/2013.04. Geneva: World Health Organization; 2013.

36. World Health Organization. Guidelines on the management of latent tuberculosis infection. WHO/HTM/TB/2015.01. Geneva: World Health Organization; 2015.
37. Dara M, Gushulak BD, Posey DL, et al. The history and evolution of immigration medical screening for tuberculosis. Expert Rev Anti-Infect Ther. 2013;11(2):137–46.
38. Migrant Clinicians Network. Health network. Austin, TX, USA: MCN; 2016. http://www.migrantclinician.org/services/network.html. Accessed March 2017.
39. Tschampl C A, Cynthia A, Zuroweste E, et al. Cost-effectiveness of bridge case management for a mobile population undergoing treatment for tuberculosis infection. In: 19th annual meeting of the international union against tuberculosis and lung disease, North American Region, Vancouver, BC, Canada, 27 February 2015.
40. WHO Representative Office Papua New Guinea. Joint external review of the national tuberculosis programme of Papua New Guinea. Port Moresby: WHO; 2014. http://www.wpro.who.int/papuanewguinea/mediacentre/who_review_tb_program/en/. Accessed March 2017.
41. George SA, Ko CA, Kirchner HL, et al. The role of chest radiographs and tuberculin skin tests in tuberculosis screening of internationally adopted children. Pediatr Infect Dis J. 2011;30(5):387–91.
42. Walls HL, Vearey J, Modisenyane M, et al. Understanding healthcare and population mobility in southern Africa: The case of South Africa. S Afr Med J. 2015;106(1):14–5.
43. National Bureau of Statistics in China. Statistical Bulletin on the National Economic and Social Development in 2017. Beijing: National Bureau of Statistics in China, 2018 (2018-2-28). http://www.stats.gov.cn/tjsj/zxfb/201802/t20180228_1585631.html.
44. Department of migrating Population Service and Management, National Population and Family Planning Commission of P. R. China. 2017 report of migrating population development in China. Beijing: Chinese Population Press; 2017.
45. Technical Guidance Team for the 5th National Epidemiological Sampling Survey for Tuberculosis & Managing Office of the 5th National Epidemiological Sampling Survey for Tuberculosis. The report of the 5th national epidemiological sampling survey in 2010. Chin J Anti-tuberc. 2012;8:485–508.
46. Tobe RG, Xu L, Song P, et al. The rural-to-urban migrant population in China: gloomy prospects for tuberculosis control. Biosci Trends. 2011;5(6):226–30.
47. Li XF, Huang PS. Treatment and management of migrating population with tuberculosis in Huicheng district of Huizhou. Chin J Trop Med. 2015;15(3):304–7.
48. Yang C, Lu L, Warren JL, et al. Internal migration and transmission dynamics of tuberculosis in Shanghai, China: an epidemiological, spatial, genomic analysis. Lancet Infect Dis. 2018;18(7):788–95.
49. Ding SH, Shao WR, Wan QL, et al. Treatment and management of patients with TB in migrating population and local residents in Huai'an during 2009 to 2014: a comparative study. Pract Prevent Med. 2016;10:1196–8.
50. An J, Gao M, Chu N, et al. Transregional movement of multidrug-resistant tuberculosis in north China: an underlying threat to tuberculosis control. Sci Rep. 2016;6:29727.
51. Managing Office of the Global Funding Program for TB Control in China. The stage II planning in the 5th round of global funding for TB control in migrating population in China. Beijing: Management Office of the Global Funding Program for TB Control in China; 2008.
52. Center for Disease Control of China. Notice on the Technical Procedures in Trans-regional Management of Patients with Tuberculosis. Beijing: Center for Disease Control; 2009. http://www.chinatb.org/AnnoucementDetail.aspx?id=120.
53. Liu XQ, Li J, Jiang SW. Performance assessment on the global funding program for TB control in migrating population in China. Chin J Anti-tuberc. 2013;35(10):768–72.
54. Management Office of the Global Funding Program for TB Control in China. Stage I planning for the 5th round of the global funding program for TB control in migrating population in China (the 2nd edition). Beijing: Management Office of the Global Funding Program for TB Control in China; 2007.
55. Chen L, Zhong Q, Jiang L. Performance analysis on trans-regional management of migrating population with TB in four counties/districts of Guangdong province. Chin J Clin Pract. 2011;8:2299–303.
56. Li JW, Zhong Q, Yang YZ, et al. Performance analysis on trans-regional management in migrating population with TB and the countermeasures. Guangdong Med. 2010;15:1932–4.
57. Lin SF, Dai ZS, Wei SZ, et al. Treatment and management of migrating population with TB in Fujian province. Chin J Trop Med. 1370;2011(11):1334–5.
58. Li J, Jiang SW, Huang F, et al. Implemented procedures in trans-regional management of patients with TB in four provinces. Chin J Anti-tuberc. 2012;5:310–4.
59. Ma L, Chen YG. Trans-regional management of patients with TB in Urumqi. Mod Prevent Med. 2014;4:667–9.
60. Guan HY, Tan WG, Yang YZ, et al. Implementation of trans-regional management of migrating population with TB in Shenzhen. Chin J Anti-tuberc. 2015;5:498–503.
61. Guo XJ, Wang J. Survey on non-arrival of transfer-out patients with TB in migrating population and its intervention. J Trop Med. 2016;16(7):951–5.
62. Guo XJ, Wang J, Zhu MM. Trans-regional management of patients with TB in migrating population in Nanshan district of Shenzhen: analysis of 6 years data. Chin J Anti-tuberc. 2015;37(5):514–9.
63. Yang N, Wang DX, He JG, et al. Detection and treatment of patients with TB in migrating population in Sichuan province. Dis Surveill. 2017;32(7):563–7.
64. Zhang Y, Ye JJ, Yang CF, et al. Trans-regional management and treatment of patients with TB in migrating population in Hubei province. Chin J Anti-tuberc. 2016;38(5):405–10.
65. Guo XJ, Wang J, Zhong T, Lu JJ. Factors analysis on re-registry of transfer-in patients with TB in migrating population against the regulation. J Trop Med. 2011;11(9):1069–72.
66. Guo XJ, Wang J, Zhu MM, et al. Performance assessment of trans-regional management of patients with TB in migrating population. J Trop Med. 2012;12(9):1154–6.
67. Zhao MG, Guo L, Zhao AG, et al. Trans-regional transfer-out patients with TB in migrating population in Baoan district of Shenzhen. Chin J Anti-tuberc. 2011;33(7):442–4.
68. Chen SH, Wang XM, Zhong JM, et al. Trans-regional management of patients with TB in migrating population. Chin J Prevent Med. 2014;15(3):230–4.
69. Zhou Y, Zhu LG, Zhu YF, et al. Trans-provincial management and treatment of patients with TB. Chin J Dis Contr. 2012;16(10):874–6.
70. Guan HY, Yang YZ, Tan WG, Lv JW, Wu QF. Performance assessment on trans-regional management of patients with TB in migrating population in Shenzhen. Chin J Trop Med. 2011;11(10):1192–4.
71. Wang YX, Zhao MG, Guo L, Zhao AG, Huang Z, Ouyang X. Factor analysis on arrival of transfer-out patients with TB in Baoan district of Shenzhen. Chin J Pract Med. 2015;15:282–4.
72. Zhu M, Wang J, Dib HH, et al. Enhancing the management of cross-regional transfer of migrating tuberculosis cases by active follow-up and communication. Eur J Pub Health. 2012;22(4):577–82.
73. van Hest R, Story A. Tuberculosis control in homeless persons in European Union: more than words alone. Pneumologia. 2009;58(2):84–7.
74. Segal-Maurer S. Tuberculosis in enclosed populations. Microbiol Spectr. 2017;5(2):TNMI7-0041-2017.
75. Mindra G, Wortham JM, Haddad MB, et al. Tuberculosis outbreaks in the United States, 2009-2015. Public Health Rep. 2017;132(2):157–63.

76. Dias M, Gaio R, Sousa P, et al. Tuberculosis among the homeless: should we change the strategy? Int J Tuberc Lung Dis. 2017;21(3):327–32.
77. Heuvelings CC, de Vries SG, Greve PF, et al. Effectiveness of interventions for diagnosis and treatment of tuberculosis in hard-to-reach populations in countries of low and medium tuberculosis incidence: a systematic review. Lancet Infect Dis. 2017;17(5):e144–58.
78. Cooper C, Levay P, Lorenc T, et al. A population search filter for hard-to-reach populations increased search efficiency for a systematic review. J Clin Epidemiol. 2014;67(5):554–9.
79. US homeless people numbers rise for first time in seven years. BBC 2017.
80. Hammond J. Homelessness in China. GB Times 2012.
81. Lee Y. CityU NewsCentre - CityU study finds main reason for homelessness is housing affordability. 2014. https://newscentre.cityu.edu.hk/media/news/2014/03/31/cityu-study-finds-main-reason-homelessness-housing-affordability.
82. Slockers MT, Nusselder WJ, Rietjens J, et al. Homeless adults' most frequent cause of death is suicide or murder. Ned Tijdschr Geneeskd. 2018;162:D2626.
83. Tornero Patricio S, Fernandez Ajuria A, Charris Castro L. Characteristics of hospitalizations of homeless persons in Seville, Spain. Rev Esp Salud Publica. 2016;90:E12.
84. Bamrah S, Yelk Woodruff RS, Powell K, et al. Tuberculosis among the homeless, United States, 1994-2010. Int J Tuberc Lung Dis. 2013;17(11):1414–9.
85. Wang L, Zhang Z, Yan Q, et al. Diagnostic dilemma of pulmonary tuberculosis among adults with severe mental illness in Beijing, China. BMC Infect Dis. 2017;17(1):83.
86. Anderson C, Anderson SR, Maguire H, et al. Tuberculosis in London: the convergence of clinical and social complexity. Eur Respir J. 2016;48(4):1233–6.
87. WHO Guidelines Approved by the Guidelines Review Committee. Guidelines on the management of latent tuberculosis infection. Geneva: World Health Organization; 2015.
88. Romaszko J, Cymes I, Draganska E, et al. Mortality among the homeless: causes and meteorological relationships. PLoS One. 2017;12(12):e0189938.
89. Stock D. National position statement for the management of latent tuberculosis infection. Commun Dis Intell Q Rep. 2017;41(3):E204–8.
90. Isler MA, Rivest P, Mason J, et al. Screening employees of services for homeless individuals in Montreal for tuberculosis infection. J Infect Public Health. 2013;6(3):209–15.
91. Jimenez-Fuentes MA, Auge CM, Gomez MN, et al. Screening for active tuberculosis in high-risk groups. Int J Tuberc Lung Dis. 2014;18(12):1459–65.
92. Kmietowicz Z. NICE advises screening for TB in hostels and prisons to reduce UK cases. BMJ. 2012;344:e2309.
93. Linas BP, Wong AY, Freedberg KA, et al. Priorities for screening and treatment of latent tuberculosis infection in the United States. Am J Respir Crit Care Med. 2011;184(5):590–601.
94. Janssens JP, Wuillemin T, Adler D, et al. Screening for tuberculosis in an urban shelter for homeless in Switzerland: a prospective study. BMC Infect Dis. 2017;17(1):347.
95. He XX. Tuberculosis in homeless population in London: an effective model for screening and treatment of tuberculosis. J Tuberc Lung Dis. 2000;1:40–6.
96. Worrell MC, Kramer M, Yamin A, et al. Use of activity space in a tuberculosis outbreak: bringing homeless persons into spatial analyses. Open Forum Infect Dis. 2017;4(1):ofw280.
97. Xu M, Yang HD, Zhang LX, et al. Spread of tuberculosis at multiple places by homeless patient with TB. Int J Tuberc Lung Dis. 2006;3:128–34.
98. Mugwagwa T, Stagg HR, Abubakar I, et al. Comparing different technologies for active TB case-finding among the homeless: a transmission-dynamic modelling study. Sci Rep. 2018;8(1):1433.
99. Sandul AL, Nwana N, Holcombe JM, et al. High rate of treatment completion in program settings with 12-dose weekly isoniazid and rifapentine (3HP) for latent mycobacterium tuberculosis infection. Clin Infect Dis. 2017;65(7):1085–93.
100. Connors WJ, Hussen SA, Holland DP, et al. Homeless shelter context and tuberculosis illness experiences during a large outbreak in Atlanta, Georgia. Publ Health Action. 2017;7(3):224–30.
101. WHO, Health topics Health promotion. [2016-6-20]. http://www.who.int/topics/health_promotion/en/.
102. Hu XG, Cao CX, Li YF. Application of health promotion in the strategy of Healthy China. Med Soc. 2017;30(4):64–7.
103. Wan JJ, Zhong H. Characteristics of, reasons for and strategies towards migrating population in recent decade: comparison of data from the 5th and 6th national census of population. Consult Policy. 2014;1:64–8.
104. Zheng YT, Ji Y, Chang C. Development and characteristics of health promotion policies in migrating population in China. Chin J Health-care Manage. 2017;34(4):310–2.
105. Wan LY. Brochure for drug-resistant tuberculosis control. Beijing: Peking Union Medical College Press; 2010.
106. Bureau of Disease Prevention and Control, Ministry of Health. Technical guideline for implementation of TB control planning in China (edition of 2008). Beijing: Peking Union Medical College Press; 2009.
107. Li SQ. Strategies for TB control in migrating population. Chin J Rural Health. 2017;4:38.
108. Wang H. Health education for TB control. Basic-level Med Forum. 2016;20(13):1805.
109. Wang LX, Cheng SM, Chen W. Brochure for tuberculosis control in schools. Beijing: Military Medical Science Press; 2012.
110. Aldridge RW, Hayward AC, Hemming S, et al. High prevalence of latent tuberculosis and bloodborne virus infection in a homeless population. Thorax. 2018;73(6):557–64.

TB Control in Schools

6

Xiao-ling Che, Chun-rong Lu, Wei-guo Tan, and Qiu Zhong

1 Current Prevalence of TB in Schools

Schools are highly populated. The communal living and studying in schools render long-term close contacts between students. In addition, for teenagers in the adolescent development period whose body immune function are not adequate, coupled with learning pressure, mental stress and less physical exercise, once there is emergence of infectious tuberculosis patients with improper treatment, it is easy to cause the spread of tuberculosis on campus epidemic. Thus, aggregating outbreak of TB may occur.

According to the data of the national economy and surveys in 2017 released by the National Statistics Bureau of China, the number of students in schools of China has reached 256.814 million by the end of 2016, including 1.981 million postgraduates, 26.958 million undergraduates, 83.274 million middle school students, 99.963 million primary school students, and 44.638 million in preschool education, special education, and reform school education. The population of students accounted for 18.57% of the whole population in China (256.814 million/1382.71 million).

In the year 2015, there were totally 864,015 cases of TB in the on-line reporting system of infectious diseases, including 34,260 students, which accounted for 3.97% of the total reported cases of TB [1]. In 2017, the new cases of TB in students reached more than 40 thousand, accounting for 4.87% of all the reported new cases of TB nationwide [2]. In reported student cases of TB, the age group of 13–15 years accounted for 16.3%, the age group of 16–18 years accounted for 39.3%, and the age group of 19–22 accounted for 32.5%. The age group of 16–18 shows the highest incidence of TB, which is also the time of hard-studying to prepare for the College Entrance Exam. Therefore, the high incidence in the age group may be related to insufficient sleep, psychological stress, and health examination before the College Entrance Exam. In the *Guideline for TB Control in Schools* (*2017*), the screening of TB in health examination, health examination before enrollment in schools, and annually routine health examination have been emphasized. These measures play important role in early active detection of TB in schools. Since then, the reported incidence of TB in students has been decreasing. In the years from 2011 to 2015, the incidence of TB in schools in China was 18.79 per 0.1 million, 16.63 per 0.1 million, 15.71 per 0.1 million, 16.63 per 0.1 million, and 15.88 per 0.1 million, respectively. And the differences showed no statistical significance ($\chi^2 = 0.35$, $P > 0.05$). During the 5 years, the incidence of TB in schools has decreased by 15.49% (Fig. 6.1).

Despite the tendency of decreasing incidence, aggregating epidemic of TB frequently occurs and its occurrence annually increases. During 2006–2016, there were 53 aggregating epidemics of TB in students, with 36 in high schools (67.9%) and 49 in boarding schools (92.5%). During 2010–2015, there were 2, 3, 6, 6, 8, and 10 aggregating epidemics of TB in schools of China, respectively, with a tendency of annual increase. Chen et al. analyzed the epidemics of TB in schools of China from 2008 to 2012 [3]. They found that the epidemics of TB in schools of China are characterized by large scale of schools, boarding high school in rural area, occurrence in winters and springs with cold weather, poorly ventilated classrooms and dormitories with closed windows, and insufficient knowledge about TB control in students. Due to insufficient knowledge about TB control, the students with suspected symptoms rarely present to hospital for diagnosis and treatment in time, which further causes persistent spread of TB in

X.-l. Che (✉) · C.-r. Lu
Shenzhen Center for Chronic Disease Control, Shenzhen, Guangdong, China

W.-g. Tan
Department of Tuberculosis, The Shenzhen Center for Chronic Disease Control, Shenzhen, Guangdong, China

Q. Zhong
Chinese Antituberculosis Association, Guangzhou, Guangdong, China

W.-y. Yu et al. (eds.), *Tuberculosis Control in Migrating Population*, https://doi.org/10.1007/978-981-32-9763-0_6

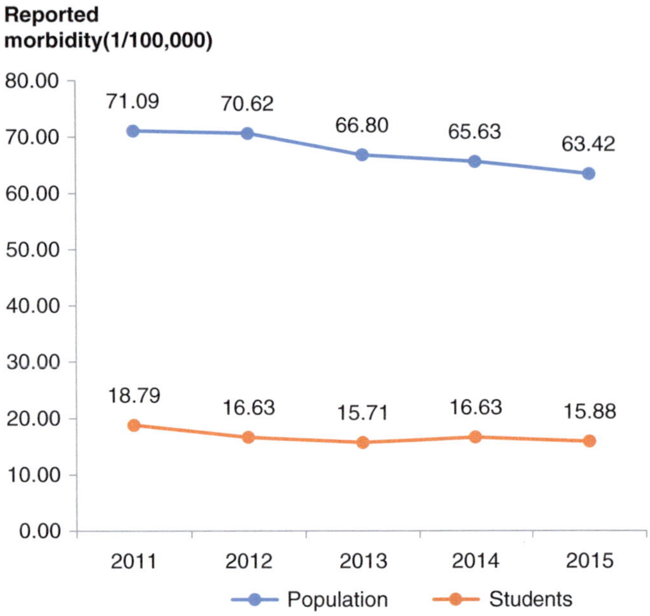

Fig. 6.1 Trends of TB morbidity among Chinese students. *Source*: China infectious diseases network direct reporting system, 2017 China statistical yearbook

students. The student patients show obvious aggregation, with multiple cases in one classroom or one dormitory. And the epidemiological correlation between student patients is definitive. Most of the student patients are detected via large-scale active screening after the initial onset in one student patient. Therefore, TB control in schools should be paid close attention. Health education and environmental hygiene play important role in TB control in schools.

In November 2017, there was one aggregating epidemic of TB in the Fourth Middle School of Taojiang County, Yiyang City, Hunan Province of China. Totally, 81 defined cases and 7 suspected cases of TB were reported. All of the patients were high school students at the 12th grade, who were working hard to prepare for the College Entrance Exam. After being exposed by mass media, TB control became a hot topic attracting social attention [4]. The painful lesson from Taojiang County has been always remembered in TB control in Shenzhen. To prevent spread of TB and minimize adverse effects of TB in schools in Shenzhen, routine and sentinel surveillance of TB have been conducted, and the procedures for field epidemiological survey have been standardized. During 2012–2018, more than 20,000 students with suspected symptoms of TB in Shenzhen were monitored, and 1151 cases of TB were detected. The screening of TB was conducted in students with close contact to patient with TB during epidemic of TB in schools of Shenzhen, and 54 cases were defined. By the end of 2018, sudden public health event has never occurred in Shenzhen.

2 Strategies for TB Control in Schools

2.1 To Establish a Working Mechanism for Joint Prevention and Control

To Establish and Improve a Working Mechanism

Organization and Management

Collaborative efforts of all levels of education administrations and health administrations should be made to establish a leadership team for health and disease control in schools. Joint meetings for heath and disease control in schools should be regularly held to discuss and solve the problems in TB control in schools. And strategies and measures for TB control applicable in the administrative area should be formulated. The health and disease control in schools should be regularly assessed to strengthen the implementation of the strategies and measures, especially those for TB control. The emergency management of TB epidemic in schools should be guided and collaborated by the leadership team.

A managing office should be established for organizing, managing, collaborating, communicating, and information collecting as well as emergency management and logistic service during sudden epidemics.

Regular Health Examination for Teachers and Students

Health examination for students before enrollment and regular health examination for teachers are important. And investigations for TB should be listed as compulsory item for early detection and early control of TB.

Regulations for TB Control in Schools

Regulations for TB control in schools should be formulated based on the characteristics of each school. And in the regulation, the responsibilities should be clearly defined and a system of accountability should be established to respond to sudden epidemics and scattering epidemics of TB in schools.

Technical Procedures for Surveillance of Epidemics, Detection, and Reporting of TB Cases

In each school, a staff responsible for reporting TB cases should be designated. Under the leadership of the working team on health in the school, the designated staff is responsible for reporting suspected epidemics and cases of TB. The staff should also be responsible for guiding the morning examination, registry of absence in the school, and data collection and analysis.

Morning Examination and Absence Due to Illness in Schools

In each school, morning examination and trace for absence due to illness should be implemented. The class teacher is the person of chief responsibility for conducting morning examination as well as registry and trace of absence due to illness in the class.

A Working Mechanism for Joint Control of TB Epidemic in Schools

Based on the principle of localization management, the collaborative efforts by multisections should be strengthened. And a working mechanism for joint control of TB epidemics in schools should be established. Regular meetings of the administrations of health and education should be held for communication and collaboration in TB control in schools [5].

The administration of education should closely communicate with the local administration of health to improve the surveillance system of TB in schools. Round and selective inspection should be conducted in the schools of the administered area.

The administration of health should also formulate an emergency plan for sudden major public health events. Meanwhile, the administration of health should also inform timely about the epidemic of TB in schools. And TB control measures should be implemented in all-level TB control agencies.

The administration in schools should closely communicate with the TB control agency. And morning examination as well as registry and trace of absence due to illness should be regularly conducted. If suspected and defined cases of TB are detected, the school administration should actively communicate with the local TB control agency. Meanwhile, the school administration should also assist to manage the epidemic of TB. And the management of suspended schooling and reentry should be strictly implemented.

The TB control agency is responsible for epidemic surveillance, field epidemiological survey, and screening of individuals with close contact. And the information about epidemic surveillance, field epidemiological survey, and screening of individuals with close contact should be timely feedback to the school. Meanwhile, the TB control agency should also guide the management of patients and infection control in schools.

Definitive Responsibilities for TB Control

Responsibilities of the Education Administration

(1) The education administration should pay close attention to TB control in schools. The management and leadership for TB control in schools should be strengthened. The education administration should also collaborate with the health administration to formulate policies on TB control in schools.
(2) The health and disease control in schools should be listed into the performance assessment on schools. Joint inspection by the education and health administrations should be regularly performed for formulation and implementation of disease control measures.
(3) Joint efforts by the education and health administrations should be made to monitor occurrence of TB in schools of the administered area. And the schools should be informed with tips for health.
(4) Epidemics of TB in schools should be investigated and managed jointly by the education and health administrations.

Responsibilities of Schools

(1) Guided by the education and health administrations, TB control should be enlisted into the work plan of the schools.
(2) A leadership team for disease control should be established in schools. The principal of the school should be the person with chief responsibilities for disease control. And a working mechanism that the principal is generally responsible for disease control and a deputy principal is responsible for implementation of measures for disease control should be established. A network with the principal, medical practitioner in school or health-care teacher, and class teacher should be established for control of infectious diseases. And a specific person should have specific responsibilities to implement the measures.
(3) The reporting system of epidemics in schools should be established. And a specific person should be designated to take the responsibility for reporting the epidemics.
(4) Collaborating with the health administration, schools are responsible for training of principals, health-care staffs in schools and class teachers about TB control.
(5) The schools are also responsible for health education about TB control.
(6) The schools are responsible for collaborating with health administration to investigate and manage epidemics of TB.

Responsibilities of Health-Care Institutions in Schools

The health-care institutions in schools include school hospitals, school clinics, and school health-care clinics. Under the leadership of the working team on disease control in school, the health-care institutions in schools have the following responsibilities:

(1) The health-care institutions in schools are responsible for formulating and implementing the working plan for TB control in the school.

(2) The health-care institutions in schools are responsible for detecting, registering, reporting, referring of patients with TB as well as surveillance of TB epidemics. And the health-care institutions in schools are responsible for DOT of patients with TB and individuals with prophylactic medication.
(3) The health-care institutions in schools are responsible for tracing the cases or suspected cases of TB.
(4) The health-care institutions in schools are responsible for health education and health promotion about TB control in schools.
(5) The health-care institutions in schools are also responsible for collaborating with TB control agency to conduct screening for individuals with close contact to patient with TB.

Responsibilities of Health Administration

(1) The health administration is responsible for enlisting TB control in schools into the local plan for disease control. And goal-oriented assessment on performance should be conducted for TB control in schools.
(2) The health administration is responsible for collaborating with the education administration to formulate TB control measures in schools.
(3) The health administration is responsible for organizing the TB control agency to provide technical guidance for TB control in schools.
(4) The health administration is responsible for formulating emergency responding plan during epidemics of TB and organizing the investigation and management during sudden public health events of TB epidemics.
(5) The health administration is responsible for informing the education administration about the epidemics of TB in schools.
(6) The health administration is also responsible for collaborating with the education administration to supervise the implementation of TB control measures in schools.

Responsibilities of TB Control Agency

Responsibilities of City-Level TB Control Agency

(1) The city-level TB control agency is responsible for formulating TB control plan in schools of the city, establishing the regulations for TB control in schools of the city, and organizing their implementation by all the TB control agencies in the city.
(2) The city-level TB control agency is responsible for providing technical training and service for all the TB control agencies in the city, and providing technical guidance for the county/district-level TB control agencies.
(3) The city-level TB control agency is responsible for collecting and reporting information about epidemics of TB in schools as well as the related field epidemiological survey and management reported by the county/district-level TB control agency to the health administration.
(4) The city-level TB control agency is responsible for supervising and assessing the TB control in schools of the city. The discovered problems should be urged for rectification.
(5) The city-level TB control agency is responsible for assisting county/district-level TB control agency to conduct field epidemiological survey and management during sudden public health events of TB epidemics in schools.
(6) The city-level TB control agency is responsible for assisting county/district-level TB control agency to conduct health education about TB control in schools.

Responsibilities of County/District-Level TB Control Agency

(1) Based on the localization management, the county/district-level TB control agency is responsible for assisting schools to formulate TB control plan, and improve the joint TB control mechanism, responsible system, and regulations on TB control in the school. In addition, the county/district-level TB control agency is responsible for providing technical training and support for TB control in schools, providing technical guidance regularly in schools, and understanding the implementation of TB control measures in schools.
(2) The county/district-level TB control agency is responsible for formulating TB control plan for schools each year, and organizing the implementation of the plan.
(3) The county/district-level TB control agency is responsible for diagnosing, reporting, registering, treating, managing the patients with TB and their health education about TB control.
(4) The county/district-level TB control agency is responsible for browsing the Information System of Infectious Diseases about cases or suspected cases of TB from schools, and confirming their presentation in health-care institutions for diagnosis and treatment. For cases with no presentation in health-care institutions, the county/district-level TB control agency is responsible for contacting with the school to trace the case.
(5) The county/district-level TB control agency is responsible for collecting and analyzing the data about TB epidemics in schools, predicting the occurrence and prevalence of TB in schools, and reporting the information to the health administration, education administration, superior TB control agency, and schools. In addition, TB control measures should be simultaneously proposed.
(6) Once patient with active TB is detected, the county/district-level TB control agency is responsible for conducting field epidemiological survey and management of TB epidemic in the school. And the management of the TB epidemic should be reported to the health and education administrations as well as superior TB control agency.

(7) When sudden public health event of TB epidemic occurs, the county/district-level TB control agency is responsible for establishing an emergency management team to manage and assess the TB epidemic. The responsibilities include verifying the TB epidemic, conducting the epidemiological survey, assessing the range of its spread, screening the individuals with close contact to patient, diagnosing, treating, and managing the patients, conducting health education, predicting the development of TB epidemic, reporting the event and management to the health and education administrations as well as superior TB control agency, and proposing specific measures to stop its further spread.

(8) The county/district-level TB control agency is responsible for conducting health education about TB control in schools. Targeting different populations in schools, such as administrators, teachers, school health-care staffs, students, patients with TB, and individuals with close contact to patient with TB, health education should be conducted about TB control policies, TB control measures, and TB control knowledge. The health education is intended to raise their awareness about TB control and self-protection against TB in schools.

Responsibilities of Health-Care Institutions

(1) The health-care institutions are responsible for diagnosis, registry, reporting, and referral of the suspected cases. It is important for the first consulted physician to take notes about the defined and suspected cases of TB in teachers or students in schools. The recorded information includes the name of school (with specified department for teachers or students from universities), grade, and class. If hospitalization is not necessary, the patient is referred to the TB control agency according to localization management. If the health-care institution is so poorly equipped that the diagnosis of TB cannot be diagnosed, after registry and reporting, the patient is referred to TB control agency.

(2) The health-care institutions are responsible for treatment and standardized management of critically and acutely ill patients with TB. Any health-care institution is responsible for active treatment of critically and acutely ill patients with TB, and standardized management of inpatients with TB. After being discharged, the patient is referred to local TB control agency according to localization management for consecutive treatment and management.

(3) During the diagnosis and treatment of teacher or student patients with TB, the health-care institutions are also responsible for their health education about TB control. To secure the uniform detection, treatment and management in the local TB control agency according to localization management, or standardized treatment during hospitalization, the physician is responsible for health education for 10 min about TB control policies and measures.

Health Surveillance Institution

(1) Health surveillance institution is responsible for supervising and inspecting the implementation of TB control measures in schools. The local health surveillance institution is responsible for active, scientific, and effective supervision and inspection of TB control measures in schools.

(2) Health surveillance institution is also responsible to urge the schools to establish and improve the TB control measures according to the policies formulated and issued by the health and education administrations. Based on its supervision and inspection, the TB control measures should be implemented for early detection, early reporting, and early management of TB patients.

2.2 Detection of Patients

Active Detection of Patients

Active early detection of patients with TB is an important measure to prevent spread of TB in schools. Health examination is the important way for early detection of TB, which plays important role in forward shift of TB control procedure. Morning examination and trace of absence due to illness are important components of TB control in schools, and are the most important measures for early detection of TB to avoid aggregation epidemic of TB and stop spread of TB in schools. Via early detection, early quarantine, and early treatment of patient with active TB, especially communicable TB, the spread of TB in school can be timely stopped.

Health Examination

According to policies formulated and issued by the health and education administrations, detection of TB is compulsory in health examination before enrollment of students and annual routine health examination of teachers. The health examination is performed by qualified institution that is well equipped for detection of TB. And the results of health examinations are filed into the health documents of students and teachers.

The TB control agency is responsible for technical support and guidance in health examination of teachers and students.

The health examination institution is responsible for reporting the defined or suspected cases of TB to the school. And the school is responsible to inform the student (or parents) or the teacher to receive further management in local TB control agency, and to trace the results of management.

During health examination, the students migrating to the city from the regions with recent occurrence of natural disasters, such as earthquake and flood, or from seriously affected region of TB are paid close attention. Such attention facilitates early detection of infection source to decrease the risk of its spread.

In the health examination, TB is detected via inquiry about history of BCG vaccination, inquiry about history of contact to patient with TB, inquiry about suspected symptoms of TB, PPD skin test, and chest X-ray. If necessary, γ interferon release assay and chest CT scan are performed to detect TB.

Morning Examination

The schools are responsible for establishing a surveillance network for suspected symptoms of TB. A working staff is designated to be responsible for morning examination and reporting of infectious disease epidemic. The class teacher or a student responsible for health surveillance in the class conducts the morning examination. And the health-care staff in schools is responsible for reporting epidemic of infectious disease.

(1) The school hospital or health-care clinic is responsible for training the students responsible for health surveillance in their classes.
(2) The class health inspector is responsible for morning examination of the students in the class. And each student in the class should be known about the presentation of suspected symptoms such as cough, expectoration, and hemoptysis.
(3) If any student shows suspected symptoms of TB, such as cough and expectoration for above 2 weeks, hemoptysis or with blood-stained sputum, the class health inspector is responsible for registering and reporting the case to the school hospital or school health-care clinic.
(4) After reception of the reporting, the school hospital or school health-care clinic is responsible for further registry and referral of the suspected patient to the local TB control agency for further diagnosis and treatment. For suspected patients in kindergartens, primary schools, and middle schools, the parents have also been informed.
(5) After referral, the school hospital or health-care clinic is responsible for tracing the student about the presentation in the TB control agency and the defined diagnosis.

Trace of Absence Due to Illness

(1) The class health inspector is responsible for paying attention to the absence due to illness. For students with absence to the class, the reason for absence should be known. If the absence is due to illness, the symptoms, the presenting health-care institution, and the diagnosis should be further inquired.
(2) If the absence lasts for above 2 days due to suspected symptoms of TB, the absent student should be timely reported to the school hospital or school health-care clinic. The school hospital or school health-care clinic is then responsible for tracing the absent student about the diagnosis and treatment as well as registering the related information about the student.

Reporting and Referral

Recommendation of Presentation

If the school hospital or school health-care clinic is not so well equipped for preliminary diagnosis of TB, the suspected cases of TB detected by health examination, morning examination, or trace of absence should be recommended to receive investigations in the local TB control agency. And the school hospital or school health-care clinic is responsible for tracing the case about the presentation, diagnosis, and treatment.

Reporting and Referral

If the school hospital or school health-care clinic is so well equipped to perform preliminary diagnosis of TB, chest X-ray and sputum bacteriology test should be performed for the suspected cases detected in the health examination, morning examination, and trace of absence. The school hospital or school health-care clinic is responsible for filling the infectious disease reporting card and forwarding the card on-line or to the local TB control agency within 24 h. Meanwhile, the school hospital or school health-care clinic is also responsible for referring the suspected patient to the local TB control agency for further diagnosis and treatment, and tracing the suspected patient about the diagnosis and treatment in local TB control agency.

Passive Detection of Patient

TB Control Agency

(1) If a patient defined with TB by TB control agency is from a school, the TB control agency is responsible for recording the name of the school (the name of department for university student), address of residence, and contact number. Meanwhile, the TB control agency is also responsible for informing the school and the local TB control agency according to localization management.
(2) The county/district-level TB control agency is responsible for browsing the information about on-line reporting of TB according to localization management. The population aged under 25 years, patient from school, or identity as student or teacher, should be paid close attention.
(3) After receiving report or detecting defined or suspected case of TB in schools of localization management, the county/district-level TB control agency is responsible for designating a staff to follow up the case within 3 days.
(4) The county/district-level TB control agency is responsible for routine surveillance of aggregation TB epidemic by close attention on multiple cases from one school. If occurrence of at least three cases of TB in one school is detected, tendency of aggregation epidemic of TB is recorded, reported, and confirmed. If necessary, field survey is conducted to confirm the occurrence of aggrega-

tion epidemic. The field survey mainly includes trace of multiple cases in one school to define or exclude the diagnosis of TB, screening of the individuals with close contacts, understandings about epidemiological association between the defined cases. If epidemiological association between the defined cases is detected, the event should be reported and feedback to the local health administration, superior TB control agency, and the school.

(5) The staff responsible for TB control in schools in county/district-level TB control agency pays close attention to the information and clues on aggregation epidemic of TB in schools via various information channels. If occurrence of aggregation epidemic of TB in school is reported via any information channel, staffs are designated to confirm the information. And the confirmed information is reported and feedback to the related institutions.

Health-Care Institution

The health-care institution is highly alert to the suspected cases of TB from schools. Standardized chest X-ray and sputum bacteriology test should be performed. For student patient with defined diagnosis of TB, reporting card of infectious disease should be filled according to the related standards. The name of school, grade, major, address of residence, and contact number should be filled in detail. And the information should be informed to the local TB control agency according to localization management.

For hospitalized student patient with defined diagnosis of TB, the reporting card of infectious disease should be filled and reported. For discharged student patient, the triplet referral sheet should be filled. And the patient should be referred to the local TB control agency according to the address of the school and the address of residence.

2.3 Health Education About TB Control

Objective

The health education about TB control in schools is intended to raise students' and teachers' awareness about TB control. Based on the increased knowledge about TB control, the students and teachers are promoted to keep environment of school, change unfavorable hygienic habit, keep healthy behaviors, actively monitor TB, and early detect TB for effective treatment. Therefore, spread of TB can be stopped in schools.

Methods

The ways of health education about TB control are diversifying. Appropriate way of health education about TB control should be selected according to the need and cognitive capability of specific groups of students. Both traditional lectures and innovative new media can be adopted.

Health Education on Enrollment and Health Education Class

During freshmen education in junior middle schools, high schools, and universities, health education about TB control is conducted in classes or grades. Alternatively, brochures on TB control are spread in freshmen. Otherwise, health education classes are regularly held to spread the knowledge about TB control. The health education about TB control is to spread the core information about TB control and other popular science about TB control and health promotion.

Campus Activities on Health Education

Various campus activities are conducted to spread knowledge about TB control, such as speeches, a letter to parents, campus broadcast, hand-written newspaper, blackboard newspaper, class meeting, lectures, quiz show, and essay competition.

Print Media for Health Education

The print media, including brochure, leaflet, poster, panels, and blackboard newspaper, is applied for health education about TB control.

Audio and Video for Health Education

The audio and video products, including cartoon, allegro, and public service advertisement, are played to spread knowledge about TB control.

Other New Media for Health Education

Other new media, including official account of Wechat, Wechat group, school official website, and Weibo, is applied to spread knowledge about TB control.

Content of Health Education

Core Knowledge of TB Control in School Health Education

(1) Pulmonary TB is a chronic infectious disease with serious long-term threats to the health of human being.
(2) Pulmonary TB mainly spread via respiratory tract and everyone may be infected.
(3) Cough and expectoration for above 2 weeks are suspected symptoms of pulmonary TB. And the suspected patients should present to health-care institution for diagnosis and treatment as early as possible.
(4) No spitting, covering the mouth and nose when coughing and sneezing, and wearing face mask help decreasing the spread of TB.
(5) By standardized whole course treatment, most patients with TB can be cured and interpersonal spread of TB can be avoided.

(6) When TB is suspected or defined, active reporting to the school is recommended. Keeping the suffering of TB as a secret and presence to class as a patient with TB should be avoided.
(7) A habit of opening window for ventilation is favorable.
(8) Sufficient sleep, well-balance diet, and more physical exercise are recommended for protection against diseases.

Popular Science for Health Education about TB Control

The lectures on popular science of TB control include the following contents:

(1) What is TB?
(2) How is TB spread?
(3) Who are susceptible to TB?
(4) Why are students susceptible to TB?
(5) What are the common symptoms of TB?
(6) What should be done if TB is suspected?
(7) What are recommended during treatment for TB?
(8) What are the consequences of non-standardized treatment of TB?

Emphasis on TB Control in School

Control of Infection Source

The main source of infection is patient with active TB, especially bacteriologically positive TB. A sputum smear-positive TB patient during excretion of bacteria can infect 10–15 persons each year. Therefore, early detection and cure of TB is the key for TB control and protection of healthy populations.

Break of the Spreading Routes

The Mtb is mainly spread via droplets inhaled by the respiratory tract. Favorable ventilation is important to stop its spread, especially in densely populated places. Do not talk to others at a short distance, cover the mouth and nose when coughing and sneezing, wear a face mask, and do not spit are recommended. The daily necessities of patient, such as his/her beddings, should be exposed to sunlight for sterilization.

Protection of Susceptible Population

The infants and young children aged under 3 years should be inoculated with BCG vaccine, which decreases the incidence of serious TB and tuberculous meningitis. And sufficient sleep, well-balanced diet, and more physical exercise are recommended for children aged above 4 years and adults to strengthen their immunity against disease.

Assessment

The conduct of health education in schools and its effects should be regularly inspected and assessed and the assessment should be enlisted as a routine in TB control in schools. Meanwhile, before and after health education, surveys on the core information awareness and the route of knowledge acquisition should be conducted to compare the coverage rate and awareness rate of knowledge about TB control as well as changes of their beliefs and behaviors. By such comparison, the effects of health education are assessed. In addition, targeting the weaknesses in health education and its assessment, changes are made to improve the effects of health education.

2.4 Environmental Health in Schools

According to the standards and requirements in the National Basic Standards on Sports and Hygiene in Schools of China and the Standards on Construction and Management of Life and Hygiene Equipments in Rural Boarding Schools of China, the per capita area for study and life should be guaranteed. Meanwhile, the densely populated areas, such as classrooms, dormitories, libraries, and canteens should be well ventilated. The campus should be regularly cleaned. And the ventilation includes natural ventilation and mechanical ventilation. The natural ventilation should be persistent if the condition permits. Otherwise, ventilation for above 10 min/h or once ventilation for above 70 min should be secured [6].

2.5 Vaccination

BCG vaccine is the suspension of attenuated bovine mycobacterium tuberculosis. It is capable of strengthening the activities of macrophages to kill tumor cells and activating T lymphocytes to strengthen the cellular immunity. BCG vaccination is to artificially trigger a mild non-hazardous primary infection of Mtb for specific immunity against Mtb infection. So far, BCG vaccine has been developed for more than 80 years. In 182 countries and regions, approximately 4 billion children have been inoculated with BCG vaccine. However, BCG vaccination cannot kill the Mtb that has invaded the human body and cannot stop the onset of the disease. It only acts to stop the spread of re-infected Mtb within human body. Therefore, it plays certain role in preventing serious TB disseminated along with blood, such as tuberculous meningitis and miliary pulmonary TB [7].

3 Control and Management

3.1 Management of Patient with TB in School

Treatment Management of Patient with TB

To guarantee the correct and regular medication and completion of the therapeutic course for cure, the patients receiving treatment should be effectively managed.

Whole Course DOT

For patients with communicable pulmonary TB or serious bacteriologically negative TB and hospitalized student patients, directly observed treatment is conducted during the whole course of treatment.

Whole Course Management

For patients with non-serious bacteriologically negative TB, student patients with TB for whom suspended schooling is unnecessary, and patients with TB receiving continual treatment after discharge, the whole course management is conducted. Health education is strengthened for such patients. Regular medications and regular follow-ups are urged by the health-care staff in school hospital or school health-care clinic, chief class teacher, or parents. The TB control agency is responsible for regular visits of the patients, review of the medications, and delay (including no presentation or no dispensary) recovery to secure correct and regular medication of the patients.

Management of Suspended Schooling and Reentry

Management of Suspended Schooling

For student patients with at least one of the following conditions, a certificate for suspended schooling is provided by the county/district-level TB control agency or designated hospital for TB after reviewed by the local county/district-level TB control agency of the school. And the school is responsible for suspended schooling management of the student patients based on the certificate of suspended schooling provided by local county/district-level TB control agency of the school.

(1) Bacteriologically positive TB is diagnosed, including sputum smear positive, sputum culture positive, or molecular biologically positive.
(2) Bacteriologically negative TB is diagnosed, and chest X-ray demonstrates extensive lesions in lung and/or accompanying cavity.
(3) The patient shows obvious symptoms of TB.
(4) The patient has other conditions for which suspended schooling is recommended by TB control agency.

For student patient with TB who returns to his/her permanent registered residence for treatment during schooling suspension, the information about his/her diagnosis and treatment is transferred by the local TB control agency of the school to the TB control agency of his/her permanent registered residence. And the TB control agency of the permanent registered residence is responsible for standardized management during the treatment. During schooling suspension for treatment, school health-care staff, patient, local TB control agency of the school, and local TB control agency of the permanent registered residence closely communicate with each other. The school health-care staff and the local TB control agency of the school are informed about the presentation, treatment and management, improvement of the condition, and the therapeutic outcome of the patient.

For patients receiving quarantine and treatment in school, local TB control agency of the school and the school are responsible for the treatment and management of the patient. The school is responsible for places of quarantine and treatment. The school health-care staff is responsible for whole course DOT. For patients with suspended schooling for quarantine and treatment, the school health-care staff, patient, and the local TB control agency of the school keep close communication. The school health-care staff is responsible for reporting the medications and adverse reactions after medications to the local TB control agency of the school. The local TB control agency of the school timely informs the school health-care staff about the subsequent presentations, the condition of the patient, and the therapeutic outcome.

Management of Reentry

After standardized treatment with improved condition, if the patient is in accordance to the following conditions, a certificate of diagnosis is provided by the county/district-level TB control agency. And a certificate of reentry is provided by the local TB control agency of the school after reviewing the certificate of diagnosis. With the certificate of reentry, the student is permitted to go back school. The school is then responsible for reentry procedures and continual treatment and management.

(1) For patients with bacteriologically positive TB or serious bacteriologically negative TB (including patients with cavity, large flake of caseous necrosis, miliary pulmonary TB), the standardized treatment is completed. Standards of cure or successful treatment are reached in the initially treated, re-treated, and drug resistant patients (including single drug resistance, multidrug resistance, and extensive drug resistance).
(2) For patients with bacteriologically negative TB, the standardized treatment persists for 2 months and the patients show alleviated or no symptoms, obvious absorption of lesions by chest X-ray. In addition, the subsequent sputum smear test shows negative for twice (with an interval of at least 1 month), and the sputum culture shows negative at least once.

Management of Teacher Patient

The schooling suspension and reentry management in teacher patients with TB refers to the requirements for student patients.

2. Screening of individuals with close contact and management of high-risk populations

Screening of Individuals with Close Contact

If a patient from school is clinically diagnosed with TB, screening of individuals with close contact is necessary, which has great significance in preventing aggregation epidemic of TB in school. Via screening, more patients with active TB can be timely detected for quarantine and treatment to stop further spread of TB. And patients with latent TB infection can be detected and subsequent intervention can stop its further progression into active TB.

Definition of Individuals with Close Contact

Individuals with close contact refer to the individuals who live together with the patient, such as roommates and family members, classmates in the same classroom in middle and primary schools. In addition, schoolmates with consecutive and direct contact to the patient for above 8 h or accumulatively for above 40 h within 3 months prior to the definitive diagnosis of TB at universities or other schools with non-fixed classrooms.

Screening of Individuals with Close Contact

Coverage of Screening

Once a patient with active TB in school under the jurisdiction was detected, the TB control agency is responsible for contacting the school for case study. And the TB control agency is also responsible for screening of TB in classmates, roommates, and teachers of the patient. If above one case of TB is detected by screening, the screening of TB is extended to the schoolmates on the same floor of the classroom building and on the same floor of the dormitory building. Meanwhile, based on the case study and filed study, the coverage of screening can be appropriately extended. And the family members of the patients are also covered by the screening of TB.

Methods of Screening

After the coverage of screening is defined, all of the individuals with close contact are inquired about suspected symptoms of TB.

All of the individuals with close contact should receive PPD skin test. According to the National Health-care Service Standards for Diagnosis of Tuberculosis (WS288-2017), demonstration of hard nodule with an average diameter of ≥15 mm, or local double rings, blister, necrosis, and lymphangitis in PPD skin test indicates strong positive. For individuals contraindicated to PPD skin tests, such as patients with fever, history of allergy to vaccination, serious skin disease, asthma, and other serious illnesses, interferon γ release assay can be an alternative.

As a way of screening suspected cases of TB, chest X-ray is performed for individuals under 15 years old with close contact showing suspected symptoms of TB or strong positive in PPD skin test (positive in interferon γ release assay). In addition, chest X-ray is performed for all the individuals above 15 years old with close contact.

For individuals with suspected symptoms of TB, strong positive in PPD skin test (or positive in interferon γ release assay), or suspected lesion of TB by chest X-ray, three specimens of sputum (instant sputum, morning sputum, and night sputum) are collected for acid-fast staining and Mtb culture. If necessary, molecular biological examination of sputum is performed simultaneously. For cases of sputum culture positive, strain identification and drug sensitivity test are performed. In economically well-developed regions, Mtb strains pool of school is established to safely preserve the isolated strains of Mtb for review and molecular epidemiological study.

Management of High-Risk Populations

Suspected Cases of TB

The suspected case of TB detected by screening is referred to the local TB control agency for further definitive diagnosis.

Patients with Mtb Infection

(1) For individuals with close contact showing strong positive in PPD skin test (nodule diameter ≥5 mm in patients with HIV positive or receiving immunosuppressant for above 1 month) and with no abnormality by chest X-ray, prophylactic drug is administered based on informed consent [8].
(2) For individuals with close contact showing non-strong positive in PPD skin test and with no abnormality by chest X-ray, the PPD skin test is performed again after 2–3 months. If the PPD skin test converse to strong positive and active TB is excluded by chest X-ray, recent Mtb infection is more likely. Based on informed consent, prophylactic drug is administered.
(3) For individuals with close contact but no prophylactic medication, health education and following medical observation are reinforced. Once suspected symptoms of TB are detected during medical observation, presentation to TB control agency is necessary for diagnosis. Generally, the medical observation lasts for 1–2 years. It is recommended that the individuals with close contact present to TB control agency for relevant investigation of TB at 3, 6, 12, and 24 months after initial screening.

Prophylactic Treatment

Objects of Treatment

The main objects of prophylactic medication are high-risk individuals of TB onset in population with Mtb infection. For those in accordance with the criteria of prophylactic treatment, prophylactic drug is administered based on informed consent. Specifically, the subjects include:

(1) Children in kindergarten who have close contact to patient with sputum smear-positive TB.
(2) Children in kindergarten and students in universities, middle and primary schools who show nodule with diameter ≥15 mm or blister in PPD skin test.
(3) Individuals with recent conversion from negative to positive in PPD skin test or individuals with enlarged nodule in PPD skin test by ≥10 mm in diameter within 2 years.
(4) Patients with HIV/AIDS and PPD skin test positive.
(5) Individuals with PPD skin test positive and receiving glucocorticoid or another immunosuppressant for above 1 month.

Treatment Regimen

(1) Only isoniazid is administered at a dosage of 10 mg/kg body weight, once a day. And the total daily dosage should not exceed 300 mg. Six months constitute one therapeutic course. The regimen shows relatively less adverse reactions but the therapeutic course lasts for a long period of time. During medication, patient needs to be well managed. In regions with high occurrence of isoniazid resistance, the regimen is not recommended.
(2) Only rifampicin is administered at a dosage of 10 mg/kg body weight, once a day. And the total daily dosage should not exceed 600 mg. Four months constitute one therapeutic course. The regimen is indicated to patients intolerant to isoniazid and those with poor compliance to long-term medication.
(3) Isoniazid and rifampicin are administered. The dosage of isoniazid is as the above, oral intake once a day. The dosage of rifampicin is 10 mg/kg body weight, oral intake once a day, and the total daily dosage should not exceed 600 mg. Three months constitute one therapeutic course. The regimen shows more adverse reactions but the therapeutic course lasts for a short period of time. The patients thus show favorable compliance with the regimen.
(4) Isoniazid and rifapentine are administered. The dosage of isoniazid is as the above, oral intake once a day. The dosage of rifapentine is oral intake of 450–600 mg, twice a week. Three months constitute one therapeutic course. The regimen shows less adverse reactions and the therapeutic course lasts for a short period of time. The dosage and adverse reaction for children under 15 years old remains unknown.

Precautions During Prophylactic Medication

(1) Prophylactic medication is voluntarily based on informed consent. And the physician prescribes appropriate regimen according to specific conditions.
(2) Before prophylactic medication, active TB is excluded.
(3) There are no contraindications to the prophylactic medication, such as drug allergy, psychiatric disorder, liver, and kidney insufficiency.
(4) Prophylactic medication is recorded in detail. And DOT strategy is applied by the school health-care staff or family member to ensure regular medication and completion of therapeutic course.
(5) The liver and kidney functions are closely monitored during prophylactic medication. The adverse reactions are timely managed.
(6) Health education about significance, methods, and precautions of prophylactic medication is conducted before and during prophylactic medication.

3.2 Infection Control

After TB is detected, the patient with communicable TB is quarantined and treated. Meanwhile, environment control measures are implemented for the densely populated places, such as classroom, dormitory, library, and canteen to control the infection of TB.

Quarantine of Patient with Communicable TB

If sputum bacteriologic positive TB, serious bacteriologic negative TB, or obvious symptoms of TB is detected in teachers or students, the patients should be quarantined immediately for treatment to cut off their close contact with other teachers and students. In such a way, the spread of Mtb can be stopped in teachers and students.

Environment Control Measures

Generally, classrooms, dormitories, and other public places have comparatively close space which is poorly ventilated. If patient of TB is detected, his/her classroom and dormitory should be managed in the following ways.

Natural or Mechanical Ventilation

Natural ventilation is the simplest measure of environment control with the lowest cost. If natural ventilation is not favorable or possible, mechanical ventilation is an alternative. The daily ventilation should last for at least 70 min.

Air Sterilization

Air sterilization should be performed in an environment with no person, with doors, and windows closed. After the air sterilization, the doors and windows can be opened for ventilation. The air sterilization includes:

(1) Ultraviolet radiation is a way of air sterilization. The average radiation energy should be at least 1.5 W/m^3 for at least 30 min.
(2) Another way of air sterilization is aerosol fumigation or spray of chemical disinfectant. Peroxyacetic acid solution at a concentration of 0.5–1.0% can be selected for aerosol fumigation for 2 h. Hydrogen peroxide compound air dis-

infectant or quaternary ammonium disinfectant solution can be selected for spray sterilization for 30 min.

Sterilization of Floors and Object Surface

For sterilization of floors, peracetic acid solution at a concentration of 0.1% or effective chlorine disinfectant at a concentration of 1000–2000 mg/L can be applied to mop or spray the floor. For sterilization of object surface, such as desks, chairs, cabinets, doors, and windows, effective chlorine disinfectant at a concentration of 1000–2000 mg/L can be applied to wipe the object surface.

3.3 Management of Sudden Public Health Event of TB

At least ten cases of TB with epidemiological association within a certain period of time in one school or occurrence of death from TB in one school are potentially a sudden public health event. And sudden public health event is defined and verified by the county/district-level health administration according to the National Emergency Planning for Sudden Public Health Event in China and other regulations. Based on technical procedures, sudden public health event of TB can be directly defined by county/district-level health administration. And the technical procedures for management of sudden public health event of TB are shown in Fig. 6.2.

Detection

Via active surveillance, telephone reporting, and screening of individuals with close contact, patient with TB is detected by county/district-level TB control agency. The defined case of TB is then compared with the defined cases of TB with the same workplace, school, and residence address to explore the possible epidemiological association.

Confirmation

The epidemiological association between the cases of TB is preliminarily confirmed by county/district-level TB control agency to define sudden public health event. And the event is immediately reported.

Field Survey

Management and Informing

The school with sudden public health event of TB should be informed about the occurrence of event and the time of field management. The individuals who should receive screening of TB are preliminarily defined and informed about the consecutive management. The patients with communicable TB are suspended of schooling or working. Ventilation and sterilization are performed. The place for field survey and management, and the time of survey are defined. The basic information of the individuals with close contact is recorded and registered. The basic information includes name, gender, date of birth, nationality, relationship with patient, contact number, duration and frequency of contact, and place of contact.

Preparation of Working Staffs and Materials

Field survey is prepared. A working team for management of sudden public health event of TB is established with professionals of epidemiology, radiology, physician, and nurse. Vehicles and drivers are appointed. And materials for inspecting, sterilization, self-protection, and emergency rescuing as well as questionnaires and cameras are prepared for field survey.

Field Survey

Health Education Before Field Survey

The school with occurrence of sudden public health event of TB is informed about the occurrence of the event and its control measures. And health education about TB control is conducted for collaborative efforts of the school and elimination of fears.

Content of Field Survey

The process of event, arrangement of buildings, environmental hygiene, implementation of routine health control measures, quarantine of the patients, and the mood of school personnel are known by field survey. Based on the field survey, the severity of the event is comprehensively assessed, based on which the time of field management and range of screening are defined. The contents of field survey include:

(1) Process of event

The cases of TB are actively searched. All the information about patients of TB within target area, population, and health-care institutions are collected. And their diagnosis is confirmed case by case. In chronological order, the defined and suspected cases of TB are analyzed. And the initial case and consecutive cases are known about their onset, consultation, diagnosis, treatment, and management.

(2) Epidemiological survey of the defined cases

The survey is to understand the basic condition, onset, diagnosis, treatment, and activities after onset of the patients.

(3) Information about school

The information about school includes address, surrounding environment, organizational framework, total amount of teachers and students, distribution of buildings, numbers and professions of health-care staffs, implementation of routine health control measures, field sterilization, implementation of suspension, and quarantine measures.

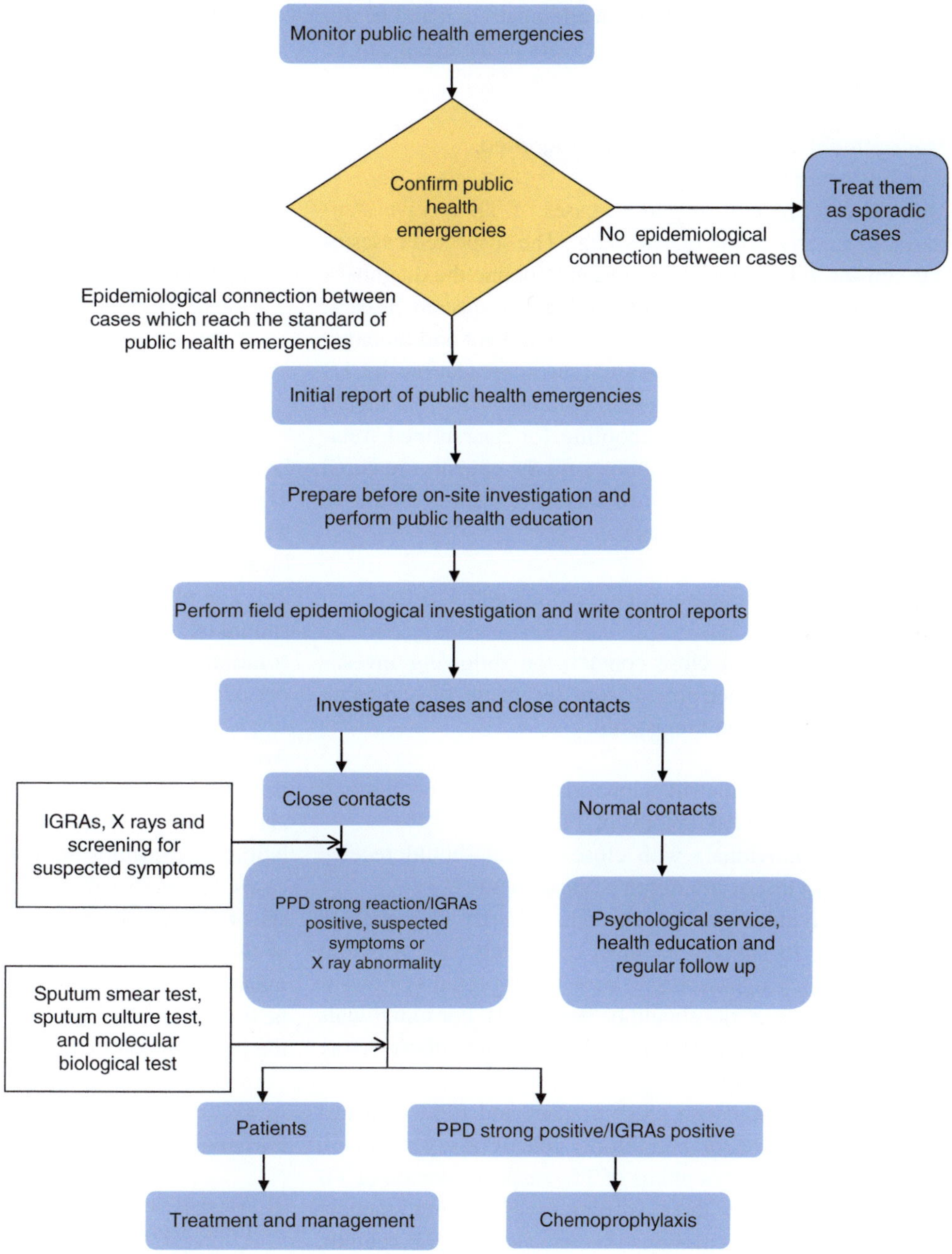

Fig. 6.2 Emergency response when TB breaks out

(4) Offices/classrooms

The number of working teachers or studying students in one office or classroom, location, surrounding environment, ventilation, hygiene, air-conditioner, ultraviolet radiation, exhaust fan, distribution of seats, and changes are known in the field survey.

(5) Individuals with close contact

Individuals with close contact refer to those who have close contacts to patient with TB, especially those live or study with patient of sputum smear-positive TB at the same floor or in the same classroom for a long period of time. Based on the facts analysis, other individuals may also be included as individuals with close contact. The field survey includes the contact, their knowledge about epidemic of TB, self-protection measures, and mood.

(6) Reporting

After field survey, the working team finishes survey report according to the findings in the field survey.

Field Control

Health Education

In the school with occurrence of sudden public health event of TB, health education by TB control agency is strengthened under the guidance of health administration and health education institute. And emotional fears of the event can be eliminated via health education.

Management of Defined, Clinically Diagnosed, and Suspected Case of TB

Defined or clinically diagnosed cases of TB receive standardized treatment and management. The suspected cases of TB consult in health-care institution to define the diagnosis. All the defined, clinically diagnosed, and suspected cases of TB should rest and cooperate to the treatment and management according to the professional recommendations by TB control agency. The patients with communicable TB should suspend their working or schooling for quarantined treatment according to the regulations until the patients are cured or significantly improved for reentry. The reentry should be approved by TB control agency.

Screening and Management of Individuals with Close Contact

For individuals with close contact, the following investigations should be performed. And the result of screening should be recorded and registered.

(1) All the individuals with close contact should be inquired about suspected symptoms of TB.
(2) All the individuals with close contact should receive PPD skin test or interferon γ release assay.
(3) For individuals with close contact under 15 years old showing strong positive in PPD skin test (or positive in interferon γ release assay) or with suspected symptoms of TB, chest X-ray should be performed. For individuals with close contact above 15 years old, chest X-ray should be performed.
(4) For individuals with close contact and PPD skin test strong positive (or interferon γ release assay positive), with suspected symptoms of TB, suspected lesion of TB by chest X-ray, three specimens of sputum, namely instant sputum, morning sputum, and night sputum, should be collected for sputum smear test and sputum Mtb culture. For those with positive finding in sputum Mtb culture, strain identification, drug sensitivity test, and homologic analysis of DNA are performed. For those with negative finding in sputum Mtb culture, molecular biological examination is performed.
(5) After screening of individuals with close contact, the newly detected cases of active TB, cases of simple PPD skin test positive, or interferon γ release assay positive are correspondingly managed.
(6) The cases of simple PPD skin test positive or interferon γ release assay positive should receive prophylactic medication voluntarily based on informed consent.
(7) Other individuals with close contact who do not receive prophylactic medication should receive health education and medical follow-ups. If suspected symptoms of TB are detected during medical follow-ups or medical diagnosis is traced, the cases should be recorded and reported to the local TB control agency. Generally, the medical follow-ups last for 2 years. Cohort follow-ups refer to medical investigations in TB control agency at 3, 6, 12, and 24 months after occurrence of sudden public health event of TB for individuals with close contact but no suspected symptoms of TB. The data from medical follow-ups should be collected and analyzed monthly by the local TB control agency to screen cases with suspected symptoms of TB for active treatment. Any abnormalities should be recorded and reported to the superior TB control agency.

Environment Hygiene and Sterilization

The sputum of defined and suspected patients of TB should be strictly sterilized according to addition of one fifth unit bleaching powder to one unit sputum for sterilization of 2 h. The place at which the patient lives, works, and studies should be regularly sterilized by fumigation of peracetic acid solution at a concentration of 0.5–1.0%, spray of hydrogen peroxide compound air disinfectant, or ultraviolet radiation.

Analysis of Cause and Effect

Based on epidemiological case study and survey of individuals with close contact, the chronological, spatial, and population relationships between the initial case and consecutive cases are analyzed. In addition to the homological analysis of DNA, the source of infection and chain procedures of the whole event are defined. Within 3 months after field management of the event, a written report of the event should be finished in detail by the working team of management and the participating sections (Fig. 6.2).

References

1. National Statistics Bureau. Statistical yearbook of China. Beijing: China Statistics Press; 2017.
2. Zhong Q, Cheng SM, Zhou L. Technical handbook for tuberculosis screening in schools. Beijing: People's Medical Publishing House; 2018.
3. Chen W, Chen QL, Xia YY, et al. Analysis of national epidemics of TB in students during 2008 to 2012. Chin J Anti-tuberc. 2013;35(12):949–54.
4. Bai LQ. Crisis or opportunity: reflection on aggregating epidemic of TB in a school in Taojiang of Hunan province. Pract Prevent Med. 2018;25(1):1–2,61.
5. Wang LX, Cheng SM, Chen W. Technical brochure on TB control in schools. Beijing: Military Medical Science Press; 2012.
6. Department of Disease Prevention and Control, Ministry of Health. Technical guideline for implementation of TB control planning in China (edition of 2008). Beijing: Peking Union Medical College Press; 2009.
7. Lu ZY, Zhong NS. Internal medicine. 7th ed. Beijing: People's Medical Publishing House; 2008.
8. Health and Family Planning Commission of P. R. China. National Health-care Service Standards: Criteria for Diagnosis of Tuberculosis (WS 288-2017).

Control of Drug-Resistant TB

7

Fan Zhang, Wei-ye Yu, Hong-Jun Li, Chun-fa Song, Zheng Yang, Bu-dong Chen, Pu-Xuan Lu, Tao Chen, Guo-fang Deng, Le-cai Ji, and Qiu-ting Zheng

1 Overview of Drug-Resistant TB

Drug-resistant TB (DR-TB) refers to the infection of Mtb that is resistant to at least one anti-tuberculosis drug. The occurrence of DR-TB is caused by non-standardized treatment and/or insufficient management of patient with TB. Most of initially treated patient with non DR-TB can be cured by regular treatment of first-line anti-tuberculosis drug for 6 months. But inappropriate medication of anti-tuberculosis drugs (such as intermittent medication or inappropriate dosage) or early retrieval of anti-tuberculosis drug can induce resistance to anti-tuberculosis drug. And Mtb resistant to anti-tuberculosis drug further causes spread of DR-TB. The spread of drug-resistant Mtb in patients with DR-TB is an important way for spread of DR-TB. The prevalence and spread of drug-resistant Mtb present challenges to the global TB control. Especially along with the formation of global village, diversified flowing of populations for business, travelling, and purchase aggravates the prevalence of DR-TB.

F. Zhang (✉) · C.-f. Song
Shenzhen Nanshan Center for Chronic Disease Control, Shenzhen, Guangdong, China

W.-y. Yu
Department of Tuberculosis, The Shenzhen Center for Chronic Disease Control, Shenzhen, Guangdong, China

H.-J. Li
Department of Radiology, Beijing You'an Hospital, Capital Medical University, Beijing, China

Z. Yang · L-c. Ji · Q.-t. Zheng
Shenzhen Center for Chronic Disease Control, Shenzhen, Guangdong, China

B.-d. Chen
Department of Radiology, Beijing Ditan Hospital, Capital Medical University, Beijing, China

P.-X. Lu
Department of Radiology, The Shenzhen Center for Chronic Disease Control, Shenzhen, Guangdong, China

T. Chen · G.-f. Deng
The Third People's Hospital of Shenzhen, Shenzhen, Guangdong, China

1.1 Types and Definition of DR-TB

In 2006, the Guideline for the Programmatic Management of drug-resistant TB was issued by the WHO. In the guideline, the concept of DR-TB is standardized that infection of Mtb that is resistant to one or more anti-tuberculosis drugs in vitro confirmed by laboratory drug susceptibility testing (DST) [1]. In March 2006, extensive drug resistance (XDR) was firstly proposed by the CDC of the USA. In October 2006, the concept of extensive drug resistance was revisited by the WHO. And in 2014, rifampicin-resistant TB (RR-TB) was firstly proposed by the WHO [2].

(1) Monoresistant tuberculosis (MR-TB)
    The infected Mtb is confirmed by in vitro DST to be resistant to any one of the first-line anti-tuberculosis drugs.
(2) Polydrug resistant tuberculosis (PDR-TB)
    The infected Mtb is confirmed by in vitro DST to be resistant to two or more first-line anti-tuberculosis drugs. And concurrent resistance to isoniazid and rifampicin is excluded.
(3) Multidrug-resistant tuberculosis (MDR-TB)
    The infected Mtb is confirmed by in vitro DST to be resistant to at least isoniazid and rifampicin.
(4) Extensive drug-resistant tuberculosis (XDR-TB)
    Based on MDR-TB, the infected Mtb is also resistant to any one of the fluoroquinolone antibiotics (such as moxifloxacin and levofloxacin) and is resistant to at least one of the second-line injections (such as amikacin, capreomycin sulfate, or kanamycin).
(5) Rifampicin resistant tuberculosis (RR-TB)
    The infected Mtb is confirmed by in vitro DST to be resistant to rifampicin.

According to the report on global surveillance of Mtb drug resistance (third edition) jointly implemented by the WHO and the International Union for Anti Tuberculosis and Lung Disease (IUATLD), drug-resistant TB is classified into

W.-y. Yu et al. (eds.), *Tuberculosis Control in Migrating Population*, https://doi.org/10.1007/978-981-32-9763-0_7

new DR-TB and re-treated DR-TB based on medication history of anti-tuberculosis drug [3].

(1) New DR-TB
New DR-TB is also known as primary DR-TB. It refers to the drug resistance in patients who have never received anti-tuberculosis drugs or have received anti-tuberculosis drugs for less than 1 month.
(2) Re-treated DR-TB
Re-treated DR-TB refers to the drug resistance in patients who have received anti-tuberculosis drugs for more than 1 month.

There are three reasons for the occurrence of re-treated DR-TB:

(1) Re-infection
The occurrence of re-treated DR-TB is caused by infection of drug-resistant Mtb during or after re-treatment of TB, which is actually primary DR-TB.
(2) Mixed infection
Mixed infection is also known as multiple infection of TB, which is caused by infection of two or more than two strains of Mtb in re-treated patient with TB, including drug-sensitive Mtb and drug-resistant Mtb. During re-treatment, the strain of drug-sensitive Mtb is killed by anti-tuberculosis drug, while the strain of drug-resistant Mtb duplicates. The drug-resistant TB during re-treatment is still caused by primary infection of drug-resistant Mtb, which is also categorized into primary DR-TB.
(3) Acquired drug resistance
Acquired drug resistance refers to survival of Mtb with mutation of drug resistance from previous medication of anti-tuberculosis drug in re-treated patient. Based on phenotype of Mtb (morphology of Mtb colony), different strains can hardly be identified. Therefore, it is inappropriate to conclude that DR-TB in patient who has received anti-tuberculosis drug for more than 1 month is acquired drug-resistant TB.

1.2 Occurrence of DR-TB

In 1940s of the twentieth century, shortly after application of streptomycin monotherapy into treatment of TB, the strain of Mtb resistant to streptomycin emerged. During medication of single anti-tuberculosis drug, the drug-sensitive strain of Mtb is killed but the drug-resistant mutants multiply with further development into predominant strain to cause failed treatment. Along with successive developments of aminosalicylic acid, isoniazid/pyrazinamide, ethambutol, and rifampicin, combined medication of multiple anti-tuberculosis drugs is clinically recommended to prevent emergence of selective drug-resistant strain of Mtb. The combined medication can improve the therapeutic efficacy, kill various Mtb strains in the lesion via cross bacteriocidal effect, and decrease or prevent drug resistance.

Currently, the cure rate of initially treated patients with TB has been above 90%. However, drug-resistant strains have been increasing. Complex reasons contribute to the occurrence of DR-TB and the main reasons are as follows [4–6].

Therapeutic Reason

Unreasonable Medication

The unreasonable medication that contributes to the occurrence of DR-TB includes: unreasonable combination of drugs, resistance to one or multiple anti-tuberculosis drugs in the regimen, insufficient dose of anti-tuberculosis drug, shorter therapeutic course than the standardized treatment, and incomplete absorption of anti-tuberculosis drug.

Irregular Medication

Due to insufficient knowledge about diagnosis, therapeutic outcome, and necessity of treatment, the patient shows poor compliance to the medication. Or in other cases, the patient is intolerant to anti-tuberculosis drugs. And the medication is interrupted due to economic difficulty or travelling.

Concurrence of Pregnancy, Alcoholism, Drug Abuse, or Other Basic Disease

If the patient with TB experiences concurrent pregnancy, alcoholism, drug abuse, or other basic disease, such as HIV/AIDS, diabetes, neurological and psychiatric disorder, liver or kidney insufficiency, the anti-tuberculosis treatment can be affected. The resultant irregular medication also causes the occurrence of DR-TB.

Mtb Itself

Primary Drug Resistance of Mtb

The infected Mtb has never been exposed to any anti-tuberculosis drug but is naturally resistant to anti-tuberculosis drug.

Spontaneous Mutation of Mtb

During reproduction of wild-type Mtb, it can spontaneously, slowly, and persistently produce a few drug-resistant strains. However, the mutation frequency of each drug resistance is different. The mutation frequency of streptomycin resistance is 3.8×10^{6}, the mutation frequency of isoniazid resistance is 3.5×10^{-6}, the mutation frequency of rifampicin resistance is 1.2×10^{-8}, and the mutation frequency of ethambutol resistance is 3.1×10^{-6}. Spontaneous mutation of Mtb commonly produces drug resistance to one anti-tuberculosis drug. And the possibility of spontaneous mutation of Mtb that produces multidrug resistance is extremely rare.

Acquired Drug Resistance of Mtb

During treatment of TB with anti-tuberculosis drug, the primary sensitive Mtb is killed but rarely found strains with spontaneous drug resistance survive, which gradually grow into predominant strains and produce acquired drug resistance to anti-tuberculosis drug.

Persister of Mtb

Mtb is in temporary dormancy or slow growth, which is thus tolerant to high concentration of anti-tuberculosis drug. However, the drug resistance is non-hereditary. When cultured again, most persisters of Mtb still remain sensitive to anti-tuberculosis drug.

Sociological Factor

Education Background

Due to different education background, the beliefs of health and way of life are different in patients with TB. The knowledge about TB is closely related to TB control.

Occupation

Peasant workers and workers are the high-risk populations of TB. Most of them participate in labor work, with overcrowded and poor hygienic housing, which increase the risk of Mtb infection.

Family Income

A study has demonstrated that the occurrence of TB is related to family income. The population in poverty, refugees, miners, and other populations living at high-risk environment are more susceptible to TB. Due to their high stress on survival, overcrowded housing, and poor hygiene, they are more susceptible to onset of TB after Mtb infection. In addition, the non-standardized treatment or insufficient therapeutic course resulted from low family income further increase the occurrence and spread of DR-TB.

Generally speaking, unreasonable regimen of anti-tuberculosis drugs, quality problem of anti-tuberculosis drugs, and poor compliance of patients may induce the occurrence of TB during treatment. Meanwhile, the patients with DR-TB may spread the disease to others via direct contact to cause primary DR-TB. Therefore, reasonable treatment and management of TB reduce the occurrence of DR-TB. For detected patient with DR-TB, to interrupt its spread is the key for control of DR-TB.

Nowadays, the global economy has developed rapidly, with increased flow of populations internationally and inter-regionally, which also increases the spread of DR-TB. Especially in China, the migrating population is at the high risk of DR-TB. In China, most migrating population is peasant workers, with poor awareness about health, low socioeconomic status, poor housing condition, and far less coverage by the national basic health-care formulary, which increase the risk of DR-TB.

Therefore, the occurrence of DR-TB is caused by unreasonable regimen of anti-tuberculosis drugs in initial treatment of TB, the infected Mtb itself, and sociological factors. There have been also reports about relationship between host gene polymorphism and occurrence of DR-TB. However, a comprehensive data analysis based on large-scale multi-regional survey is needed to confirm the relationship.

2 Epidemiology of Drug-Resistant TB

DR-TB persistently threatens the health of human being, especially the occurrence of MDR-TB has been one of the major global public health problems. The global TB report issued by the WHO in 2018 indicated that the global cases of latent TB infection have reached about 1.7 billion in 2017, with an infection rate of 23%. It has been estimated that the global new cases of TB are ten million, with an incidence of 133 per 0.1 million, including 5.8 million males, 3.2 million females, and one million children. In that, the adult patients above 15 years old and the patients with HIV/AIDS account for 90% and 9% (72% in Africa) of the new cases, respectively. And the new cases in India (27.4%), China (8.9%), Indonesia (8.4%), and Philippines (5.8%) account for 50% of the global new cases. In the 30 countries with high TB burden, the new cases of TB account for two-thirds of the global new cases [7]. The global TB report issued by the WHO in 2017 indicated that the global new cases of TB are 10.4 million in 2016, with adults accounting for 90%, males for 65%, carriers of HIV for 10% (74% in Africa). The new cases in 7 countries account for 64% global new cases. In the 7 countries, India has the newest cases of TB, followed by Indonesia, China, Philippines, Pakistan, Nigeria, and South Africa [8].

In addition, MDR-TB persistently threatens the health of human being. According to the estimate by the WHO in 2018, the global new cases of RR-TB have estimated to reach about 0.56 million, with MDR-TB accounting for 82%. The new cases of MDR/RR-TB in India (24%), China (13%), and Russia (10%) account for half of the global new cases of MDR/RR-TB. In 2017, in patients with MDR-TB, about 8.5% suffers from XDR-TB (95% CI: 6.2–11%). In 2016, the new cases of RR-TB are 0.6 million, with 0.49 million with MDR-TB and 47% in India, China, and Russia. Based on the released data, China ranks the second in the incidence of DR-TB. The prevalence and spread of DR-TB is a great challenge in TB control in China.

2.1 Global Prevalence of DR-TB

In 2016, the survey conducted by WHO was reported, which summarized the global prevalence of DR-TB targeting on MDR/RR-TB and isoniazid/second-line anti-tuberculosis drugs resistant TB.

MDR/RR-TB

It has been estimated that the morbidity of DR-TB in 2017 is 3.5% (95% CI: 2.5–4.7%), and the morbidity of re-treated DR-TB (MDR/RR-TB) is 18% (95% CI: 6.3–34%). That is to say, there have been about 0.558 million cases of MDR/RR-TB in the world (0.483 million–0.639 million), with MDR-TB accounting for about 82% (0.46 million–0.56 million) and about 0.11 million (7.4%) cases of rifampicin resistance but sensitive to isoniazid. In addition, 47% of MDR/RR-TB is distributed in China, India, and Russia. In 2017, 0.23 million (0.14 million to 0.31 million) cases of death occurred from MDR-RR-TB.

Isoniazid/Second-Line Anti-Tuberculosis Drugs Resistant TB

During 2003–2017, the isoniazid resistance (sensitive to rifampicin) in patients with TB has been assessed in 149 countries. In all cases of TB, the global average of isoniazid resistance is 8.5% (95% CI: 7.4–9.7%). In the new cases of TB and previously treated cases of TB, the global average of isoniazid resistance is 7.1% (95% CI: 6.2–8.0%) and 7.9% (95% CI: 5.9–10%), respectively.

By the end of 2017, reports on XDR-TB had been submitted by 127 member countries of WHO. Based on the reported data, patients with MDR-TB account for 8.5% (95% CI: 6.2–11%) of the patients with XDR-TB, which is higher than 6.2% (95% CI: 3.6–9.5%) in 2016 but lower than 9.5% in 2015, 9.7% in 2014, and 9.0% in 2013. In 40 countries with high TB or MDR-TB burden, resistance to second-line anti-tuberculosis drugs is monitored in 22 countries. The resistance to any fluoroquinolones (including ofloxacin, levofloxacin, and moxifloxacin) in patients with MDR-TB/RR-TB is about 22% (95% CI: 17–28%).

2.2 Prevalence of DR-TB in China

China is one of the countries with high prevalence of DR-TB across the world. Since 1996, consecutively 13 provinces of China have participated in the global drug resistance surveillance program initiated by WHO/IUATLD. The results indicated that the prevalence of DR-TB is high in some provinces of China, such as Henan, Liaoning, and Inner Mongolia. According to the estimate by WHO in 2017, the incidence of DR-TB in China is only lower than that in India and the patients with MDR-TB in China account for one fourth of the global cases of MDR-TB.

In China, 5 national epidemiological sampling surveys of TB have been conducted in 1979, 1984–1985, 1990, 2000, and 2010, respectively [9–13]. The results of previous 4 national surveys indicated that the drug resistance rate in initially treated patients is 26.2%, 47.8%, 28.1%, and 18.6%, respectively, and the acquired drug resistance rate is 68.1%, 64.1%, 41.1%, and 46.5%, respectively. However, in the four previous national surveys, resistance to 6 anti-tuberculosis drugs was detected, including 4 first-line anti-tuberculosis drugs of isoniazid, streptomycin, rifampicin, and ethambutol, and 2 second-line anti-tuberculosis drugs of sodium aminosalicylate and thiosemicarbazide. In the national survey of 2010, resistance to 11 anti-tuberculosis drugs was detected, including 4 first-line anti-tuberculosis drugs and 7 second-line anti-tuberculosis drugs (sodium aminosalicylate, kanamycin, amikacin, capreomycin, prothionamide, ofloxacin, and levofloxacin). The resistance rate to any one of the 11 anti-tuberculosis drugs is 42.1%, and 42.7% in initially treated patients and 38.5% in re-treated patients. Because different anti-tuberculosis drugs are detected in the national survey in 2010, the drug resistance cannot be directly compared (Table 7.1).

2.3 Reasons of High Prevalence of DR-TB in China

It is necessary to define the reason of DR-TB in one region. Is it caused by anti-tuberculosis treatment or direct interpersonal spread of DR-TB? Only if the reason is defined, appropriate measures for control can be formulated and adopted. A study by Gao et al. [14, 15] has demonstrated that the main reason for high prevalence of DR-TB in China is direct interpersonal spread of DR-TB.

Percentage of Initially Treated DR-TB Patients Is Higher than Re-Treated DR-TB Patients

The fifth national epidemiological sampling survey on TB in 2010 indicated that in 103 cases of drug resistance to first-line anti-tuberculosis drugs, 89 cases (86.4%) are initially treated patients, and 14 cases (13.6%) are re-treated patients. In addition, in 69 cases of drug resistance to second-line anti-tuberculosis drugs, 62 cases (89.9%) are initially treated patients and 7 cases (10.1%) are re-treated patients. A study conducted in Shanghai has demonstrated that in 1401 cases

Table 7.1 Changes of initial drug resistance rate of monodrug-resistant in four epidemiological sample surveys

	Initial drug resistance rate (%)			
Resistant drugs	1984–1985	1990	2000	2010
INH	28.0	23.5	11.0	8.7
RFP	10.1	10.9	10.3	1.2
EMB	10.8	4.5	1.5	0.4
S	23.3	20.0	12.2	6.2
T	21.1	6.3	1.9	–
PAS	17.3	4.4	2.7	2.5
Km	–	–	–	0
Am	–	–	–	0
Cm	–	–	–	0.8
Pto	–	–	–	3.7
Ofx	–	–	–	0.4
Lfx	–	–	–	0.4

of drug resistance to first-line anti-tuberculosis drugs during 2000–2006, 1016 cases (72.5%) are initially treated patients and 385 cases (27.4%) are re-treated patients. And in 333 cases of drug resistance to second-line anti-tuberculosis drugs, 199 cases (59.8%) are initially treated patients and 134 cases (40.2%) are re-treated patients.

Based on the above data, it can be concluded that the percentage of initially treated DR-TB patients is far higher than that of re-treated DR-TB patients. Therefore, primary drug resistance is more common and direct interpersonal spread of DR-TB is the main reason for high prevalence of primary DR-TB.

Recent Spread of DR-TB Is the Main Reason for High Prevalence of Primary DR-TB

In patients with latent TB infection, 5% shows symptoms within 1–2 years after infection. And such patients are known as TB of recent spread. And another 5% patients with latent TB infection may show symptoms during their life due to compromised immunity. And such patients are known as TB of distant spread or endogenously re-activated TB.

Based on the genotyping of Mtb, researchers have found that in 135 strains of drug-resistant Mtb at the 5 places for field survey across the country, 59 cases (43.7%) are caused by recent spread of TB. And further study has demonstrated that drug-resistant strains of Mtb more commonly induce drug-sensitive strains of Mtb.

Generally speaking, appropriate treatment and management of initially treated patients with TB facilitate to decrease the incidence of acquired drug resistance. But if the patients with DR-TB fail to be detected, diagnosed, and treated early to control spread of drug-resistant Mtb, the prevalence of DR-TB cannot be controlled. Therefore, based on standardized treatment of TB and strengthened DOTS strategy, early detection and diagnosis of DR-TB are effective measures for DR-TB control.

3 Strategies for DR-TB Control

3.1 Strengthened Leadership, Policy Making, and Financial Funding for DR-TB Control

The responsibilities of government officials are defined and emphasized. The corresponding laws and regulations are formulated and issued. A mechanism for trans-regional management of patients with DR-TB is established and has been gradually improved. The quantity of health-care staffs in basic level TB control agencies is appropriately increased. All these measures are intended to meet the demands in TB control [16]. Meanwhile, the incentive mechanism has been established and improved to encourage commitment to control of TB in basic level TB control agencies. Health education about DR-TB control is strengthened, especially targeting on the high-risk populations of migrating population, the elderly, patients with diabetes, and individuals with close contact.

Persistent financial funding for management of TB in migrating population is secured by governments of all levels [16]. On one hand, the coverage of national basic health-care formulary is extended. And feasibility of the coverage of critical illness insurance program on definitive diagnosis and treatment of TB is explored. Financial funding is persistently invested into health-care service to alleviate economic burden in patients with DR-TB. Thus, more patients receive standardized treatment. On the other hand, social organizations, institutions, companies, and public institutions are encouraged to further study on the pathomechanism of TB.

3.2 Strengthened Detection of Patients with DR-TB

Early detection, diagnosis, and treatment are vitally important for control of DR-TB. And general hospitals play key role in preventing and treating DR-TB. Early detection and referral are important principles and responsibilities of general hospitals in the control of DR-TB. The clinical experience has demonstrated that in patients with delayed diagnosis of DR-TB, along with increased number of exudative and necrotic lesions, the quantity of Mtb in sputum of patients has been increasing. In such patients, the therapeutic efficacy is commonly unfavorable, and resistance to anti-tuberculosis drugs is more likely [17].

In China, about 70–80% patients with TB initially present to a general hospital for diagnosis and treatment. But some patients, especially young and middle-aged adults with no obvious symptom, are detected by private clinics or health examination institutions [18]. Collaborative efforts of health-care institutions and TB control agencies should be emphasized and standardized for bi-directional referral of patients with TB and surveillance of DR-TB. The defensive line against DR-TB should be elongated with private clinics and health examination institutions integrated into the network of DR-TB control. And the on-line reporting of infectious diseases should be implemented and optimized. For newly detected patients with TB, the National Technical Guideline for Implementation of TB Control Planning in China should be strictly observed. Monthly sputum bacteriological test should be performed. For patients with sputum bacteriologically positive, the drug sensitivity test should be timely performed to define or exclude DR-TB.

In addition, screening of DR-TB should be performed in high-risk populations. The high-risk populations include patients with HIV/AIDS; individuals with close contact to recently diagnosed patient with DR-TB; children with no inoculation of BCG vaccine and tuberculin test positive; tuberculin test positive patients with diabetes, silicosis, and those receiving long-term medication of adrenal corticosteroids; patients with non-active TB lesion shown by chest X-ray but receiving no treatment; and those with tuberculin test strong positive [19].

3.3 Improved Accuracy in Diagnosis and Standardized Treatment

Community-based clinic plays an important role in detecting and managing patients with TB. However, the diagnosis and treatment of TB in community clinic need to be improved. Training of the health-care staff is necessary to improve their capabilities in diagnosing and treating TB. Emphasis on community-based clinic is important to strengthen detection of patients with TB and their convenient consultation. Based on community clinic, the risk of spreading TB during transportation of patients can be decreased.

Formulating reasonable and standardized treatment regimen for treatment of TB is one of the basic responsibilities of a physician, especially, a physician specialized in respiratory disease. However, the capability of physicians is still limited. When individualized treatment regimen is formulated, the body weight of patient should be taken into consideration for sufficient dosage of anti-tuberculosis drugs. While the route of administration is changed or another anti-tuberculosis drug is added, the great dosage variance resulted from different body weight of patient should not be neglected. A study has demonstrated that insufficient dosage of anti-tuberculosis drug is common in China, which may be one of the reasons for high incidence of DR-TB [20]. The therapeutic course should not be arbitrarily elongated, otherwise the resultant poor compliance may increase the risk of DR-TB.

The occurrence of adverse reaction should be decreased and a physician should adopt correct management measures when adverse reactions occur. Currently, the awareness of patient about whole course regular medication of anti-tuberculosis drugs has been increased. However, the patients have to interrupt medication due to the occurrence of adverse reactions, which further increases the risk of DR-TB [21]. Therefore, adverse reactions should be detected as early as possible for retrieval of medication. After the adverse reactions subside, medication can be continued after regulation of regimen. Drug allergy that may seriously impair patients should be avoided. The basic measure adopted to avoid drug allergy is to simplify treatment regimen and not to prescribe unnecessary drug.

3.4 Standardized Management of Patient with DR-TB

DOTS strategy should be strictly observed. After the treatment regimen is formulated, health education and consecutive DOTS should be conducted for regular medication and favorable compliance of patient. For completion of therapeutic course, whole course DOTS is necessary [19]. The physical should establish favorable relationship with his/her patients to improve communication, which plays favorable role in promoting completion of therapeutic course. The trust from patients improves their compliance and cooperation to the treatment. For outpatients and patients discharged from hospital, follow-ups at least once a month are important, which promotes the patients to receive regular chest X-ray and sputum smear test. Based on the investigations, the therapeutic efficacy can be assessed and the adverse reactions can be detected and managed. Meanwhile, the follow-ups facilitate implementation of DOTS strategy and regulation of treatment regimen for more favorable therapeutic outcome.

For trans-regional patients with DR-TB, collaborative efforts should be made between TB control agencies in different regions for standardized whole course management of patient. The referral-in TB control agency should be assessed due to its important role in consecutive treatment, management, and therapeutic assessment. Based on favorable collaborative efforts of trans-regional TB control agencies, the regional health-care resources should be well utilized for control of DR-TB. Meanwhile, control of DR-TB nationwide should be taken into consideration instead of only one region. Only if the departments, regions, and institutions are well collaborated, the prevalence of DR-TB in migrating population can be controlled [22].

3.5 Application of New Technologies in TB Control

Nowadays, due to regional difference in economic development, the technologies applied in TB control show great variance. After verified by practice, the new technologies should be widely promoted for application in TB control [23]. For instance, in some regions of China, GPS has been applied in home quarantined treatment or hospital quarantined treatment of TB. In some regions with advanced infrastructure of information technology (IT), Wechat-based or smart phone APP-based DOTS system has been developed, which authentically records the medication of patient and facilitates health-care service. The IT-based DOTS system is an effective supplement to traditional DOTS strategy. In some other regions, geography-based epidemic surveillance system has been developed, which traces, represents, and analyzes daily trajectory of patient for prediction of epidemic of TB. In addition, DR-TB has been enlisted into the Critical Illness Insurance Program in some regions of China, which further decreases the expenses of patients on DR-TB and improves the compliance of patients.

4 Laboratory Test

Laboratory test for TB is an important part of the national TB control planning (NTP) and is necessary for diagnosis, treatment, and control of TB [24]. The laboratory test for TB is the main way of etiologically detecting the source of infection. Meanwhile, it is also the main basis for definitive diagnosis and formulating treatment regimen of TB, and provides reliable criteria for assessing the therapeutic efficacy and performance of TB control. The result of laboratory test is an important basis for definitive diagnosis of TB, and the drug sensitivity test to anti-tuberculosis drugs is important basis for definitive diagnosis of DR-TB. The laboratory test for DR-TB is almost the same as the routine laboratory test for TB. And the sputum smear test and sputum culture are necessary for definitive diagnosis of TB. After diagnosis of TB is defined, rapid drug sensitivity test, such as GeneXpert is commonly performed for preliminary diagnosis of rifampicin-resistant TB. If resistance to rifampicin is detected, purified strain of Mtb is harvested for drug sensitivity test of the first-line and second-line anti-tuberculosis drugs or drug-resistant gene mutant detection. The detected strain with drug resistance plays auxiliary role in clinical treatment and control of DR-TB. Since May 1st, 2018, molecular biology has been enlisted for definitive diagnosis of TB in China. In gradually promoted Stop TB strategy in China, bacteriology and molecular biology (holistically as etiology), in combination with chest X-ray, play important role in detecting TB [25]. The laboratory tests for TB include sputum smear for staining and microscopy (sputum smear), sputum culture for Mtb (sputum culture), sputum TB-PCR, preliminary identification of Mtb strain, identification of non tuberculosis mycobacteria (NTM) strain, drug sensitivity test of Mtb, drug-resistant gene mutant detection, and immunological assay for Mtb.

4.1 Sputum Smear for Staining and Microscopy

The external layer of the mycobacterial cell wall contains large quantity of lipid, which surrounds the peptidoglycan. The mycobacteria can thus be hardly stained. In common Gram staining, mycobacteria fail to preserve the crystal violet and look like a poorly defined shell after staining. In combined use of carbolic acid, aniline and other commonly applied staining agents can penetrate the wax-like cell wall of mycobacteria. In 1882, Robert Koch applied basic stain containing methylene complex staining solution to stain mycobacteria tuberculosis. After that, Ehrlich discovered acid-fastness of mycobacteria tuberculosis. After improved by Ziehl and Neelsen, the presently applied acid-fast staining came into being. Acid-fastness is a physical property of mycobacterial cell, specifically its resistance to decolorization by acids during laboratory staining procedures. For identification of mycobacteria, Ziehl–Neelsen acid-fast staining is commonly applied. Via heating, the mycolic acid binds to carbolfuchsin to form complex, which can hardly be decolorized by treatment of 3% hydrochloric ethanol. After addition of alkaline methylene for re-staining, the mycobacteria are stained red, while other bacteria and background materials are stained blue, based on which acid-fast bacteria is differentiated from other common bacteria.

In fluorescent staining, auramine O is commonly applied as the initial stain agent. As acid-fast bacteria is resistant to re-staining of potassium permanganate, the acid-fast bacteria shows yellowish fluorescence under a fluorescence microscope, while other bacteria and background materials show dark yellow. With no heating, fluorescent staining is safer. In addition, with low power microscopy, acid-fast bacteria can be detected within a shorter period of time. And fluorescent staining is more sensitive than Ziehl–Neelsen staining [26, 27].

Sputum smear for staining and microscopy is a bacteriological test with optimal cost-benefit ratio. Compared to other clinical and laboratory tests, high-quality sputum smear for staining and microscopy has its advantages:

(1) As a diagnostic technology, it is superior to chest X-ray in accurate diagnosis of communicable TB.
(2) As a laboratory test, it has simple operational procedures, and standardized procedures can be completed with simple operations.
(3) Its cost is low and is commonly performed.
(4) Less sophisticated equipments are needed for sputum smear test.
(5) The result can be obtained within a shorter period of time. In the most rapid cases, the result can be obtained within the same day of specimen collection.
(6) It can be applied to assess the therapeutic efficacy in patients with bacteriologically positive TB. However, due to its less sensitivity (positive when bacteria quantity is above 5×10^3/mL) and poor quality of sputum specimen, the positive rate of sputum smear test in patients

with TB remains about 30% in China, which is far less than the desired positive rate of 50%. In addition, the laboratory staffs are required with interpretation experience in sputum smear for staining and microscopy. Therefore, improved quality of sputum specimen and training of the laboratory staffs are important to decrease false positive rate, false negative rate, and quantifying error [28, 29].

4.2 Sputum Culture for Isolation of Mtb

Sputum culture for isolation of Mtb is the most reliable way to define the diagnosis of TB. Meanwhile, it is also basis for strain identification, drug sensitivity test, and other biological studies. Presently, improved Lowenstein–Jensen medium is commonly applied to isolate and culture Mtb in China. And its sensitivity is higher than sputum smear test. When the quantity of microorganism is above 100 bacteria per 1 mL specimen, it shows positive. But due to slow growth of Mtb, solid culture commonly consumes more than 4 weeks, which negatively affects the diagnosis and treatment of TB. In many laboratories, liquid culture is applied, which significantly shortens the time of waiting. In liquid culture, rapid culture instrument, such as MIGT, BacT/Alert, and ESP, is applied to identify growth of Mtb via detection of bacterial growth and metabolism. Take ABCTEC MGIT960 as an example, if there is growth of Mtb in inoculated MGIT culture tube, the nutrients and oxygen in the tube are persistently consumed and the fluorescent display agent in the MGIT culture tube releases fluorescence along with changes of oxygen concentration in the tube. The fluorescence intensity memory detector successively detects the fluorescence intensity in the culture tube at an interval of 60 min, and monitors the growth of Mycobacteria in the tube. In the liquid culture medium, there are abundant nutrients. And the detector is capable of consecutive monitoring. Therefore, liquid culture improves the sensitivity of sputum culture for isolation of Mtb, and shortens the time consumed [30]. To ensure the reliability of sputum culture for isolation of Mtb, the Mtb rapid culture and detection system is equipped with corresponding equipments, reagents, and standardized procedures including pretreatment of the clinical specimen, inoculation, detection, and result reporting. Therefore, repeatability of the procedures and comparability of the results are more favorable. In rapid culture of mycobacteria, before inoculated, the specimen is decontaminated to decrease the contamination rate. When the system reports positive, the culture liquid of corresponding specimen is firstly performed microscopy for acid-fastness and positive finding is reported after detection of acid-fast bacilli. Liquid culture and isolation of mycobacteria has many advantages, such as advanced design, short period of time for detection of positive finding, high positive rate, and wide range of specimens. In addition, the built-in quality control system is automatic, which greatly reduces the working load of laboratory staffs and improves the safety in operations.

4.3 Polymerase Chain Reaction for Mycobacteria Tuberculosis (TB-PCR)

With the rapid development of molecular biology in the medical field, the technology has formally been included in the diagnostic criteria of TB since 2018. Fluorescent quantitative polymerase chain reaction (FQ-PCR) is a highly sensitive and specific diagnostic technique for TB. Its value in the diagnosis of TB has been widely recognized worldwide in recent years. FQ-PCR amplification and results display are fully automated. The contamination probability of FQ-PCR is smaller than that of the traditional PCR, but it cannot be ignored. It is necessary to pay close attention to every procedure during the detection to ensure the accuracy of the detection results. All other fluorescent quantitative PCR detection reagents for the diagnosis of TB, such as the nucleic acid detection kit of Mtb developed by Daan Gene Corporation, Ltd., involve extraction of DNA from sputum specimen. Therefore, for the specimen with low sputum bacteria content or high impurity ratio, the quality control during DNA extraction in sputum specimen is extremely important for the sensitivity of subsequent PCR amplification. GeneXpert MTB/RIF (for rapid detection of Mtb and diagnosis of rifampin-resistant TB) has been recommended by WHO for twice as an innovative technology, and in the third edition of International Standard for Tuberculosis Care (2014), it is recommended for initial diagnosis of TB in various situations. GeneXpert MTB/RIF technology is based on fluorescence quantitative PCR. Its amplification products include Mtb specific sequence and rpoB locus sequence which determines rifampicin resistance. The advantages of GeneXpert technology are as follows:

(1) Sputum from patient as the specimen for detection of Mtb DNA within as soon as 2 h;
(2) Simultaneous detection of rifampicin resistance related mutation in sputum specimen;
(3) Addition of sputum into a fully enclosed specimen processing box after simple pretreatment for DNA extraction.

However, GeneXpert MTB/RIF technology is not perfect. Its reagent consumables cost nearly RMB ¥400 yuan per test, which limits its application in screening of TB [31].

4.4 Preliminary Identification of Mycobacteria Strain

By traditional identification of Mycobacterium strain, the specimen undergoes the growth test of p-nitrobenzoic acid (PNB), the growth test at 28 °C, thermo-contact test, observation and recording of bacterial growth rate, colony morphology, and colony color to differentiate Mycobacterium tuberculosis complex (MTC) or non-tuberculosis Mycobacteria (NTM). Take the growth test of PNB as an example, because NTM can reduce PNB to bacterial available p-aminobenzoic acid (PABA), it can grow on modified Roche medium (L-J) containing 500 μg/mL PNB. However, MTC is incapable of the reduction, and cannot grow on culture medium containing PNB. Based on the growth variance, NTM and MTC can be differentiated. Meanwhile, due to intolerance of Mycobacterium bovis to thiophene-2-carboxylic hydrazine (TCH), the modified Roche medium containing 5 μg/mL TCH is applied to categorize the laboratory isolated MTC into Mtb or Mycobacterium bovis. The preliminary identification of Mycobacteria strain by culture medium containing PNB and TCH is shown in Table 7.2.

Mycobacterium strain identification based on biochemical experiments has gradually been abandoned due to the complex operational procedures. The application of rapid liquid culture shortens the time for laboratory diagnosis of TB. However, being similar to solid culture, BD MGIT™960 liquid culture positive cannot differentiate Mtb from NMT. Further identification is needed. In order to save time consumed in identification, combination of acid-fast staining with antigen detection is applied to preliminarily identify strains in many laboratories. For specimen with liquid culture positive, MPB64 antigen detection (colloidal gold method) and acid-fast staining are performed for review to exclude contamination and preliminarily identify Mtb (acid-fast staining positive, MPB64 positive) and NTM (acid-fast staining positive, MPB64 negative). In addition, TB-specific primer amplification-based FQ-PCR (developed by Daan Gene and Xiamen Zhishan, China), gene chip-based microarray (developed by Boao Biology, China), reverse dot hybridization-based GenoType MTBDR for drug resistance detection (developed by Hain Lifesciences, Germany), and gene sequencing can all achieve the preliminary identification of Mycobacteria strains.

Table 7.2 Observation results and records

	PNB	TCH	L-J
Mycobacterium bovis	–	–	+
Mycobacterium tuberculosis	–	+	+
Non-mycobacterium tuberculosis	+	+	+

4.5 Identification of NTM Strain

Most strains of NTM are saprophytic, and only a few are conditional pathogenic to human. However, NTM has an extensive natural resistance to commonly used anti-tuberculosis drugs, and different strains of NTM show different resistance spectrum. Therefore, identification of NTM strains helps in selection of clinical therapeutic drugs. Currently, the methods to identify NTM strains are as follows:

(1) The Mycobacteria identification kit developed by Hain Lifesciences in Germany based on reverse dot hybridization technology is capable of identifying 16 strains of NTM [32]. With its upgraded version and GenoType CM direct kit, NTM strains can be directly identified from sputum specimen. In addition, GenoType Mycobacterium CM/GenoType Mycobacterium AS kit is capable of identifying up to 27 clinically common NTM strains.
(2) The microarray kit for Mycobacterium identification based on gene chip technology developed by Beijing Boao Biotechnology Co., Ltd., China is capable of distinguishing 17 clinically common NTM strains.
(3) The NTM identification reagent based on gene sequencing developed by Shenzhen Yasheng Biotechnology Co., Ltd., China is capable of accurately identifying 22 strains of mycobacteria.

4.6 Drug Sensitivity Test of Mycobacteria

Drug sensitivity test of Mtb is indispensable in control of DR and MDR TB. It plays an active role in the diagnosis of DR-TB, the selection and adjustment of treatment regimen, surveillance of DR-TB, and control of patients with DR-TB [33]. Currently, drug sensitivity tests of Mtb are classified into the following types: (1) drug sensitivity tests based on solid medium (proportional method and absolute concentration method); (2) drug sensitivity tests based on liquid medium (BACTEC, MGIT); and (3) rapid drug sensitivity tests (Microplate assays/MIC, FASTPlaque, and E-test).

Drug Sensitivity Tests Based on Solid Medium

Drug sensitivity tests based on solid Roche culture medium mainly consist of proportional method and absolute concentration method, which were first proposed by G. canetti, and J. Grossete from France and G. Meissner from Germany in 1960s, respectively. The proportional method is currently adopted in epidemiological surveillance and MDR-TB control planning and management programs in China. Drug sensitivity tests can be divided into direct method and indirect method. Direct drug sensitivity test is performed by pretreatment of clinical specimen, dilution according to the amount of Mtb examined by smear for microscopy, and direct inoculation into control and drug-containing medium. It is applicable for specimens with large quantity of Mtb verified by microscopy. And its advantage is that culture for isolation and drug sensitivity test are carried out simultaneously, and the results can be reported 3–4 weeks ahead of the indirect drug sensitivity test. However, its disadvantage is that the amount of inoculation can hardly be quantified, and difficulty controlling contamination. The indirect drug sensitivity test is to culture clinical specimen for isolation of Mtb, followed by drug sensitivity test after the purified culture of Mtb is visible to the naked eyes. The indirect drug sensitivity test consumes more time than the direct method, but the operation based on the purified culture facilitates to control the amount of Mtb. Therefore, the results are accurate with lower contamination rate. The basic procedures of proportion method (indirect method) are as follows: The tested bacteria of 10^{-4} mg and 10^{-6} mg is inoculated for culture on the slope of modified Roche (L-J) medium containing or without drugs (control) for 4 weeks. And the drug resistance ratio is then calculated by comparing the difference of colony number between the cultures with the same amount of inoculated bacteria on medium containing no drugs.

The percentage of drug resistance = (number of colonies on drug-containing medium)/(number of colonies on control medium) × 100%. If the percentage of drug resistance is above 1%, the tested bacteria are considered to be resistant to the anti-tuberculosis drug.

The basic procedures of absolute concentration method (indirect method) are as follows: The tested bacteria of 10^{-3} mg is firstly inoculated and cultured on the slope of the improved Roche medium containing high concentration, low concentration, and no (control) drugs for 4 weeks. The number of colonies is observed by examining the culture medium, and the growth of colonies is recorded. On the premise of favorable growth of colonies on the control medium, observation of more than 20 colonies on the drug-containing culture medium is considered as drug resistance.

Drug Sensitivity Test-Based Liquid Medium

The BD BACTEC™ MGIT™960 liquid drug-sensitive test system is for rapid drug sensitivity test based on the BD960 culture device. Its underlying mechanism is similar to that of BACTEC MGIT960. When oxygen is consumed in the culture tube, the concentration of CO_2 increases. The fluorescent indicator in the culture tube releases fluorescence under the activation of a specific light source, and fluorescence intensity in the culture tube is continuously measured at an interval of 60 min by a fluorescence intensity memory detector. The system can detect the sensitivity of up to 14 anti-tuberculosis drugs, including 4 first-line drugs of rifampicin, isoniazid, ethambutol, and streptomycin as well as 5 second-line drugs of amikacin, capreomycin, kanamycin, ofloxacin, and pyrazinamide. The results can be obtained within 13 days. And the results of sensitivity to PZA can be obtained within 21 days. The shorter period of time in waiting results is beneficial to the early diagnosis and treatment of patients. The liquid drug sensitivity test system is also based on the proportional method. When drug sensitivity to anti-tuberculosis drugs is detected, the threshold value is 1%. When the GU value of the control tube containing no drug reaches 400, the system detects the MGIT culture tube. The GU value in the drug-containing tube being less than 100 is considered drug sensitive, and the value being above 100 is considered drug resistant. In some laboratories in China, BD BACTEC™ MGIT™960-based drug sensitivity test has been performed. In order to test the consistency of BACTEC-MGIT960 automatic rapid drug sensitivity test with Roche proportional method, Yang et al. parallelly detected sensitivity of 245 clinically isolated strains of mycobacterium from inpatients to rifampicin (RFP), isoniazid (INH), streptomycin (SM), and ethambutol (EMB). They found that BACT-MGIT960 automatic drug sensitivity test system is capable of detecting the sensitivity of Mycobacterium to RFP, INH, SM, and EMB within 4–13 days, with an average of 7.8 days. The consistency rates with Roche proportional method are 98.78%, 97.55%, 96.73%, and 96.73%, respectively, with an average consistency rate of 97.45%. Therefore, BACTEC-MGIT 960 drug sensitivity test system can rapidly and accurately test the drug sensitivity, especially for rapid drug sensitivity screening of clinical isolates [34]. However, the cost of reagents and instruments for liquid drug sensitivity test is high, and the flux is limited by equipment. Therefore, its application in community-based clinic can hardly be promoted.

Rapid Drug Sensitivity Test

Compared with Roche culture, the minimum inhibitory concentration (MIC) method only needs addition of certain quantities of culture medium and bacterial suspension due to the use of pre-prepared plate for drug sensitivity test, which greatly shortens the period of time consumed in manual operations. Most importantly, the MIC method can provide results within 7–21 days, which greatly reduces the reporting time of drug sensitivity test. In addition, the inclusive quantitative QC range can provide immediate quality assurance for the test. However, the results obtained by MIC are the lowest inhibitory concentration, and reference criteria are necessary for determination of drug sensitivity. The MIC of Mtb by microplate culture has been promoted in some hospitals of China (such as Beijing Thoracic Hospital). Drug sensitivity of Mtb to 12 first-line and second-line anti-tuberculosis drugs is tested with Thermo Sensititre™ MIC platform [35].

4.7 Detection of Drug-Resistant Mutations of Mycobacterium

There are four main types of detection techniques for drug-resistant mutations of Mycobacterium: (1) fluorescence quantitative PCR (developed by Saipei); (2) melting curve technology (developed by Zhishan Biology and Lifescience); (3) reverse hybridization technology (developed by Hain Lifescience); and (4) gene chip technology (developed by Boao Biology). These techniques are based on the analysis of identified drug resistance-related mutations (including insertion, deletion, and SNP) of Mtb. The drug resistance-related mutations include rpoB/C gene mutation that mediates rifampicin resistance, inhA, katG, ahpC gene mutations that mediate isoniazid resistance, embA/B/C/R gene mutation that mediates ethambutol resistance, RRs and rpsL gene mutations that mediate streptomycin resistance, gyrA and gyrB gene mutations that mediate fluoroquinolones resistance, ethA/R and inhA gene mutations that mediate ethionamide resistance, pncA, rpsA, and panD gene mutations that mediate pyrazinamide resistance. As the discovery and validation of drug-resistant genes is a developing process, the gene mutations detected by kits do not and cannot cover all phenotypic drug resistance-related mutations. In addition to complex relationships between phenotypes and genotypes of drug-resistant genes, inconsistency or partial consistency between phenotypes and genotypes is possible in clinical practice.

Based on fluorescence quantitative PCR, GeneXpert MTB/RIF platform directly extracts DNA of Mtb from sputum specimen by using fully enclosed automatic DNA extraction kit. Mtb specific sequence and rpoB gene locus sequence responsible for rifampicin resistance are amplified. Presence of Mtb and rifampicin resistance can be reported within as short as 2 h. Researchers from Xiamen University (Zhishan Biology, http://www.zsandx.com/) applied Melt-Pro platform based on melting curve technology to detect drug-resistant mutations of Mtb (with independent intellectual property rights). It is capable of detecting the mutations of Mtb responsible for drug resistance to rifampicin, isoniazid, ethambutol, streptomycin, and fluoroquinolones. Meanwhile, they also developed a one-stop service platform integrating procedures from DNA extraction to result report, which successfully avoids the potential risks of cross-contamination caused by complex molecular hybridization and tube opening. In addition, the one-stop service platform helps to save labor and time with automated result reporting. The sensitivity, specificity, and total coincidence rates of Melt-Pro detection and linear probe MTBDRplus MDR were 71.43%, 94.21%, 92.97% and 71.43%, 98.35%, 96.88%, respectively. The sensitivity and specificity of Melt-Pro detection and linear probe MTBDRplus MDR for diagnosis of INH-resistant, RIF-resistant, and MDR-TB in sputum smear-positive specimens were similarly high [36]. GenoType MTBDRplus developed by Hain Lifescience in Germany is capable of detecting Mtb and obtaining gene mutation information related to rifampicin and isoniazid resistance in TB-positive sputum specimen/culture by using PCR amplification and reverse hybridization. GenoType MTBDRsl kit can obtain gene mutation information related to fluoroquinolones and aminoglycosides resistance or fluoroquinolones, cycloserine, and ethylamine resistance [37]. With the rapid development of genome-wide sequencing technology, the cost of sequencing is greatly reduced, the ability of information analysis is rapidly improved, and the database for drug resistance of Mtb is increasingly improved. Drug resistance based on genome-wide sequencing can definitely be predicted in clinical practice in the near future.

4.8 Immunological Assay for Mycobacterium

Immunological assays for Mycobacterium mainly include interferon γ release test, antibody detection, and antigen detection. Interferon γ release assay (IGRA) can be applied to diagnose latent TB infection, especially for patients with major diseases or severe malnutrition. There are two commercially available kits for IGRA, QuantiFERON-TB Gold (QFT, Qiagen) and T. SPOT-TB (Oxford Immunotec). The former one is based on enzyme-linked immunosorbent assay (ELISA) for detection of Mycobacterium, while the latter one is based on enzyme-linked immunodot assay (ELISPOT) for detection of Mycobacterium. QFT is to quantitatively detect the total amount of interferon γ produced by mononuclear cells in peripheral blood after stimulated by TB antigen (ESAT-6 and CFP-10). And T. SPOT-TB is to detect the number of cells that secrete interferon γ. Although both kits are expensive, they can provide objective and accurate results compared with tuberculin skin test.

Antibody detection to assist the diagnosis of TB remains controversial due to its unstable sensitivity and specificity. Since 2012, serum antibody detection has not been recommended by WHO for diagnosis of TB infection [17]. However, with the development of technologies in identifying and detecting new TB antigens, chemiluminescence detection based on multi-antigen targets tends to be applied in detection of blood antibody for diagnosis of TB. The potential of kit has also been gradually improved. Concerning antigen detection, the detection of antigen in blood for diagnosis of TB has always been difficult because of its low level and the low sensitivity of routine detections. In 2017, scholars in the USA successfully applied time-flight mass spectrometry (MALDI-TOF MS) to detect cfp10 and esat6 antigens in blood specimens. Its sensitivity and specificity for patients with TB, extrapulmonary TB, and latent TB infection have reached the level of clinical recognition. Its promotion in clinical practice is thus valuable. The detection of Mtb specific antigen MPB64 can be applied as an assistant way for preliminary identification of Mtb strains with liquid culture-positive MGIT tube as specimen.

4.9 Other Molecular Biological Detections for Mtb

With rapid development of molecular biology in the field of medicine, researchers have also introduced the principles of molecular biology into the field of tuberculosis. Polymerase chain reaction (PCR) is a diagnostic technology based on nucleic acid biochemistry, which is one of the most valuable methods in the field of biomedicine. Currently, the molecular biological detections for Mtb with high sensitivity and specificity include: nucleic acid amplification (such as Amplicor MTB, MTD Gen-Probe, and SDA), nucleic acid hybridization, 16S ribosome gene sequencing, high performance liquid chromatography (HPLC) for cell wall lipid (mycobacterium acid) analysis, mass spectrometry (MS) technology for detection and analysis of Mtb protein in plasma of patients.

Based on molecular biology, biomarker of Mtb has been explored. Based on the determination of its genotype, the prevalence and distribution of Mtb with different phenotypes in populations can be analyzed. Under certain conditions, the source of infection can be traced. The molecular biology provides reliable reference indicators for the molecular epidemiological study of TB. Currently, the widely applied genotyping methods include restriction fragment length polymorphism (IS6110-RFLP), variable number of tandem repeats (VNTR), mycobacterial interspersed repetitive units (MIRU), spacer oligonucleotide typing (spoligotyping), single nucleotide polymorphism analysis (SNPs), and deletion mapping.

5 Diagnostic Imaging of Drug-Resistant Tuberculosis

5.1 Radiological Demonstrations of DR-TB

Common Location with DR-TB Lesion

The intrapulmonary location of DR-TB lesion is extensive. At the location rarely with lesion of secondary pulmonary TB, the lesion of DR-TB is common. The locations commonly with DR-TB lesion include the right middle lung lobe, the lingual segment of the left upper lung lobe, and the basal segments of bilateral lower lung lobes. Involvement of more than 3 lung lobes by DR-TB is more common than drug-sensitive pulmonary TB. In 87.07% of the patients with DR-TB, the anterior segment of upper lung lobe and the basal segment of lower lung lobe are simultaneously involved. And these locations are rarely involved in patients with TB. In different types of drug resistance, the distribution and location of lesions in lungs show insignificant difference [38–40].

Imaging Demonstrations of DR-TB

DR-TB has the same imaging demonstrations as drug-sensitive secondary TB [38–40]. It is radiologically characterized by consolidation, nodules (including centrilobular nodules and acinar nodules), cavity, tree-bud sign, bronchial wall thickening, bronchiectasis, pleural thickening and/or calcification, pneumothorax and/or pleural effusion, mediastinal and/or hilar lymphadenectasis (Fig. 7.1).

Nodule and Cavity

Nodule and cavity are more common in patients with DR-TB than in patients with drug-sensitive TB. And DR-TB is radiologically characterized by multiple small nodules with accompanying cavity (Fig. 7.2), which commonly distribute within one lung lobe. That is to say, the nodules and cavities in patients with DR-TB tend to aggregate. The cavity in nodule is shown with smooth and intact inner wall, rarely with air-liquid level. Draining bronchus is sometimes observed at proximal part of the nodule with cavity. In patients with DR-TB, the incidence of nodule and cavity within one lung lobe is significantly higher than involvement of two or more lung lobes. However, no significant difference has been found in the number and distribution of nodules and cavities among different types of DR-TB [41, 42].

Tree-Bud Sign

The tree-bud sign in patients with tuberculosis is a characteristic imaging manifestation of dissemination of Mtb along bronchus, which is related to bacteriologically positive TB [43]. Therefore, the tree-bud sign is one of the characteristic signs in the imaging diagnosis of active TB. However, it has no value in the differential diagnosis of DR-TB from drug-sensitive pulmonary TB (Fig. 7.3).

Consolidation

Pathologically, consolidation is mainly exudative or proliferative lesion of pulmonary TB, which is one of the main signs indicating active pulmonary TB. Consolidation may be accompanied by cavity formation. The consolidation opacity is non-specific to both DR-TB and drug-sensitive pulmonary TB. The finding of multiple consolidations involving multiple lobes and multiple segments at the location rarely with

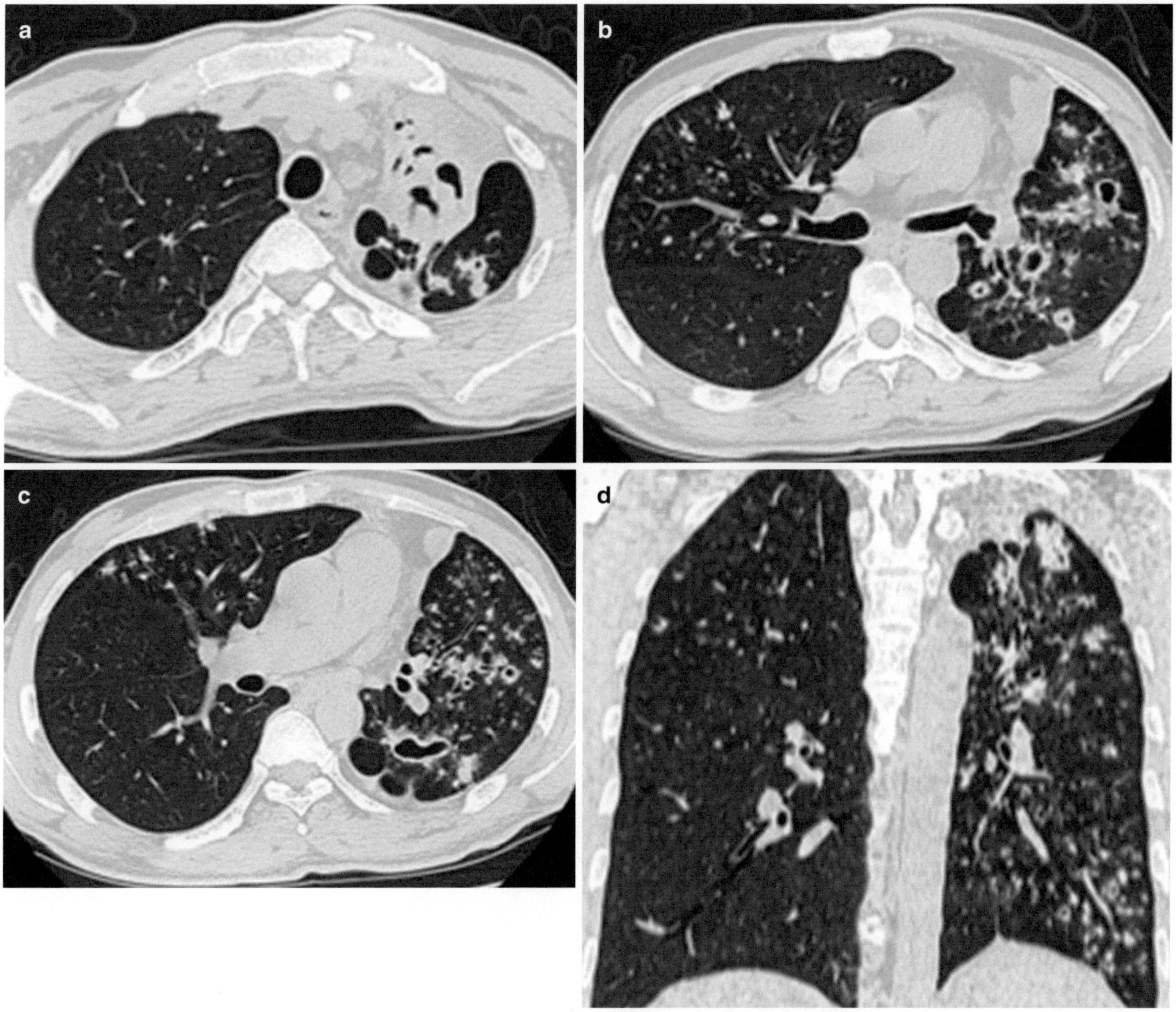

Fig. 7.1 MDR-TB in a 31-year-old male patient. (**a**). Pulmonary window of CT scanning demonstrates small cavity and nodular opacity at the apecoposterior segment of the left upper lung. (**b**). There are multiple small cavities at the left upper lobe and left lingual lobe, and scattering small nodular opacity at the right upper lung. (**c**). The left lower lung lobe is demonstrated with multiple cavitary opacities and small nodular opacity, and the right middle lung lobe is revealed with small nodular opacity. (**d**). Coronal reconstruction shows multiple cavities and nodular opacity at the left lung

lesion of secondary pulmonary TB, with cavitary nodule and/or tree-bud sign, is helpful in the diagnosis of DR-TB (Fig. 7.4).

Bronchial Wall Thickening and Bronchiectasis

DR-TB commonly induces extensive bronchial wall thickening and bronchiectasis [42]. Unlike drug-sensitive TB with bronchial TB that commonly involves major bronchus, DR-TB commonly involves intrapulmonary minor bronchial branches. By diagnostic imaging, it is revealed as wall thickening of adjacent multiple bronchioles, often accompanied by bronchiolar dilation (Fig. 7.5).

Pleural Thickening and Calcification, Pleural Effusion, and Pneumothorax

At the early stage of DR-TB, exudative pleurisy may occur to cause pleural effusion. Pneumothorax, tuberculous empyema, or empyema may occur after lesions of pulmonary TB penetrate the visceral pleura. With the prolongation of the illness course, the affected pleura continues to proliferate to cause irreversible pleural thickening and adhesion, with resultant occurrence of encapsulated empyema or empyema pneumothorax. At its advanced stage, strips of calcification occur. Therefore, extensive pleural hypertrophy, calcification, and adhesion, with accompanying encapsulated

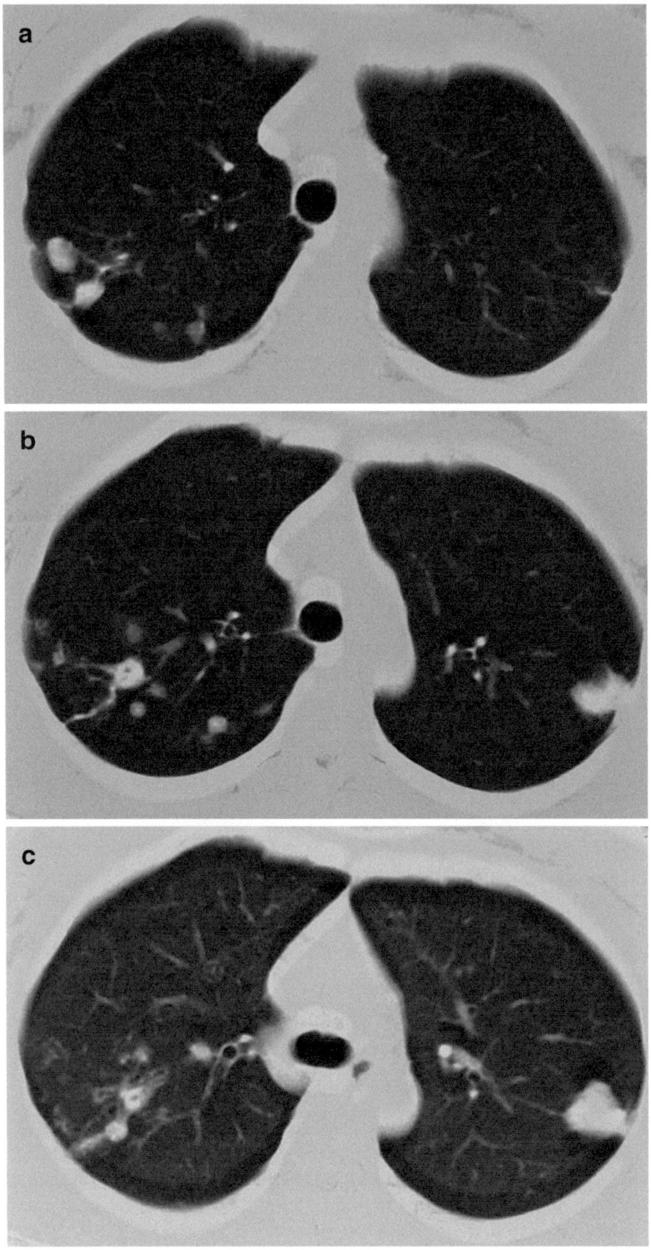

Fig. 7.2 Nodules with accompanying cavities in a 23-year-old female patient with DR-TB. She was diagnosed with drug resistance of Mtb to H, R, Ofx, and S. (**a**–**c**). The lung window of CT scanning shows multiple small nodules with cavities at the right upper lung lobe. There are consolidation opacity at the left upper lung lobe and pleural adhesion

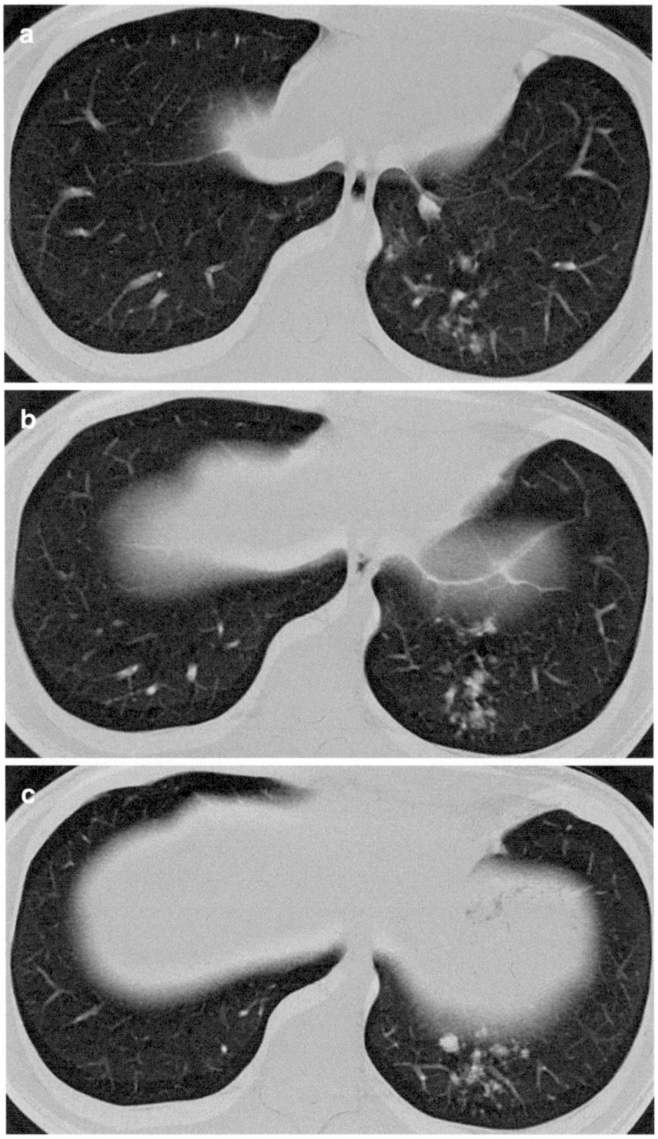

Fig. 7.3 Tree-bud sign in a 25-year-old male patient with DR-TB. He was diagnosed with drug resistance of Mtb to H, Cm, and Pto. (**a**–**c**). The lung window of CT scanning demonstrates dilatation and mucus impaction at the lobular central bronchus and its distal airway of the left lower lung lobe. The lesions combine at different cross-sections to form tree-bud sign

empyema or empyema, are helpful in the diagnosis of DR-TB (Figs. 7.6 and 7.7).

Destructed Lung

In the cases of persistent DR-TB, lung destruction is more common than in the cases of drug-sensitive TB. Tuberculous lung destruction is characterized by extensive lesions in lung lobes or unilateral lung, which are mainly bronchial collapse and atelectasis induced by extensive caseous lesions and fibrosis. There may be accompanying singular or multiple tuberculous fibrous cavity or caseous cavity, bronchiectasis, and/or bronchial stenosis. The lung tissues are severely destructed, with structural distortion and loss of lung function. Unilateral thoracic collapse and mediastinum shift towards the affected lung occur, commonly with severe pleural hypertrophy, adhesion, and calcification (Fig. 7.8).

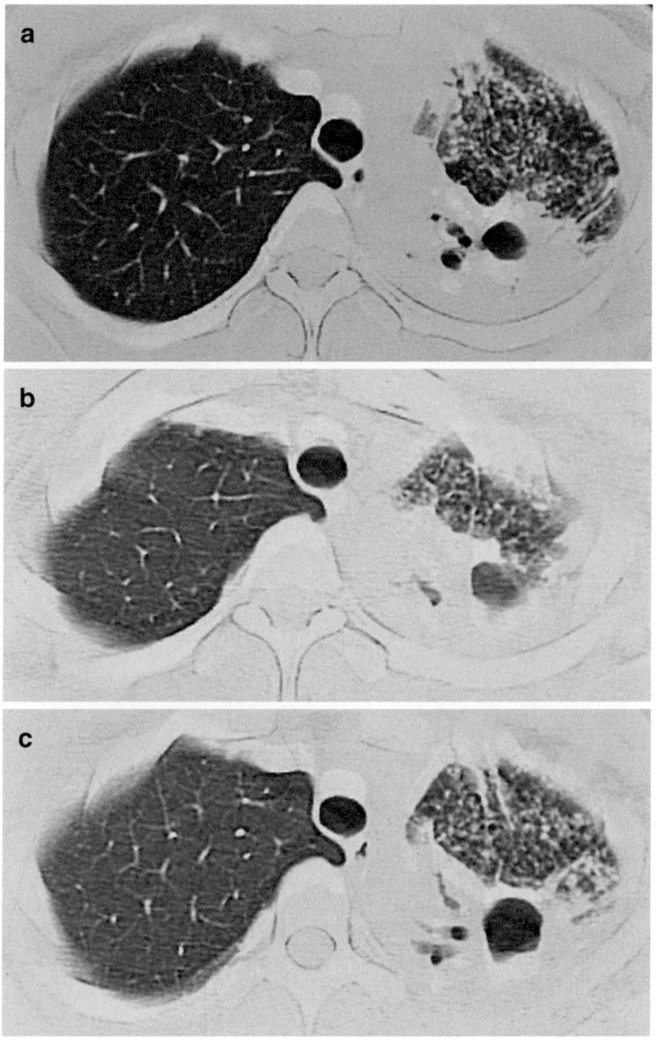

Fig. 7.4 Consolidation in a 23-year-old female patient with DR-TB. She was diagnosed with drug resistance of Mtb to H, R, and S. (**a**–**c**). The lung window of CT scanning reveals a large area of consolidation at the left upper lung lobe, accompanied by thick-wall cavities and draining bronchus. Miliary nodules and pleural thickening are shown anterior to the consolidation at the left upper lung lobe

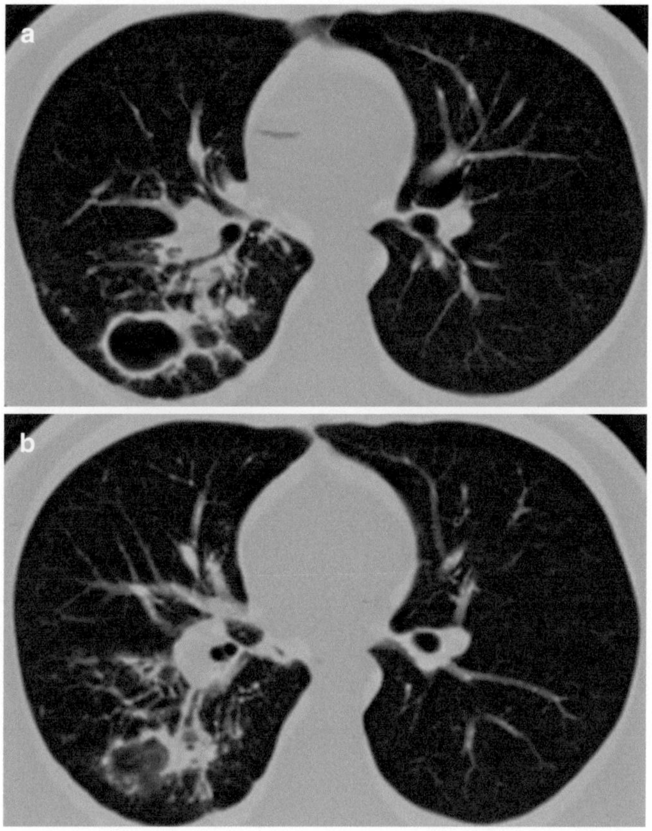

Fig. 7.5 Bronchial wall thickening with bronchiectasis in a 29-year-old male patient with DR-TB. He was diagnosed with drug resistance of Mtb to H, R, Ofx, and S. (**a**, **b**). The lung window of CT scanning shows two thick-wall cavities, draining bronchial wall thickening and bronchiectasis

5.2 Imaging Diagnosis and Differential Diagnosis of DR-TB

Imaging Diagnosis of DR-TB

DR-TB also shows radiologically characteristic signs as drug-sensitive secondary TB. When the following lesions are revealed, the diagnosis of DR-TB is indicated:

(1) The lesions of pulmonary TB cause extensive damage to the pulmonary parenchyma. And the lesions involve the location that rarely occur in the cases of secondary pulmonary TB, such as the right middle lung lobe, the lingual segment of the left upper lung lobe, and the basal segment of bilateral lower lung lobes. In addition, the lesions commonly involve more than three lung lobes.
(2) There are multiple small nodules with cavity formation, which aggregate in one lung lobe.
(3) The wall of adjacent multiple bronchioles is thickened, with dilation of bronchioles.
(4) There are extensive pleural hypertrophy, calcification, and adhesion, with accompanying encapsulated empyema or pyopenumothorax.
(5) The disease persists, with the occurrence of lung destruction.

Differential Diagnosis of DR-TB

DR-TB should be differentiated from infection of non-tuberculosis mycobacterium (NTM).

Radiologically, NTM infection is characterized by infiltration, cavity, nodules, fibrosis, and caseous lesions, among which thin-wall cavity and fibrous tissue proliferation are common. The lesions are mainly located in the upper lung lobes, and the cavity is widely distributed. Thin-wall cavity

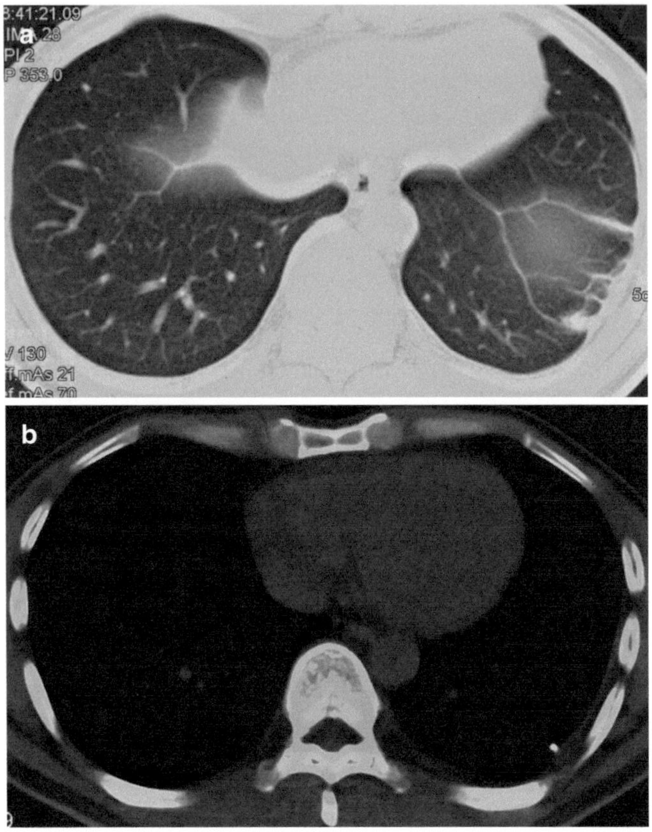

Fig. 7.6 Pleural thickening, adhesion, and calcification in a 42-year-old male patient with DR-TB. He was diagnosed with drug resistance of Mtb to H. (**a**). The lung window of CT scanning reveals pleural thickening and adhesion at the left lower lung lobe. (**b**). The mediastinal window of CT scanning demonstrates spots of pleural calcification at the left lower lung lobe

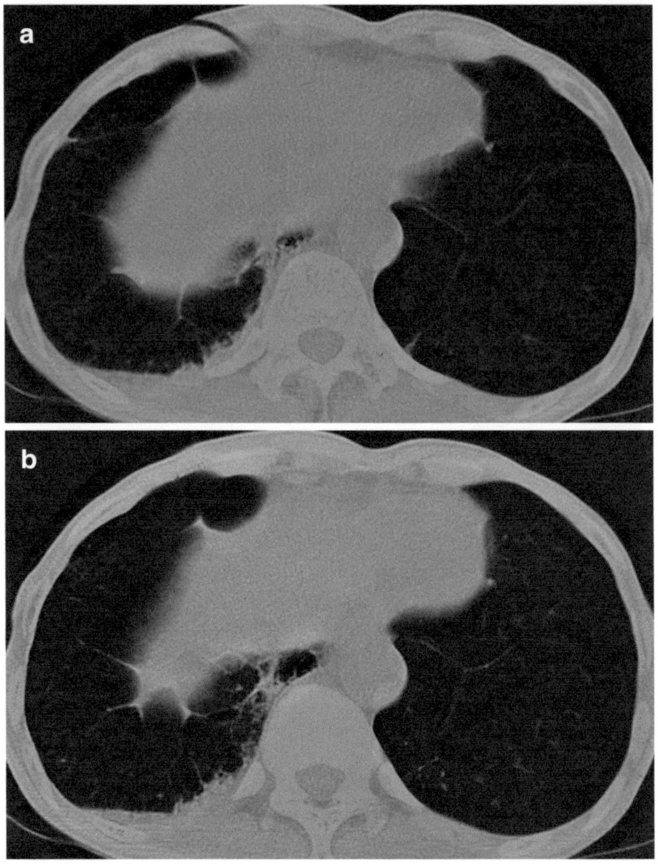

Fig. 7.7 Pleural effusion in a 69-year-old male patient with DR-TB. He was diagnosed with drug resistance of Mtb to H. (**a**, **b**) The lung window of CT scanning shows pleural effusion and pleural adhesion at the right lower lung lobe, with observable fluid level

fibrosis is more common, rarely with surrounding infiltrations. In most cases of NTM infection, bronchiectasis of varying degrees can be found, and the lesions rarely disseminate along bronchus. Hilar lymphadenectasis and calcification of lesions are rare.

NTM is an opportunistic pathogen. Therefore, it commonly complicates chronic pulmonary diseases (such as chronic obstructive pulmonary disease, bronchiectasis, pneumoconiosis, cystic fibrosis, and obsolete pulmonary TB) induced respiratory obstruction and/or airway structural destruction. Congenital or secondary immunodeficiency is also one of the high-risk factors of NTM infection.

The detection rates of bronchiectasis, lobular central nodules, and thin-wall cavities in patients with NTM induced pulmonary disease are higher than those in patients with DR-TB. However, the detection rates of acinar nodules, pulmonary consolidation, atelectasis, lung destruction, calcification within lesion, pleural thickening, and pleural effusion in patients with NTM induced pulmonary disease are lower than those in patients with DR-TB. By CT scanning, NTM induced pulmonary disease is characterized by direct spread of peribronchiolar micronodules, bronchiectasis at the right middle lung lobe and the lingual segment of left upper lung lobe, and subpleural thin-wall cavity to adjacent lung tissues, instead of dissemination along bronchus. In patients with NTM induced pulmonary disease, pleural thickening near the lesion is occasionally revealed, with rare occurrence of pleural effusion.

6 Treatment of DR-TB

To treat DR-TB is challenging, especially MDR-TB and EDR-TB. Formulation of a reasonable treatment regimen can effectively improve the therapeutic efficacy. The following recommended treatment regimens are for clinical reference. If the recommended regimen is ineffective due to drug resistance or intolerance of patient, individualized treatment regimen should be formulated based on the basic principles of the recommended regimen [2, 44, 45].

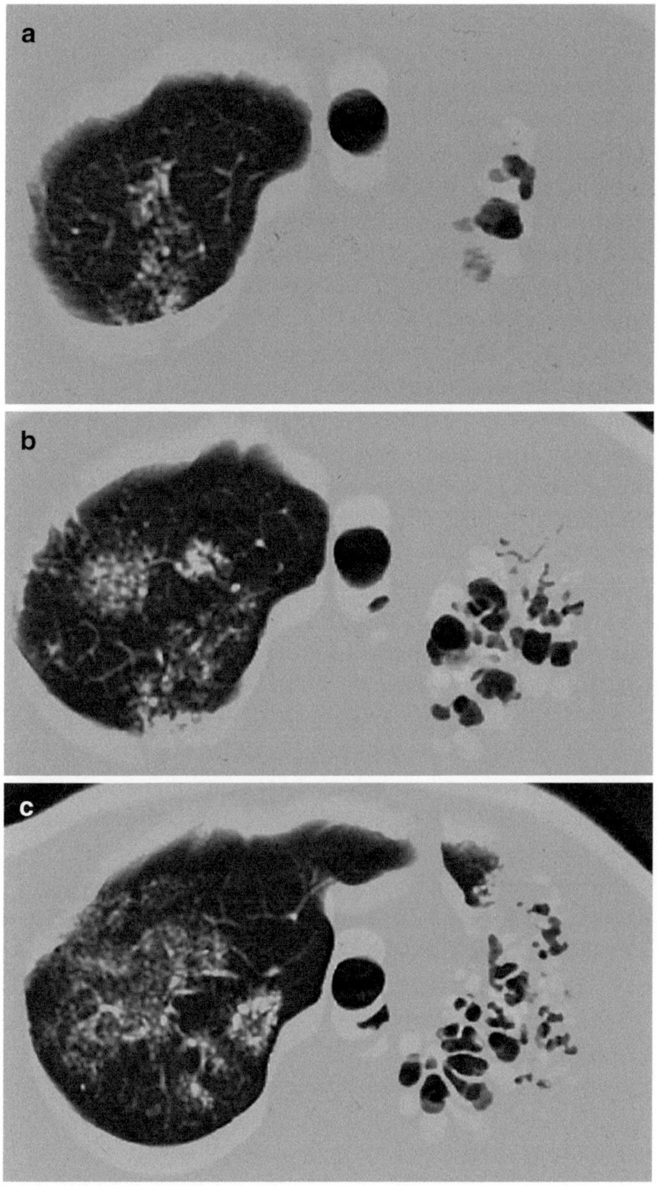

Fig. 7.8 Lung destruction in a 30-year-old female patient with DR-TB. She was diagnosed with drug resistance of Mtb to H, R, and S. (**a**–**c**). The lung window of CT scanning shows destructed left upper lung lobe with extensive multiple caseous fibrotic cavities. The lung tissues are revealed to be seriously destructed, with left thoracic collapse, mediastinal shift towards the left lung. The right upper lung lobe is demonstrated with diffuse bronchial disseminated lesions of TB

6.1 Treatment by Medication of Chemical Drug

Single Drug Resistant TB

Single drug-resistant TB refers to resistance of the infected Mtb to one first-line anti-tuberculosis drug, which is confirmed by in vitro drug sensitivity test. The most common single drug-resistant TB is isoniazid-resistant TB. And resistance of the infected Mtb to one of other first-line anti-tuberculosis drugs is also defined as single drug-resistant TB, with exclusion of rifampicin-resistant TB.

Basic Principles of Chemical Mediation Regimen for Treatment of Single Drug Assistant TB

(1) At least 4 effective first-line anti-tuberculosis drugs during the intensive phase and 3 effective first-line anti-tuberculosis drugs during the continuation phase are selected. If there is not enough effective first-line anti-tuberculosis drug for use, second-line anti-tuberculosis drugs can be selected as alternative.
(2) In principle, the Group 4 second-line oral anti-tuberculosis drugs and the Group 5 other types of anti-tuberculosis drugs are not recommended.
(3) For those with drug resistance of Mtb to isoniazid, the selection of levofloxacin from fluoroquinolones is recommended.
(4) For those with drug resistance of Mtb to streptomycin or with intolerance to streptomycin, one second-line anti-tuberculosis injection is recommended when no first-line effective drug is available. It is recommended to apply the injection for 3 months.
(5) The course of treatment generally lasts for 9–12 months.

Chemical Treatment Regimen for Single Drug Resistant TB

Chemical Treatment Regimen for Isoniazid Resistant TB

(1) Recommendation 1: 3S-R-Z-E/6R-Z-E

Applicable subjects: initially treated patients with isoniazid resistant TB who have no extensive lesions.

Notes: The total course of treatment is 9 months, including intensive phase of 3 months and continuation phase of 6 months. During the intensive phase, streptomycin, rifampicin, pyrazinamide, and ethambutol are applied each day. For the continuation phase, rifampicin, pyrazinamide, and ethambutol are applied each day.

(2) Recommendation 2: 9R-Lfx-Z-E

Applicable subjects: re-treated patients with isoniazid resistant TB; initially treated patients with isoniazid resistant TB and extensive lesions; patients with isoniazid resistant TB and intolerance to streptomycin.

Notes: The total course of treatment is 9 months, with daily use of rifampicin, levofloxacin, pyrazinamide, and ethambutol.

(3) Recommendation 3: 6R-E-Z-Lfx [46]

Applicable subjects: patients with rifampicin-sensitive and isoniazid-resistant TB.

Notes: The total course of treatment is 6 months, with daily use of rifampicin, ethambutol, pyrazinamide, and levofloxacin.

Chemical Treatment Regimen for Other Single Drug Resistant TB

Currently, the DST accuracy of other first-line anti-tuberculosis drugs is lower than that of isoniazid and rifampicin. In combination with epidemiological data and clinical conditions, a chemical treatment regimen is formulated. It is necessary to ensure that the chemical treatment regimen contains 4 effective anti-tuberculosis drugs.

Polydrug Resistant TB

Polydrug resistant TB refers to resistance of the infected Mtb to more than one first-line anti-tuberculosis drugs that is confirmed by in vitro drug sensitivity test. But resistance of infected Mtb simultaneously to isoniazid and rifampicin is excluded.

Basic Principles of Chemical Treatment Regimen for Polydrug Resistant TB

(1) At least 4 effective first-line anti-tuberculosis drugs during the intensive phase and at least 3 effective first-line and second-line anti-tuberculosis drugs are selected. When the infected Mtb is resistant to more than two first-line anti-tuberculosis drugs, pyrazinamide resistance is more likely. If there is reliable evidence supporting effectiveness of pyrazinamide, it can be applied as a core drug. In the written chemical treatment regimen, it should be the last one anti-tuberculosis drug.

(2) For polydrug resistant TB with isoniazid resistance or rifampicin resistance, levofloxacin from fluoroquinolones is recommended. Other rifamycin drugs are not recommended for polydrug resistant TB with rifampicin resistance, such as rifabutin or rifapentine.

(3) For polydrug resistant TB with streptomycin resistance or intolerance to streptomycin, capreomycin is the first choice.

(4) The administration of injections generally lasts for 3 months.

(5) The course of treatment is generally 12–18 months.

Chemical Treatment Regimen for Polydrug Resistant TB

Polydrug Resistant TB with Resistance to Isoniazid and Other First-Line Anti-Tuberculosis Drugs

Recommended regimen: 3S-R-Lfx-Z-E/9R-Lfx-Z-E

Notes: The total course of treatment is 12 months, including the intensive phase of 3 months and the continuation phase of 9 months. During the intensive phase, streptomycin, rifampicin, levofloxacin, pyrazinamide, and ethambutol are applied daily. During the continuation phase, rifampicin, levofloxacin, pyrazinamide, and ethambutol are applied daily.

Polydrug Resistant TB with Resistance to Isoniazid and Other 2–3 First-Line Anti-Tuberculosis Drugs

Recommended regimen: 3S-R-Lfx-Pto-Z/15R-Lfx-Pto-Z

Notes: The total course of treatment is 18 months, including the intensive phase of 3 months and the continuation phase of 15 months. During the intensive phase, streptomycin, rifampicin, levofloxacin, prothioisoxanthine, and pyrazinamide are applied daily. During the continuation phase, rifampicin, levofloxacin, prothioisoxanthine, and pyrazinamide are applied daily.

Multidrug-Resistant TB

Multidrug-resistant TB is resistance of the infected Mtb to isoniazid, rifampicin, and other anti-tuberculosis drugs that is confirmed by in vitro drug sensitivity tests. In patients with multidrug-resistant TB, resistance to 3, 4, or even 5 first-line anti-tuberculosis drugs is possible. And most of the patients with multidrug-resistant TB are re-treated patients.

Basic Principles of Chemical Treatment Regimen for Multidrug-Resistant TB

(1) During the intensive phase, at least 4 effective second-line anti-tuberculosis drugs (including one injection and pyrazinamide) are selected. During the continuation phase, at least 3 effective second-line anti-tuberculosis drugs are selected. And whole course administration of pyrazinamide is recommended.

(2) Second-line injection and fluoroquinolone are of first choice, with first choice of capreomycin for second-line injection, and moxifloxacin from fluoroquinolones. If bedaquinoline is selected, moxifloxacin should be avoided.

(3) In oral second-line anti-tuberculosis drugs, the order of selection is recommended to be linezolid, clofazimine, and cycloserine.

(4) The chemical treatment regimen for multidrug-resistant TB should be decided by consensus of an expert team instead of individual physician. The therapeutic efficacy of anti-tuberculosis drugs, quantity and dosage of anti-tuberculosis drugs, and routes of administrations should be considered in formulation of chemical treatment regimen for multidrug-resistant TB.

Chemical Treatment Regimen for Multidrug-Resistant TB

Recommended regimen 1: 6Cm (Am)-Lfx (Mfx)-Pto (PAS, E)-Cs (PAS, E)-Z/18 Lfx (Mfx)-Pto (PAS, E)-Cs (PAS, E)-Z

Notes: The total course of treatment is 24 months, including the intensive phase of 6 months and the continuation phase of 18 months. The intensive phase can be prolonged to 8 months. During the intensive phase, capreomycin, levofloxacin, prothionamide, cycloserine, and pyrazinamide are administered each day. For re-treated patients with extensive lesions and no negative conversion from bacteriological sputum positive at the end of the intensive phase, the intensive phase can be prolonged to 8 months, while the continuation phase is correspondingly shortened. During the continuation phase, levofloxacin, prothioisoxanthine, cycloserine, and pyrazinamide are administered daily. For those with resistance or intolerance to capreomycin, sensitive amikacin can be administered. For those with resistance to levofloxacin, sensitive moxifloxacin can be applied. For those with intolerance to cycloserine or propionamide, effective or possibly effective p-aminosalicylic acid or ethylamine butanol can be administered.

Recommended regimen 2: 8Cm (Am)-Lfx-Pto (PAS, E)-Cs (PAS, E)-Z/12 Lfx-Pto (PAS, E)-Cs (PAS, E)-Z [47]

Notes: The total course of treatment is 20 months, including the intensive phase of 8 months and the continuation phase of 12 months. During the intensive phase, capreomycin, levofloxacin, propionamide, cycloserine, and pyrazinamide are administered daily. During the continuation phase, levofloxacin, prothioisoxanthine, cycloserine, and pyrazinamide are administered daily. For those with resistance or intolerance to capreomycin, sensitive amikacin can be administered. For those with intolerance to cycloserine or prothioanisamine, effective or possibly effective p-aminosalicylic acid or ethambutol can be administered.

Recommended regimen 3: 4Km (Am)-Mfx-Pto-Cfz-Hh-Z-E/5Mfx-Cfz-E-Z [47]

Applicable subjects: Patients with MDR-TB who have not received second-line anti-tuberculosis drugs.

Notes: The total course of treatment is 9 months, including the intensive phase of 4 months and the continuation phase of 5 months. The intensive phase can be prolonged to 6 months. During the intensive phase, kanamycin, moxifloxacin, prothioanthridine, clofazimine, high-dose isoniazid, pyrazinamide, and ethambutol are administered daily. If there is no evidence supporting negative conversion of sputum smear positive, the intensive phase can be extended to 6 months, the continuation phase is correspondingly shortened. During the continuation phase, moxifloxacin, clofazimine, ethambutol, and pyrazinamide are administered daily. Amikacin can be administered to substitute kanamycin, and ethionamide can be applied to substitute propionamide.

Extensive Drug-Resistant Tuberculosis (XDR-TB)

XDR-TB refers to resistance of the infected Mtb to at least one fluoroquinolone and one second-line anti-tuberculosis injection on the basis of multidrug resistance that is confirmed by in vitro drug sensitivity test. The patients with XDR-TB are mostly re-treated patients with TB or patients with failed treatment of multidrug-resistant TB or relapsed multidrug-resistant TB.

Basic Principles of Chemical Treatment Regimen for XDR-TB

(1) At least 6 effective, possibly effective or never administered anti-tuberculosis drugs in the intensive phase and at least 4 effective, possibly effective or never administered anti-tuberculosis drugs during the continuation phase are selected to form chemical treatment regimen.
(2) A sensitive anti-tuberculosis injection is selected.
(3) Moxifloxacin is the first choice in fluoroquinolones.
(4) Effective or never administered second-line oral anti-tuberculosis drug is selected.
(5) If patient is resistant to low concentration of isoniazid, high-dose isoniazid (16–20 mg/kg) is recommended.
(6) Linezolid is categorized into group A drugs and is one of the key drugs in the chemical treatment regimen for XDR-TB, followed by clofazimine and cycloserine [47].
(7) The course of treatment is generally 30 months. The administration of anti-tuberculosis injection commonly lasts for 12 months. And the administration of injection can be appropriately extended according to the condition of patient. If necessary, the whole course administration of injection is possible.
(8) The chemical treatment regimen for XDR-TB should be based on consensus of an expert team rather than individual physician. The therapeutic efficacy of anti-tuberculosis drugs, quantity and dosage of anti-tuberculosis drugs, and routes of administration should be considered in formulating chemical treatment regimen for XDR-TB.
(9) When there are no sufficient drugs for an effective chemical treatment regimen, palliative treatment is recommended, including symptomatic treatment, nutritional support, and psychological counseling.

Chemical Treatment Regimen for XDR-TB

Recommended regimen: 12Cm-Mfx-Pto (PAS)-Cs (PAS)-Clr-"Amx-Clv"-Z/18Mfx-Pto (PAS)-Cs (PAS)-Clr-"Amx-Clv"-Z

Notes: The total course of treatment is 30 months, including the intensive phase of 12 months and the continuation phase of 18 months. During the intensive phase, capreomycin, moxifloxacin, propionamide, cycloserine, clarithromycin, amoxicillin-clavulanate potassium, and pyrazinamide are administered daily. During the continuation phase, moxifloxacin, propionamide, cycloserine, clarithromycin, amoxicillin-clavulanate potassium, and pyrazinamide are administered daily. For those with intolerance to propionamide or cycloserine, p-aminosalicylic acid is an alternative. If the conditions permit, especially when no second-line oral medication is available, linezolid and/or clofazimine is recommended.

Rifampicin Resistant TB

Rifampicin resistant TB refers to resistance of the infected Mtb to rifampicin that is confirmed by in vitro drug sensitivity test, including any type of resistance of the infected Mtb to rifampin.

Recommended regimen 1: 6Cm (Am)-Lfx (Mfx)-Pto (PAS, E)-Cs (PAS, E)-Z/12Lfx (Mfx)-Pto (PAS, E)-Cs (PAS, E)-Z

Applicable subjects: patients with all types of rifampicin-resistant TB.

Notes: The total course of treatment is 18 months, including the intensive phase of 6 months and the continuation phase of 12 months. The intensive phase can be prolonged to 8 months. During the intensive phase, capreomycin, levofloxacin, prothioanisone, cycloserine, and pyrazinamide are administered daily. For re-treated patients with extensive lesions and patients with no negative conversion of sputum bacteriologically positive at the end of the intensive phase, the intensive period can be extended to 8 months, and the continuation period is correspondingly shortened. During the continuation phase, levofloxacin, prothioisoxanthine, cycloserine, and pyrazinamide are administered daily. For those with resistance or intolerance to capreomycin, sensitive amikacin is an alternative. For those with resistance to levofloxacin, sensitive moxifloxacin is an alternative. For those with intolerance to cycloserine or propionamide, effective or possibly effective p-aminosalicylic acid or ethylamine butanol can be selected.

Recommended regimen 2: 4Km (Am)-Mfx-Pto-Cfz-Hh-Z-E/5Mfx-Cfz-E-Z [48].

Applicable subjects: patients with rifampicin-resistant TB who have not received second-line anti-tuberculosis drugs.

Notes: The total course of treatment is 9 months, including the intensive phase of 4 months and the continuation phase of 5 months. The intensive phase can be prolonged to 6 months. During the intensive phase, kanamycin, moxifloxacin, propionamide, clofazimine, high-dose isoniazid, pyrazinamide, and ethambutol are administered daily. For those with no negative conversion from sputum smear positive, the intensive phase can be prolonged to 6 months, and the continuation phase is correspondingly shortened. During the continuation phase, moxifloxacin, clofazimine, ethambutol, and pyrazinamide are administered daily. Amikacin can be selected to substitute kanamycin, and ethionamide can be selected to substitute propionamide.

6.2 Surgical treatment

Principles of Surgical Treatment for TB

Application of surgery in treatment of TB has 100 years of history in China. According to relevant data, about 5% of the patients with TB in China need surgical treatment. Surgery is still an effective way for patients with failed re-treatment, serious complications, and special types of TB in China. Therefore, surgery plays an indispensable role in eliminating sources of infection and reducing incidence. However, TB is a systemic disease, and surgical removal of all Mtb is impossible. Therefore, after surgery, administration of anti-tuberculosis drugs is important in improving the success rate of surgery as well as preventing and reducing the occurrence of surgical complications and relapse of TB.

Principles of Surgical Treatment for MDR-TB

The surgical treatment is basically to make negative conversion in patients with persistent Mtb positive possible, reduce the relapse rate, reduce the Mtb load, shorten the anti-tuberculosis treatment, and eliminate its spread. In the WHO Guideline for Treatment of Drug-Resistant Tuberculosis (Revisited in 2016), simultaneous chemical treatment for MDR-TB and partial pneumoresection (lobectomy or wedge resection) is recommended to remove unabsorbed lesions, reduce Mtb load, and thereby improve the prognosis [49].

6.3 Interventional Treatment

Transbronchoscopic Airway Interventional Treatment

Different types of interventional treatment have different characteristics. And different types of TB require different interventional treatment measures. Clinically, comprehensive interventional therapy combining multiple interventional treatments is sometimes applied.

Interventional Treatment via Percutaneous Lung Puncture

Guided by X-ray or CT scan, percutaneous lung puncture is performed for injection of anti-tuberculosis drugs or anhydrous alcohol into the cavity.

6.4 Immunotherapy for TB

T cells and B cells are involved in the humoral and cellular immune responses, respectively. Immunomodulator assisted treatment can help to improve the cellular immunity in patients with TB.

The commonly applied immunomodulators include: (1) cytokines: such as interleukin-2 (IL-2), recombinant human γ interferon, and transfer factor; (2) mycobacteria immunologic agents: such as M. vaccae vaccine, and Mycobacterium phlei; (3) other biological agents: such as BCG polysaccharide nucleic acid and thymosin. Despite the large variety of immunomodulators, only M. vaccae vaccines are widely recognized in China as an immunologic agent that plays an immunomodulatory role in patients with TB.

7 Application of DOT Strategy in Management of DR-TB

Since TB is an infectious disease, the management of patients with TB plays an important role in the global TB control strategy. In particular, the key to the successful treatment of DR-TB lies in reasonable treatment regimen, complete treatment course, and effective management. With implementation of multiple measures from multiple perspectives, the goal of TB control can be achieved [50]. The Directly Observed Treatment, Short-course (DOTS) strategy recommended by the WHO has been proven effective worldwide [51]. In Tanzania, the USA, and China, the success of DOTS strategy has proven its feasibility and effectiveness [52].

7.1 Main Contents of the DOTS Strategy

Political Commitment of the Government to the National Planning of TB Control

TB is enlisted as one of the key diseases to be controlled. Under the leadership of the government, the national planning for TB control is implemented. A national network for TB control is established and improved. And the human and financial resources needed in implementing TB control plan are supported by the government.

Detection of Communicable TB by Sputum Smear Test

To control and eliminate the sources of infection is the most effective way to control TB [53]. Currently, it is believed that only patients with sputum smear-positive TB are the main source of infection, and smear negative or culture-positive TB are less communicable. The infectivity is dependent mainly on the amount of Mtb that a patient carries. Therefore, patients with smear-positive TB are the main source of infection. And sputum smear test is the main way to detect the source of infection. The county-level TB control agency should be equipped to perform sputum smear test and its quality should be ensured. Three sputum specimens from each initially presenting patient with suspected symptoms of TB should be collected. Those with sputum smear positive are diagnosed with communicable TB.

Free-in-Charge Short Course Treatment under Direct Observation

To cure communicable TB is its best preventive measure. For each patient with defined diagnosis of communicable TB, DOTS strategy is necessary. And the treatment coverage rate of communicable TB should reach above 98%.

Regular and Continuous Supply of Anti-Tuberculosis Drugs

Regular and continuous supply of anti-tuberculosis drugs is an important measure to ensure the implementation of DOTS. A unified bidding is adopted in purchase of anti-tuberculosis drugs. And the dispense quantity, inventory quantity, and the demand of anti-tuberculosis drugs in the next quarter are registered in all-level TB control agencies to ensure the uninterrupted supply of anti-tuberculosis drugs.

Surveillance System for TB Control Planning

The surveillance system is intended to record the detection, registry, and treatment of patients with TB. Various reporting sheets are timely filled and reported. The TB control agencies are responsible for checking the reporting sheets from subordinate TB control agencies for timely feedbacks.

7.2 Experience of Successful TB Control in China

Beijing is the first city in China to implement the DOTS strategy for TB control and has achieved success. After years of implementing modern TB control strategies, the mortality from TB in Beijing has dropped significantly, from 230 per 0.1 million in 1949 to 1.7 per 0.1 million in 1997. In order to actively promote the implementation of DOTS strategy for TB control, China has launched a number of TB control programs since 1992, which extends the coverage of DOTS. In addition, detection and cure of patients with communicable TB have been emphasized, and free-in-charge treatment and whole course DOTS management have been implemented [54]. A registry and reporting system of patients with TB has been established and improved. Via unified purchase and supply, the quality of anti-tuberculosis drugs has been stabilized. Via supervision by all-level TB control agencies, DOTS strategy has been fully implemented. And all the TB control programs have been well managed. By implementation of these measures, the expense of patients on TB has been greatly reduced and their compliance to treatment has been greatly increased. The standardized treatment is guaranteed to increase the cure rate, decrease the risk of its spread, and prevent the occurrence of DR-TB [55, 56].

7.3 DOTS Strategy for Patients with TB

DR-TB is characterized by less effective therapy, more adverse reactions, and poor compliance of patients. Therefore, the treatment of DR-TB is challenging, with low cure rate. The key to improve the cure rate of DR-TB is to improve the compliance of patients for completion of whole course treatment [57]. Currently, patients with TB tuberculosis are mainly treated and managed in the following ways.

TB Control Agency-Based DOTS Strategy

DOTS strategy is recommended by the WHO for management of TB, which plays an important role in improving compliance of patients and timely managing adverse drug reactions. However, recent studies have demonstrated that DOTS strategy is more applicable for inpatients. For outpatients, DOTS strategy can hardly be implemented for timely sufficient intake of anti-tuberculosis drugs. In addition, the patients commonly have poor awareness about the hazards and seriousness of the disease, and, therefore, tend to change the treatment regimen by themselves, or even discontinue the anti-tuberculosis treatment. These behaviors finally lead to failed treatment [58, 59].

Family- or Community-Based DOTS Strategy

Family- or community-based DOTS strategy is to directly observe the medication of patient by one of the patient's family members or community workers. The selected observer is trained by health-care professionals to manage the patient from perspectives of daily life, regular medication, adverse drug reactions management, and regular review of the medication. Compared to health-care professionals for direct observation of medication, the family- or community-based DOTS strategy plays more important roles in managing the patients with TB. Because family members are in close contact with patients, the privacy of patient can be best protected and the direct observation by family member is the most acceptable by patient. However, due to different situation of each patient and the complex relationship between patient and his/her family members, some patients can hardly accept the family-based DOTS strategy. Therefore, its application should be based on analysis of the specific situation [60–62].

Public–Private Mix-Based DOTS Strategy

Public–private mix-based DOTS strategy was initially implemented in countries such as India, the Philippines, Indonesia, and Vietnam. The quality of the DOTS strategy has been greatly improved due to the introduction of private clinics [63–66]. The public–private mix-based DOTS strategy is established for collaboration of public health-care service and private clinics. Via internal collaborative mechanism, professional training, strengthened DOTS strategy, and a reward/punishment system are performed. In China, this type of DOTS strategy has been implemented since 2004. Via direct on-line reporting, and bi-directional referrals between TB control agency and private clinics, treatment and management has been integrated to increase both the treatment rate and management rate of TB [67, 68].

Telephone and Mobile Phone Text Message-Based DOTS Strategy

Direct face-to-face observed treatment has problems, such as difficulty implementing and poor compliance of patients. To solve these problems, telephone and text messages are used to supervise the treatment and management of patients with TB. Application of telephone and text message is simple to operate, which avoids the long-way transportation of patients for DOTS and effectively improves the compliance of patient. However, it has its limitations. Based on telephone and text message, the treatment cannot be fully observed and failure is possible [69–71].

QQ and WeChat-Based DOTS Strategy

The 2014 WHO Conference explicitly advocates the development of new DOTS strategies. Research and innovation are emphasized for development of new tools to improve implementation of DOTS strategy. The concept of "Internet +" was put forward by the Chinese government. Currently, China is striving to explore the TB control strategy based on the concept of "Internet +" [72]. Direct trace of patients via instant communication tools such as WeChat facilitates one-to-one health education about TB control. Via WeChat, the importance of regular medication is emphasized and the knowledge about adverse reactions of anti-tuberculosis drugs is conveniently spread. When patients encounter adverse drug reactions, dietary contraindications, and other problems, they can also receive timely guidance. Thereby the possibilities of drug withdrawal and drug reduction due to adverse reactions are decreased. Instant communication tool-based DOTS strategy improves the compliance of patient and thus improves the therapeutic efficacy. It is especially important in the treatment and management of DR-TB.

References

1. World Health Organization. Guidelines for the programmatic management of drug-resistant tuberculosis: 2006. WHO/HTM/TB/2006.361. Geneva: World Health Organization; 2006.
2. World Health Organization. Companion handbook to the WHO guidelines for the programmatic management of drug-resistant tuberculosis. WHO/HTM/TB/2014.11. Geneva: World Health Organization; 2014.
3. WHO/IUATLD. Global Project on Anti-tuberculosis Drug Resistance Surveillance. Anti-tuberculosis drug resistance in the world. Third report. Geneva: WHO; 2004. p. 343.
4. Tang SJ, Xu SF, Li L. Drug-resistant tuberculosis. Beijing: People's Medical Publishing House; 2014. p. 126–287.
5. Gao Q, Mei J. Spread is the main reason for high incidence of drug-resistant TB in China. Chin J Antituberculosis. 2015;37(11):1091–6.
6. Wang ZY. Recent development of studies on drug-resistant TB. Inf Infect Dis. 2018;31(1):19–23.
7. World Health Organization. Companion handbook to the WHO guidelines for the programmatic management of drug-resistant tuberculosis. WHO/HTM/TB/2018.09. Geneva: World Health Organization; 2018.

8. World Health Organization. Companion handbook to the WHO guidelines for the programmatic management of drug-resistant tuberculosis. WHO/HTM/TB/2017.10. Geneva: World Health Organization; 2017.
9. Ministry of Health, P. R. China. Compiled data on the national epidemiological sampling survey of TB in 1979; 1981.
10. Ministry of Health, P. R. China. Compiled data on the national epidemiological sampling survey of TB in 1984/1985; 1988.
11. Ministry of Health, P. R. China. Compiled data on the national epidemiological sampling survey of TB in 1990; 1992.
12. Ministry of Health, P. R. China. Compiled data on the national epidemiological sampling survey of TB in 2000; 2002.
13. Ministry of Health, P. R. China. Report on the national epidemiological sampling survey of TB in 2010; 2012.
14. Gao Q, Mei J. Spread is the main reason for high prevalence of DR-TB in China. Chin J Antituberculosis. 2015;37(11):1091–6.
15. Gao Q, Yang CG. Recent spread of TB in China and strategies for its control. J Tuberc Lung Health. 2017;6(13):193–8.
16. Yang HJ. Present tuberculosis control in migrating population. Med Inf. 2014;2014(19):642–3.
17. Lu W, Fu YY. Sustainable development of drug resistant TB control in China. J Tuberc Lung Health. 2016;5(4):262–6.
18. Zhou XJ. Drug resistant TB and its treatment strategies. West Med. 2017;29(1):141–4.
19. Bu QB. Epidemiology of pulmonary TB and its control measures. Healthcare Nutr China. 2015;25(10):58–9.
20. Kliiman K, Altraja A, Tang SJ, et al. Factors predicting failed treatment for multidrug resistant TB and extensive drug resistant TB. Chin J Tuberc Respir. 2009;32(8):563.
21. Du JH, Liu JC, Wang AM, et al. Research developments on drug resistant TB and its impact factors. Med Equip China. 2016;2016(s1):144.
22. Yang HJ. Present TB control in migrating population. Med Inf. 2014;2014(19):42–643.
23. Zhang T, Xi MX. Evolvement of directly observed treatment for patients with pulmonary TB. Pract Prev Med. 2017;2017(03): 382–5.
24. Zhao YL, Li L, Zhou XH. Diagnosis of tuberculosis: part I. China Med News. 2006;21(10):14–5.
25. Zhao YL, Shang M. Laboratory diagnosis of tuberculosis in China. Chin J Lab Med. 2007;30(7):725–58.
26. Steingart KR, Ng V, Henry M, et al. Sputum processing methods to improve the sensitivity of smear microscopy for tuberculosis: a systematic review. Lancet Infect Dis. 2006;6(10):664–74.
27. Yang XJ. Acid-fast staining for detection of bacillus: a comparative study. J Qiannan Med Coll Nat. 2008;21(1):6–7.
28. Alisjahbana B, Van Crevel R, Danusantoso H, et al. Better patient instruction for sputum sampling can improve microscopic tuberculosis diagnosis. Int J Tuberc Lung Dis. 2005;9(7):814–7.
29. Hirooka T, Higuchi T, Tanaka N, et al. [The value of proper sputum collection instruction in detection of acid-fast bacillus]. Kekkaku. 2004;79(2):33–7.
30. Guo J, Fan H, Kang M. Laboratory test for rapid detection of Mycobacterium tuberculosis. Int J Lab Med. 2006;27(9):807–8.
31. Steingart K R, Schiller I, Horne D J, et al. Xpert(R) MTB/RIF assay for pulmonary tuberculosis and rifampicin resistance in adults. Cochrane Database Syst Rev. 2014(1):CD009593.
32. Safianowska A, Walkiewicz R, Nejman-Gryz P, et al. [Diagnostic utility of the molecular assay GenoType MTBC (HAIN Lifesciences, Germany) for identification of tuberculous mycobacteria]. Pneumonol Alergol Pol. 2009;77(6):517–20.
33. Sun FS, Wu HN, Gu HM. Research developments on control of drug resistant tuberculosis. Med Rev. 2018;2018(1):86–9.
34. Yang SL, Bu HL, Fan MB. Drug sensitivity test by BACTEC-MGIT 960 and Roche proportional method: a comparative study. Clin Pract. 2015;2015(12):919–21.
35. Zheng Y, Xia H, Zhao YL. Sensitivity test of Mycobacterium tuberculosis to first-line and second-line anti-tuberculosis drugs by TREK Sensititre MYCOTB. Chin J Antituberculosis. 2015;37(6):597–602.
36. Li H, Wang SH, Zhu YK. Diagnosis of multidrug-resistant tuberculosis based on two different molecular biological detections for multidrug-resistant genes. Chin J Health Lab Technol. 2015;25(15):2567–9.
37. Makinen J, Marttila HJ, Marjamaki M, et al. Comparison of two commercially available DNA line probe assays for detection of multidrug-resistant Mycobacterium tuberculosis. J Clin Microbiol. 2006;44(2):350–2.
38. Committee of Infectious Disease Radiology in Branch of Radiology, Chinese Medical Society. Consensus on imaging diagnosis for grading of pulmonary tuberculosis. Electron J Emerg Infect Dis. 2018;3(2):118–27.
39. Zhang ZX, Ren GY, Tan YC, et al. CT scanning demonstrations of Rifamycin resistant pulmonary tuberculosis. Guide China Med. 2015;13(25):64–5.
40. Chen GM, Cheng GX, Zhu SQ, et al. CT scanning demonstration of initially treated patients with single drug resistant pulmonary tuberculosis. Electron J Emerg Inf Dis. 2018;3(2):111–4.
41. Li CH, Lv SX, Wang HQ, et al. CT scanning demonstrations of multidrug resistant pulmonary tuberculosis and their relationship with CD4 cell count. Chin J Antituberculosis. 2017;39(6): 597–603.
42. Wang YX, Chung MJ, Skrahin A, et al. Literature analysis on radiological demonstrations related to multidrug resistant pulmonary tuberculosis. Electron J Emerg Inf Dis. 2018;3(3):244–53.
43. Yu WY, Tan WG, Zhong FX, et al. Categorization and typing of drug resistant pulmonary tuberculosis and their diagnostic imaging. Electron J Emerg Inf Dis. 2019;4(1):52–6.
44. Chinese Anti-tuberculosis Society. 2015 Guideline for chemical treatment of drug resistant tuberculosis. Chin J Antituberculosis. 2015;37(5):421–69.
45. World Health Organization. WHO guideline for treatment of isoniazid resistant tuberculosis: supplement to the WHO guideline for treatment of drug resistant tuberculosis. Geneva: World Health Organization; 2018.
46. Companion handbook to the 2014 WHO guidelines for the programmatic management of drug resistant tuberculosis. Chin J Antituberculosis. 2015;37(7):800–2.
47. Aung KJ, Van Deun A, Declercq E, et al. Successful '9-month Bangladesh regimen' for multidrug-resistant tuberculosis among over 500 consecutive patients. Int J Tuberc Lung Dis. 2014;18(10):1180–7.
48. WHO. Rapid communication: key changes to treatment of multidrug- and rifampicin-resistant tuberculosis (MDR/RR-TB). Geneva: World Health Organization; 2018.
49. World Health Organization. WHO treatment guidelines for drug-resistant tuberculosis. 2016 update. Geneva: World Health Organization; 2016.
50. Dai ZC, Xiao DL, Wan LY. The history of anti-tuberculosis in China. Beijing: People's Medical Publishing House; 2013. p. 58.
51. World Health Organization. Global tuberculosis report 2014. Geneva: World Health Organization; 2014.
52. Zhou L, Xue X, Wang F, et al. Implementation of tuberculosis management. Chin J Antituberculosis. 2013;35(2):120–4.
53. Disease Control Bureau of Health Ministry, Medial Administration Department of Health Ministry, Center for Disease Control, China. Technical guideline for implementation of tuberculosis control planning in China. Beijing: Peking Union Medical College Press; 2009. p. 20.
54. Chen J, Wang Y, Hu DY. Effects of directly observed treatment on tuberculosis control. Med Foreign Countries: Social Med. 2005;22(4):166–70.

55. Huang CY, Song JD, Li GZ, et al. DOTS in management of outpatients with sputum smear positive pulmonary tuberculosis. Popul Health. 2014;8(24):114.
56. Jiang L. Research developments on compliance of patients with tuberculosis to medication. Inf Infect Dis. 2012;25(1):55–7.
57. Ma HX, Wang JY. Effects of health education on patients with pulmonary tuberculosis. China Med Innov. 2012;9(13):147–8.
58. Guo WR. Family based DOT strategy in 155 patients with sputum smear positive tuberculosis. Chin J Antituberculosis. 2010;32(4):202–3.
59. Wen K, Ma J. Effects of family based DOT strategy on compliance of initially treated patients with sputum smear positive pulmonary tuberculosis. China Med Innov. 2015;12(3):124–6.
60. Zhu J. On nursing of patients with pulmonary tuberculosis. China Med Innov. 2012;9(1):85–6.
61. Xu GB, Liu FY, Feng QM, et al. New strategy on tuberculosis control in rural areas of Guangxi Zhuang autonomous region of China. Chin J Antituberculosis. 2011;45(1):30–5.
62. Wang YX. Community based DOT strategy in 56 patients with pulmonary tuberculosis. Anhui Med. 2012;16(11):1720–1.
63. Li JW, Wu WF, Han DL. Comprehensive survey on pulmonary tuberculosis in peasant workers. China Med Innov. 2011;8(2): 26–8.
64. World Health Organization. Public-private mix for DOTS—global progress. Geneva: World Health Organization; 2004. p. 2–9.
65. Lal SS, Sahu S, Wares F, et al. Intensified scale-up of public-private mix: a systems approach to tuberculosis care and control in India. Int J Tuberc Lung Dis. 2011;15(1):97–104.
66. Haq Z, Khan W, Scita A. Promoting public-private mix for TB-DOTS: a multi-country study from the WHO Eastern Mediterranean Region. East Mediterr Health J. 2012;18(5):410–6.
67. Technical Guidance Team of the national epidemiological sampling survey for tuberculosis. Report on 2000 National Epidemiological Sampling Survey on tuberculosis. Chin J Antituberculosis. 2002;24(2):86–96.
68. Zhu LY, Zhang QY, Zhong CQ, et al. Implementation of PPM-DOTS tuberculosis control program in urban area of Lianyungang, China. J Nanjing Med Univ (Nat Sci). 2008;28(12):1690–3.
69. Yang HL, Bao CL, Bai LQ, et al. Telephone based DOTS and traditional DOTS in rural areas of Hunan province, China: a comparative study. Chin J Antituberculosis. 2011;33(10):646–50.
70. Lu F, Xu H, Fu J. Effects of mobile phone text message based DOTS on compliance of patients with pulmonary tuberculosis. Chin J Antituberculosis. 2012;34(10):651–4.
71. Bao CL, Bai LQ, Tang Y, et al. Effects of telephone based DOTS and traditional DOTS on therapeutic efficacy of pulmonary tuberculosis. Pract Prev Med. 2012;19(12):1803–6.
72. Xi MX, Qin Q, Zeng YL, et al. Application of internet based collaborative nursing in management of patients with MHD. J Changsha Univ. 2015;29(1):58–61.

Control of TB/HIV Coinfection

8

Wei-guo Tan, Zhi-peng Zhuo, Zheng Yang, Pu-Xuan Lu, Yu-xin Shi, Ru-Ming Xie, Bu-dong Chen, Hui Wang, and Yang Zhou

1 Overview of TB/HIV Coinfection

Due to immunodeficiency in patients with HIV infection and AIDS, their immunity is compromised and they are vulnerable to infection of pathogenic bacteria. Mtb is mainly transmitted via the respiratory tract and is highly tolerant to the external environment. Therefore, Mtb constitutes one of the major opportunistic pathogenic bacteria to patients with HIV/AIDS. Studies have shown that the prevalence of TB in HIV-positive patients is 19 times as high as that in HIV-negative patients [1]. When patients with HIV/AIDS are infected by Mtb, they are coinfected with TB and HIV/AIDS (abbreviated as TB/HIV coinfection).

Currently, the new cases of TB each year in the world have been decreasing, and the incidence of TB in China has also been decreasing [2]. However, the patients with HIV/AIDS have been increasing, and a significant proportion of patients with HIV/AIDS are not detected and registered. Due to the large population of patients with TB and its long course of treatment, the patients with HIV/AIDS are vulnerable to repeated infection of Mtb. TB/HIV coinfection may progress into DR-TB, MDR-TB, or even XDR-TB. Our experience has warned us that the prevalence of TB/HIV coinfection is directly threatening the achievements of TB control in recent decades. In sub-Saharan Africa, the incidence of TB has been rising, which can be largely attributed to the HIV epidemic. It is compulsory and urgent for TB control agencies and HIV/AIDS control agencies to strengthen collaborative efforts on control of TB/HIV coinfection. When the prevalence of TB/HIV coinfection remains at a low level, effective measures should be implemented to prevent aggravation of the epidemic [3].

2 Epidemiology of TB/HIV Coinfection

2.1 Epidemiology of TB/HIV Coinfection

According to the data in the 2018 Global Tuberculosis Control Report, the patients with TB are estimated to be ten million across the world in 2017, including 1.01 million children, 3.68 million females, and 6.36 million males. Patients with TB/HIV coinfection amount up to 0.920 million (9% of the total patients with TB), and patients with MDR-TB and rifampicin-resistant TB amount up to 0.56 million (with MDR-TB accounting for 82%). In 2017, the estimated number of deaths from TB worldwide is 1.57 million, including 0.203 million children, 0.606 million females, and 0.968 million males. And the number of deaths from TB/HIV coinfection is estimated to be 0.3 million.

Since 2000, the absolute number of deaths from TB in HIV-negative populations worldwide has been declining, from 1.7 million in 2000 to 1.3 million in 2016. Between 2000 and 2016, the mortality of TB decreased by 37%, and by 3.4% between 2015 and 2016. In 2016, approximately 82% of deaths from HIV-negative TB occurred in WHO

W.-g. Tan (✉)
Department of Tuberculosis, The Shenzhen Center for Chronic Disease Control, Shenzhen, Guangdong, China

Z.-p. Zhuo · Z. Yang
Shenzhen Center for Chronic Disease Control, Shenzhen, Guangdong, China

P.-X. Lu
Department of Radiology, The Shenzhen Center for Chronic Disease Control, Shenzhen, Guangdong, China

Y.-x. Shi
Shanghai Public Health Clinical Center, Fudan University, Shanghai, China

R.-M. Xie
Beijing Ditan Hospital, Capital Medical University, Beijing, China

B.-d. Chen
Department of Radiology, Beijing Ditan Hospital, Capital Medical University, Beijing, China

H. Wang · Y. Zhou
The Third People's Hospital of Shenzhen, Shenzhen, Guangdong, China

W.-y. Yu et al. (eds.), *Tuberculosis Control in Migrating Population*, https://doi.org/10.1007/978-981-32-9763-0_8

Africa and Southeast Asia. Meanwhile, the number of deaths from TB in these areas account for 85% of the total number of deaths from TB in HIV-negative and HIV-positive populations. In 2016, the global mortality of TB in HIV-negative population was 17 per 0.1 million, and the global mortality of TB in HIV-positive population was 24 per 0.1 million.

In 2016, 10% (8–12%) of the estimated new cases of TB were HIV infected patients. The countries with the highest proportion of TB/HIV coinfection are in African region, and the percentage is above 50% in some southern African countries. The risk of Mtb infection in 37 million HIV infected patients is 21 times (16–27 times) as high as that in other populations in the world. The global burden of HIV/AIDS is mainly from low- and middle-income countries, with 95% of HIV infected patients living in these countries. Sub-Saharan Africa is the mostly affected region of HIV/AIDS epidemic. Nearly 70% of patients with sputum smear-positive TB in this region are HIV positive. And, to some extent, the HIV/AIDS epidemic has increased the incidence of TB in the region. Since the mid-1980s, there has been a four-fold increase in the annual registry rate of patients with TB patients in many African countries (including those with well-implemented TB control programs), with a morbidity of above 400 per 0.1 million. The number of deaths from TB/HIV has been increasing.

Nowadays, a large number of HIV infected patients in China have not been detected, and the risk of its latent transmission is high. Especially in high-risk regions and populations, the measures for its prevention, treatment, and management need to be reinforced. It is necessary to further extend the coverage of screening for HIV/AIDS to detect patients with HIV/AIDS. Therefore, further transmission can be reduced. In addition, patients with HIV/AIDS need to receive appropriate treatment to reduce the occurrence of death. It is necessary to further expand the coverage of health education and to enhance the intervention. Efforts are also needed to reduce and eliminate social discrimination towards patients with TB and HIV/AIDS. Based on these efforts, the hazards of HIV/AIDS can be diminished to effectively safeguard the population health [4].

2.2 Significance

HIV infected patients in China have been increasing. Current research indicated that HIV infection is the highest risk factor to activate latent TB infection into active TB. HIV infection accelerates the progression of new Mtb infection or latent Mtb infections into active TB. Meanwhile, 5–15% cases of Mtb infection in patients with HIV/AIDS develop into TB each year, and the chance rises to 50% during their lifetime. However, only 5–10% cases of Mtb infection in HIV-negative patients develop into TB during their lifetime. In addition, HIV infection increases the relapse rate of TB, which may be induced by endogenous activation or exogenous reinfection [5].

TB also contributes to the progression of HIV. Studies have shown that response of patient with TB/HIV coinfection to Mtb promotes replication of HIV and accelerates the progression of AIDS. In patients with HIV/AIDS who develop TB, the mortality rate at the end of anti-tuberculosis treatment is very high (about 20% in patients with sputum smear-positive TB, and nearly 50% in patients with sputum smear-negative TB) [6].

TB is one of the major opportunistic infections in patients with HIV/AIDS. Screening of HIV in patients with TB facilitates early detection of patients with HIV/AIDS to reduce its further transmission. And the screened patients with HIV/AIDS can receive effective treatment promptly to reduce occurrence of death. In addition, it is necessary to strengthen health education and behavioral intervention concerning HIV/AIDS control in patients with TB, which can reduce the hazards of HIV/AIDS and effectively safeguard the population health. Furthermore, screening for TB and health education about TB control in patients with HIV/AIDS facilitate early detection of TB, which is one of the major causes of death in patients with HIV/AIDS, to prevent spread of TB in populations. Meanwhile, the resistance rate of Mtb, incidence, and mortality of TB can be reduced [7].

3 Measures for TB/HIV Coinfection Control

3.1 Screening of TB in Patients with HIV/AIDS

Screening for Suspected Symptoms of TB

Workplace and Subjects of Screening

The workplaces for screening of TB in patients with HIV/AID include all the institutions responsible for follow-ups of HIV/AIDS, such as CDC, street disease control agency, health-care institutions, anti-viral treatment agencies, voluntary counseling and testing clinics, and methadone clinics. The subjects of the screening include all the defined cases of HIV/AIDS.

Human Resources

The health-care staffs working in above institutions and places are responsible for the screening.

Method and Frequency of Screening

During epidemiological survey and follow-up of patients with HIV/AIDS, the suspected symptoms of TB are inquired in detail. And the Case Follow-up Form is correctly filled.

Referral of Patients with HIV/AIDS

Subjects

The subjects of referral include newly reported and registered cases of HIV/AIDS, patients with HIV/AIDS who receive routine test for TB each year, patients with HIV/AIDS who show suspected symptoms of TB during follow-ups.

Procedure of Referral

The patients with HIV/AIDS are referred to the local TB control agency according to localized management. One instant sputum specimen, one-night sputum specimen, and one next morning sputum specimen are collected for sputum smear test and acid-fast staining. If the patients with HIV/AIDS cannot be referred, the above three sputum specimens and clinical data are transferred to the local TB control agency for examination.

Measures to Ensure Presentation of Referrals

The health-care staff responsible for referral should emphasize the importance of TB screening to patients with HIV/AIDS and contact the TB control agency via telephone calls. The presentation of referral to the TB control agency should feedback to the institution of referral-out. If the referral fails to present in the local TB control agency within 3 days after reception of the referral sheet by the local TB control agency, the local TB control agency is responsible for contacting with the institution of referral-out to inform the non-presentation of the referral. And the institution of referral-out is responsible to trace the patient within 3 days.

Detection and Diagnosis of TB

Sputum Smear Test and Chest X-Ray

All the patients with HIV/AIDS who are suspected with TB should receive sputum smear test and chest X-ray. All the patients with HIV/AIDS, regardless of showing the suspected symptoms of TB, should be referred by the HIV/AIDS control agency to the local TB control agency for screening of TB at least once a year. The screening examinations include sputum smear test and chest X-ray.

Isolation and Culture of Mtb

If patients with HIV/AIDS show suspected symptoms of TB or abnormality in chest X-ray, the local TB control agency is responsible to select 2 high-quality sputum specimens for Mtb culture.

Tuberculin Test

If patients with HIV/AIDS show suspected symptoms of TB but fail to be diagnosed by other examinations, tuberculin test is recommended as an auxiliary way for diagnosis.

Diagnostic Treatment

If patients with HIV/AIDS show suspected symptoms of TB but fail to be definitively diagnosed, diagnostic anti-inflammatory treatment (usually observed for 2 weeks) is an alternative for diagnosis. However, quinolones, aminoglycosides, and the other drugs with significant anti-tuberculosis activity should not be selected. For patients suspected with active TB after anti-inflammatory treatment, diagnostic anti-tuberculosis treatment is an alternative for further diagnosis. The treatment regimen for initially treated TB is recommended and the course of treatment usually lasts for 1–2 months.

Differential Diagnosis

Symptoms, signs, and chest X-ray demonstrations of TB resemble to many other thoracic diseases. Therefore, differential diagnosis is important.

Strain Identification and Drug Sensitivity Test

Strain of TB/HIV coinfection should be identified with the following drug sensitivity test to guide the formulation of treatment regimen.

Diagnostic Criteria of TB

The diagnosis of TB in patients with HIV/AIDS is based on bacteriologic test. Meanwhile, the bacteriological test should be combined with case history, clinical manifestations, chest imaging demonstrations, necessary auxiliary examinations, and differential diagnosis for comprehensive analysis.

Technical Procedures (Fig. 8.1)

3.2 HIV Antibody Detection in Patients with TB

Participation of the Patients with TB

When the Agreement on Free-in-charge Management and Treatment of Tuberculosis is signed by the TB control agency and patient with TB (especially those with high-risk behaviors of HIV/AIDS), free-in-charge HIV antibody detection is added. And the importance of HIV antibody detection is explained to patients with TB. If the patient with TB agrees to receive HIV antibody detection, an agreement on treatment and management containing free-in-charge HIV antibody detection is signed. If the preliminary screening of HIV antibody shows positive, blood specimen from the patient is collected again and two blood specimens are sent to HIV/AIDS control agency to define the diagnosis. The agreement is properly preserved by the TB control agency.

HIV antibody detection is performed after informed consent is obtained from the patient. The patient has the right to refuse HIV antibody detection, which does not affect the performance of other free-in-charge examinations and treatments. If a patient with TB refuses HIV antibody detection when the diagnosis of TB is defined, HIV antibody detection should be recommended by the TB control agency in the follow-ups for treatment and management of TB.

HIV Antibody Detection

Laboratory HIV antibody detection is conducted according to the National Technical Specification on Detection of HIV/AIDS. For patients with preliminary screening positive, HIV infection is confirmed according to relevant regulations.

Fig. 8.1 Discovery of TB patients among HIV(+)/AIDS patients

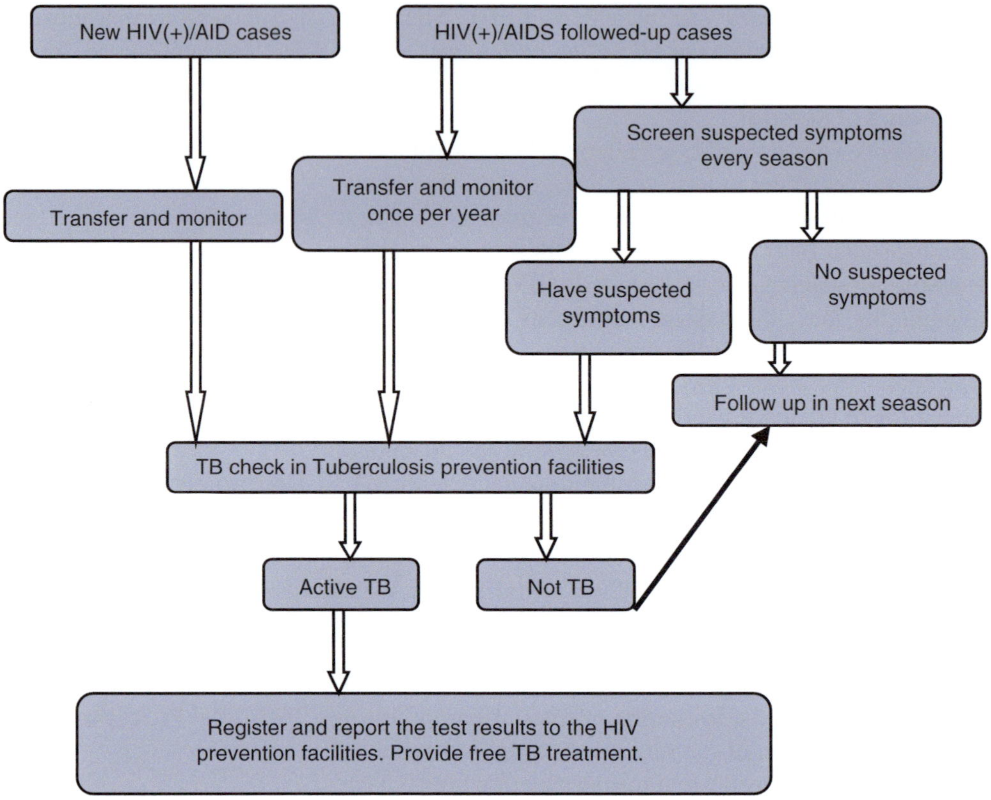

Results Report of HIV Antibody Detection

The laboratory result of HIV antibody detection in patient with TB is promptly reported to the TB control agency of localization management. And the result must be recorded in the dedicated and confidential registry book by the local TB control agency.

Consultation and Referral After HIV Antibody Detection

Consultation on HIV Antibody Negative

The health-care staffs in TB control are responsible for providing consultation for patients with TB and HIV negative. The consultation can be performed during follow-ups of TB treatment and management. If the patient has further questions, he/she can seek help in local voluntary counseling and testing (VCT) clinic.

Consultation and Referral of HIV Antibody Positive

If patient with TB is detected with HIV antibody positive, the health-care staffs in local TB control agency should immediately contact the patient for follow-up, and contact the local VCT HIV/AIDS clinic to provide consultation and anti-HIV management. In combination with the condition of the patient, the TB control agency is responsible for treatment, follow-ups, and management of TB.

Technical Procedures (Fig. 8.2)

3.3 Intervention of HIV/AIDS

In TB control agency and HIV/AIDS control agency, cross infection between patients with HIV/AIDS and patients with TB should try to be prevented [8]. In TB control agency and HIV/AIDS control agency, the National Technical Guidelines for AIDS Testing should be strictly observed for collection of blood specimen and occupational protection. Meanwhile, large quantity of interventions are needed in the field of care and support for patients with HIV/AIDS to prolong their lives and improve their quality of life.

Care and Support for Patients with HIV/AIDS

A series of measures including antiretroviral treatment should be implemented for patients with HIV/AIDS. The key elements in care of patients with HIV/AIDS include:

(1) Voluntary counseling and testing services;
(2) Prevention, screening, and treatment of opportunistic infections, including TB;
(3) Health education and health promotion, including nutrition, family planning, and prevention of further HIV transmission;

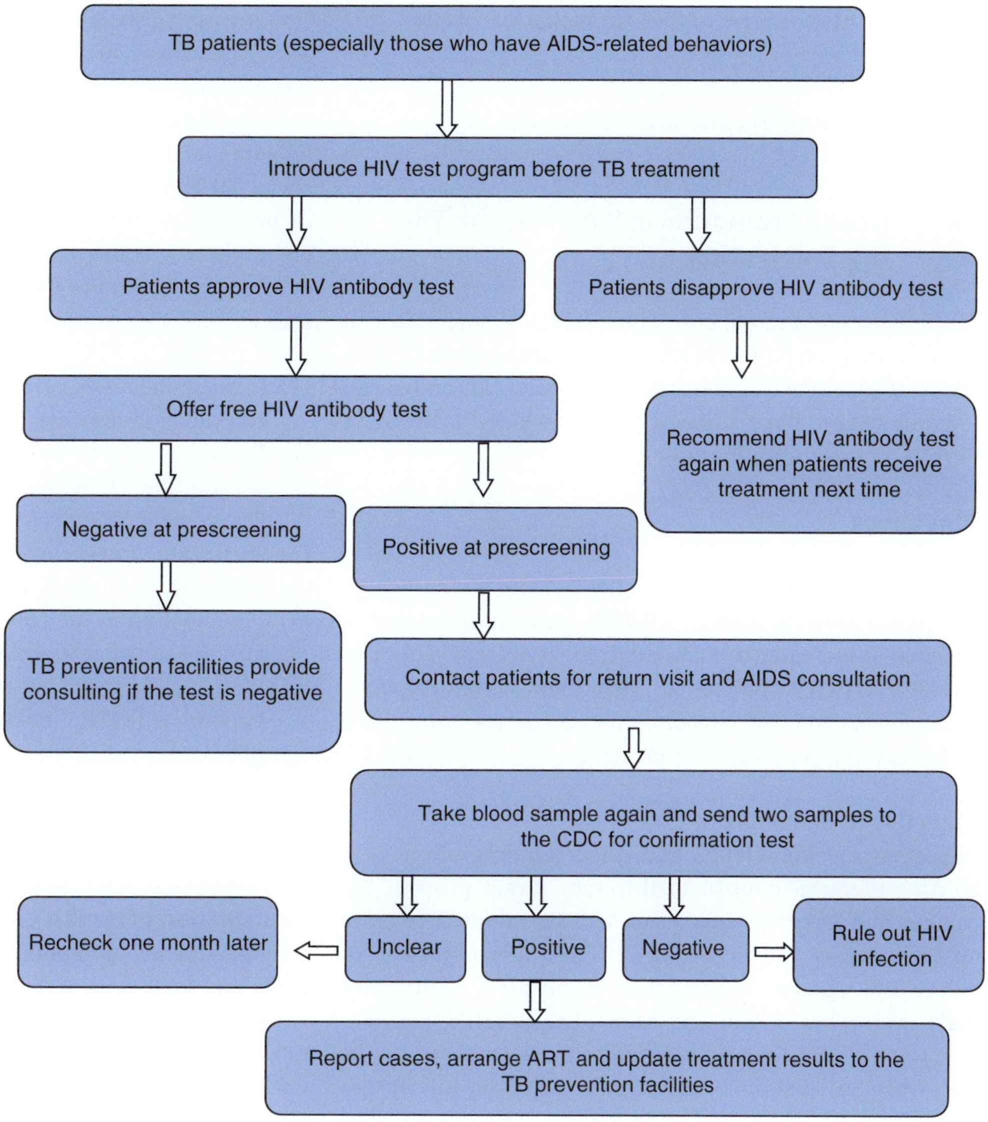

Fig. 8.2 Process of performing HIV antibody test among TB patients

(4) Social psychological support, including counseling;
(5) Social economic support and mitigation of discrimination;
(6) Symptoms and pain relief (palliative therapy);
(7) Support of orphans and care givers;
(8) Antiretroviral therapy.

Government agencies should assist in planning and establishing HIV/AIDS care centers (or similar institutions) that operate by the patients themselves. Such institution is intended to provide care, management, capacity building, coordination, and promotion. Therefore, it is a core or club of HIV/AIDS care system in a geographical area, responding to the needs of patients with HIV/AIDS. The patients, therefore, show more favorable compliance with antiretroviral therapy and prophylactic treatment for opportunistic infections. The care center should also contribute to the early detection of opportunistic infections, including TB.

Prevention of HIV/AIDS

The following interventions have been proved effective after planning, pilot project research or controlled trials in some developing countries:

Safe Sexual Behaviors

(1) 100% condom use program in high-risk groups (such as commercial sex workers);
(2) Promotion of condom use in incidental sexual behaviors;
(3) Reduction of sexual partners.

Use of Safe Injectable Drugs

Treatment of Sexually Transmitted Diseases

Uniform Prescription and Preventive Measures for Health-Care Staffs After Occupational Exposure

Prevention of Mother-to-Child Transmission of HIV/AIDS

Voluntary Counseling and Testing Service

3.4 Health Promotion in Patients with TB/HIV Coinfection

Health promotion in patients with TB/HIV coinfection is a social strategy and a social action with participation of governments and social organizations in health education and communication about policies and knowledge concerning TB/HIV coinfection control.

Objectives

Objective of Education

The health education about TB/HIV coinfection control is intended to increase the knowledge about policies and measures for TB/HIV coinfection. Therefore, the old and mistake opinions and understandings about TB/HIV coinfection in the targeted population are changed.

Objective of Behaviors

Based on the knowledge and understanding about TB/HIV coinfection control in different target groups, the correct and effective behaviors can be adopted or mistake behaviors can be changed. The main objective of behavioral change in government officials is to raise their awareness of the importance of TB/HIV coinfection control and thus increase the investments in human and financial resources. The main objective of behavioral change in patients is to promote their presentation in health-care institutions and their active cooperation to the supervision and management. The main objective of behavioral change in government agencies and social organizations is to promote their active participation in the control of TB/HIV coinfection. Behavioral changes in the target populations are more important and more difficult than knowledge and belief changes about TB/HIV coinfection [9].

Objective of TB/HIV Coinfection Control

By achieving the objectives of education and behavioral changes, strategy for TB/HIV coinfection control can be more effectively implemented to progressively achieve the ultimate goal of TB/HIV coinfection control.

Activities

Different target groups have different roles, needs, benefits, and acceptability in the control of TB/HIV coinfection. To improve the effects of health education and promotion, different health education and promotion activities should be implemented in different target groups.

Government Officials

The government officials are the formulators and implementers of government behaviors, and they play key role in ensuring the human, financial, and material resources in TB/HIV coinfection control. Meanwhile, they are also the leaders in TB/HIV coinfection control. Therefore, the objective of health education and promotion activities targeting the government officials is to obtain policy as well as human and financial support. The health education and promotion activities for government officials include:

(1) Regular meetings of the leading team or departmental coordination meetings.
(2) Regular report of the progress and difficulties encountered in the TB/HIV coinfection control to the relevant government officials.
(3) Participation in the activities on the World Tuberculosis Day and the World AIDS Day.
(4) Participation in the follow-ups of patients and visit the families of patients with TB/HIV coinfection.
(5) Participation in the supervision, inspection, and summarization of TB/HIV coinfection control and sign the new policies.
(6) Emphasis on the importance of TB/HIV coinfection control at government meetings and health-care related conferences.

Participation of Health-Care Professionals

The health-care professionals are responsible for the diagnosis and treatment of TB/HIV coinfection. They are also responsible for the reporting of the epidemic and the referral of suspected cases. Meanwhile, they are also the implementers in detecting and managing patients. Only when they have the relevant knowledge, can they achieve accurate diagnosis, treatment, and self-protection, and conduct effective health education for patients and other related personnel. Health education and promotion activities for relevant health-care professionals mainly include:

(1) Training for health-care professionals in respiratory, pulmonary, infectious diseases and preventive departments as well as health-care professionals in TB control agencies and HIV/AIDS control agencies.
(2) Giving out health education brochures on TB, HIV/AIDS, and TB/HIV coinfections, and giving lectures at regular intervals.
(3) Posting posters and bulletin boards on TB/HIV coinfection control at various levels of health-care institutions.

Patients with TB, HIV/AIDS, or TB/HIV Coinfection

For patients with TB, HIV/AIDS, or TB/HIV coinfection, the health education and promotion about TB control is mainly that TB is curable; regular treatment is the key to cure; the anti-tuberculosis treatment is free in charge; and TB can be non-communicable after treatment. In addition, patients with

TB need to wear a face mask before negative conversion of sputum bacteriological test and they should cover their nose and mouth when coughing or sneezing. And the health education and promotion about HIV/AIDS is mainly that HIV/AIDS is preventable; sexual contact is the most important route of its transmission; sharing syringes is an important risk behavior for HIV/AIDS transmission through the blood; daily life and workplace contact cannot cause infection of HIV/ AIDS. In addition, proper use of condoms prevents contraception and risks of contracting HIV/AIDS and sexually transmitted diseases. The health education and promotion about TB/HIV coinfection is mainly that TB commonly occurs in the early stage of HIV infection and TB screening is necessary when HIV infection is detected; TB is the most common and curable disease in patients with HIV/AIDS; and TB is also one of the most common causes of death among patients with HIV/AIDS. In addition, HIV infection increases the relapse rate of TB; HIV infection can change the clinical manifestations of TB, which increases spread of TB and difficulty in its diagnosis; TB infection accelerates the progress of HIV/AIDS and aggravates the condition of patient [10].

Targeted Health Promotion Activities Mainly Include

(1) When the TB/HIV coinfection is defined, the health-care professional is responsible for relevant health education about TB/HIV coinfection.
(2) Videos, album, brochure, and other methods are applied to conduct health education in all health-care institutions.
(3) Patients management team should be established. And seminars are regularly held for communication and support.
(4) Communication between health-care professionals and patients should be strengthened in clinical reexaminations and follow-ups.
(5) Health education and promotion should be conducted during hospitalization.

Participation of Common Population

The health education and promotion for common populations is mainly the threats of TB, HIV/AIDS, and TB/HIV coinfection to human health and their common symptoms. Therefore, individuals with relevant symptoms present to health-care institutions for diagnosis and treatment. In addition, free-in-charge policies for patients with TB and HIV/AIDS are implemented.

Health education and promotion activities for the common populations mainly include:

(1) Targeting on populations with different demographic characteristics, the health education and promotion is conducted.
(2) Health education is conducted in communities via videos, radio broadcasts, posters, bulletin boards, brochures, and fun questions and answers.
(3) Health education and promotion as well as training are conducted for community-based health-care professionals and community officials.
(4) The individuals with suspected symptoms but fail to present in health-care institutions are followed up and traced.

Core Information about TB/HIV Coinfection Control

When health education and promotion activities are conducted, the information imparted to the target population should be simple and accurate, instead of lengthy. The core information about TB/HIV coinfection control includes as follows.

TB

(1) TB is a chronic infectious disease that seriously threatens health for a long period of time.
(2) TB is mainly transmitted via the respiratory tract, and anyone may be infected.
(3) Cough and expectoration for more than 2 weeks are suspected symptoms of TB. And timely presentation to health-care institution is necessary.
(4) The patients with TB should not spit. And the patients with TB should cover their nose and mouth when coughing and sneezing. And the patients with TB should wear a face mask. By these ways, the spread of TB can be reduced.
(5) By whole course standard treatment, the vast majority of patients with TB can be cured, and spread to other can thus be avoided.

HIV/AIDS

(1) Observance of sexual ethics is the fundamental measure to prevent sexual transmission of HIV/AIDS.
(2) The proper use of condoms not only prevents contraception, but also reduces the risk of contracting HIV/AIDS and sexually transmitted diseases.
(3) Early treatment and cure of sexually transmitted diseases can reduce the risk of contracting HIV/AIDS.
(4) Sharing syringes is an important way to spread HIV/AIDS, and it is necessary to refuse drug abuse.
(5) Unnecessary blood transfusions and injections should be avoided. Use of blood and blood products after HIV antibody detection is necessary.
(6) AIDS is a serious infectious disease with extremely high mortality. There are no cures available yet. So far, no vaccine has been developed to prevent HIV/AIDS. But its infection can be prevented.
(7) HIV antibody can be detected from the blood after 4–8 weeks of HIV infection. But HIV infection is already infectious before it can be detected. The blood, semen, vaginal secretions, milk, and wound exudates from individuals with HIV infection contain a large amount of HIV, which is highly contagious.

(8) Via daily life and workplace contact with patients with HIV/AIDS, individuals cannot be infected with HIV/AIDS.

TB/HIV Coinfection

The core information about TB/HIV infection mainly includes:

(1) About 74–100% of patients with HIV/AIDS develop TB. And the symptoms and signs of TB/HIV coinfection can hardly be differentiated from other HIV/AIDS related lung diseases.
(2) TB commonly occurs in the early stage of HIV infection. Therefore, TB screening should be performed when HIV/AIDS is diagnosed.
(3) HIV/AIDS compromises the immunity of human body to Mtb infection. Therefore, patients with HIV/AIDS and Mtb infection rapidly show symptoms of TB. Death from TB occurs in about 50–80% of patients with HIV/AIDS.
(4) When an individual with HIV negative is infected with Mtb, the chance of progression of Mtb infection into TB is about 10% during his/her lifetime. However, when an individual with HIV positive is infected with Mtb, the chance of progression of Mtb infection into TB is about 10% within 1 year.
(5) HIV infection promotes the onset of TB. Patients with HIV infection show compromised immunity, which renders them vulnerable to reinfection of Mtb and rapid progression. Patients with TB/HIV are also more likely to spread to others.
(6) Patients with TB/HIV coinfection should actively receive anti-tuberculosis medication. Patients with HIV positive should try to avoid contact to patients with TB. Children who are congenitally HIV positive and symptomatic are not allowed to be vaccinated with BCG.
(7) TB is the most common and curable infectious disease in patients with HIV/AIDS. And TB may accelerate the progression of HIV/AIDS and aggravates the condition of patient. TB is the most common causes of death in patients with HIV/AIDS.
(8) HIV infection also increases the relapse rate of TB. HIV infection changes the clinical manifestations of TB, which increase the spread of TB and increase the difficulty in diagnosis of TB.

4 Laboratory Test

TB/HIV coinfection remains to be a major global public health challenge. TB infection is the most common opportunistic infection in patients with HIV/AIDS, with a high risk of death [11]. Along with the decline of immunity in patients with HIV/AIDS, the Mtb in patients with latent TB infection is gradually activated, and the risk of active TB is greatly increasing. Even if CD4 cell count is not lower than 200, the risk of TB in patients with HIV/AIDS is significantly higher than that in HIV-negative individuals. TB may occur at any stage of HIV/AIDS and is commonly a primary way to detect potential HIV infection. Therefore, all patients diagnosed with HIV infection should receive screening of TB to provide opportunities for timely and prophylactic treatment of TB. Both HIV screening in patients with TB and TB screening in patients with HIV positive are of great significance. Laboratory tests for TB in patients with HIV positive show no significant difference from routine laboratory tests for TB. And for screening of TB, tuberculin skin test is recommended. And if necessary, interferon γ release test (T-SPOT) can be further performed to confirm the diagnosis. For those with positive finding in TB screening test and for patients with HIV positive who have a history of close contact to patient with communicable TB (regardless of the results of screening tests), chest X-ray should be performed to exclude active TB. Even if no evidence has been found to support active TB (no active TB lesion detected by chest X-ray), patients with HIV-positive who show TB screening test positive should receive treatment for latent TB infection. Once patients with HIV/AIDS present toxic symptoms of TB, such as fever, night sweats, cough, and weight loss, their presentation to hospital is necessary to define the diagnosis.

4.1 Sputum Smear for Microscopy

Sputum smear for microscopy is still the most commonly applied test due to its low cost, high speed, and high specificity. However, sputum smear for microscopy only shows positive when the sputum bacterial content is above 10^5/mL, and its sensitivity rate in patients with HIV/AIDS is only 43–51% of the conventional sputum smear for microscopy. The sensitivity rate may even be further reduced due to the presence of other opportunistic infections. Compared with acid-fast staining, fluorescence staining can improve the sensitivity and specificity, while bacteria collection and other corresponding methods can also improve the sensitivity.

4.2 Culture-Based Detection

Mycobacterium culture is a recommended way as an assistant for diagnosis of TB infection in patients with HIV positive. Compared to sputum smear test, mycobacterium culture is more sensitive. In addition, pure culture strains can be obtained, which is the basis of the following strains identification and drug sensitivity test.

Traditional Mycobacterium Culture

Traditional mycobacterium cultures include Lowenstein–Jenson culture and Middlebrook culture. Solid culture technology is sensitive, but it consumes a long period of time, usually 6–8 weeks, which delays the treatment and resultant progression of TB/HIV coinfection. The automatic liquid culture system detects CO_2 production or oxygen consumption in the growth indicator tube (MGIT) by radioactivity detector (BACTEC 460 TB), fluorescence detector (BACTEC MGIT 960), colorimetric meter (MB/BacT), pressure detector (ESP), and reduced products detector to report the growth of bacteria in the tube. Usually positive results can be reported within 1–2 weeks, which greatly shortens the time for culture, and relatively pure mycobacterium culture can be obtained.

Microscopically Observed Drug Sensitivity Test (MODS)

MODS is a low-cost, non-commercial test, which is applied to detect microclones, cords, and early drug sensitivity. It is characterized by high sensitivity and short culture time for positive specimens, and is cheaper than Lowenstein–Jenson culture. It has also been applied for diagnosis of TB in patients with HIV positive.

Phage-Based Detection

Phage-based detection has been applied in the etiological diagnosis of TB. By using FAST Plaque TB test (developed by Biotech Laboratory), sputum specimen with 50–65% of smear-negative can be detected, with a specificity as high as 98% [12, 13]. The accuracy of FAST Plaque TB test is high in detecting cultured isolates. However, when it is applied to detect specimen from patient with TB/HIV coinfection, due to the presence of other opportunistic infections and complex microorganism components in the specimen, its sensitivity is greatly reduced and the specimen is susceptible to contamination. Therefore, its application in the diagnosis of TB/HIV coinfection is limited.

Other Rapid Diagnostic Techniques

Other rapid diagnostic techniques are also undergoing clinical assessment, such as colorimetric culture system based on recombinant bacteriophages (luciferase-based reported "Bronx-box" detection) and TK medium (Salubris) [14]. The rapid and automated culture and detection systems significantly increase the isolation rate of Mtb in clinical specimens, and significantly shorten the time required for positive reports (within 9–10 days). Rapid results promote implementation of evidence-based treatment for patients with HIV/AIDS, and improve the therapeutic efficacy and prognosis.

4.3 Molecular Biology Diagnosis

Nucleic acid amplification provides a reliable way for diagnosis of TB. With its increasing specificity and sensitivity, molecular diagnosis technology has been one of the core technologies in the diagnosis of TB.

Improved and Simplified Nucleic Acid Amplification

Some improved and simplified nucleic acid amplifications, such as loop-mediated isothermal amplification (LAMP), fluorescence in situ hybridization (FISH), and linear probe assay (LPA) have attracted more and more attention. A recent retrospective analysis showed that the sensitivity and specificity of LPA to pure cultures are as high as 95% and 100% [15]. The linear probe assay has also been adopted by WHO due to its capability in detecting Mtb complex in smear-positive sputum specimens and early positive cultures, and identifying rifampicin and isoniazid resistance. Based on linear probe assay, developed and represented by Hain Life Science in Germany, new kits have been developed to detect gene information about resistance to fluoroquinolones, aminoglycosides or fluoroquinolones, cycloserine, and ethambutol. Melt-Pro (developed by Zhishan Biology, http://www.zsandx.com/), a melting curve technology for drug sensitivity test with independent intellectual property rights in China, is capable of detecting drug resistance mutations to rifampicin, isoniazid, ethambutol, streptomycin, and fluoroquinolones.

GeneXpert MTB/RIF

Since 2011, GeneXpert MTB/RIF technology has been adopted by WHO to diagnose TB and rifampicin-resistant TB in patients with HIV/AIDS. The technology is a fully automated TB-specific module-based nucleic acid amplification system, which integrates and automates specimen preparation, PCR amplification, and result analysis. It is capable of reporting the test results within 2 h. The clinical validation experiments in 4 different laboratories have demonstrated that the detection rate of GeneXpert for positive specimen is 92.2%, while the detection rate of sputum smear is only 59.5%. In addition, its detection rate for smear-negative specimen is 72.5%. If repeated for three times, the positive detection rate increases to 90.2%. The specificity of GeneXpert MTB/RIF technology can reach up to 99%. HIV coinfection significantly reduces the sensitivity of sputum smear for microscopy, but hardly affects the performance of GeneXpert MTB/RIF technology. Its sensitivity and specificity for rifampicin-resistant TB are 99.1% and 100%, respectively. Meanwhile, concerning the detection time, GeneXpert MTB/RIF technology and sputum smear test are capable of reporting results within 1 day, while liquid culture consumes about 17 days and solid culture consumes more than 30 days. Therefore, the potential of its application is enormous, which can supplement the current diagnostic criteria for TB, improve overall sensitivity, and shorten the detection time [16].

4.4 Immunological Diagnosis

Detection of Tuberculosis-Specific Antibodies

In 2011, by cross-laboratory validation of a batch of reagents for TB antibody detection, scientists found that the sensitivity and specificity of some commercially available reagents for TB could not meet the requirements of clinical tests. Neither could they replace the sputum smear for microscopy nor could they be applied as an additional detection to exclude TB infection. Therefore, antibody detection reagent for diagnosis of TB failed to be recommended by WHO. However, with the development of new technologies for identification and detection of TB antigens, chemiluminescence detection based on multi-antigen targets has shown promising future in detection of blood TB antibody, and the performance of the kit has gradually improved. A kit based on chemiluminescent protein chip has been developed by Puruikang (Shenzhen, China. http://www.szprk.com/) for detection of specific antibodies against 16 kD, 38 kD, Lam, CFP10, and RV1636 antigens, with high sensitivity to TB infection. China has never denied the value of antibody detection reagents in the auxiliary diagnosis of TB.

Detection of Mtb Antigen

Commercially available kits for detection of MPB64 in peripheral blood (TAUNS), Esat-6 in cerebrospinal fluid (CSF), and lipoarabinomannan (LAM) in urine have been developed. The detection of LAM in urine is more effective in patients with HIV positive than in individuals with HIV negative [17]. The combination of sputum smear and LAM detection in urine needs further clinical assessment, especially in areas with high HIV burden.

Tuberculin Skin Test

Tuberculin skin test commonly shows positive in patients with HIV negative and TB. However, in patients with HIV positive and TB, the tuberculin skin test commonly shows negative, which is related to HIV-induced immunodeficiency. In areas with high prevalence of TB, the tuberculin skin test may also underestimate the prevalence of latent TB infection. Therefore, health-care professionals with rich clinical experience and sufficient knowledge on the tuberculin skin test are needed for correct operations of the test and accurate readings of the test results. In addition, the second presentation of the patients is necessary. But for patients with HIV positive, the tuberculin skin test indicates the diagnosis of TB. Prophylactic treatment administered to patients with tuberculin skin test positive can significantly reduce the mortality rate [18].

Interferon γ Release Assay (IGRA)

IGRA can be applied to diagnose latent TB infection, especially for patients with major diseases or severe malnutrition. There are two commercially available kits for IGRA: QuantiFERON-TB Gold (QFT, Qiagen) and T. SPOT-TB (Oxford Immunotec). QuantiFERON-TB Gold (QFT, Qiagen) is based on enzyme-linked immunosorbent assay (ELISA), while T. SPOT-TB (Oxford Immunotec) is based on enzyme-linked immunodot assay (ELISPOT). QFT is to quantitatively detect the total amount of interferon γ (IFN-γ) produced by monocytes in peripheral blood after stimulation by TB antigen (ESAT-6 and CFP-10). And T. SPOT-TB is to detect the number of cells secreting IFN-γ. Both kits are relatively expensive, but their sensitivity and specificity are higher than those of tuberculin skin test. However, IGRAs fails to differentiate latent TB infection from active TB, and fails to differentiate immune reconstitution inflammatory syndrome (IRIS) from reconstruction failure. IGRAs results are independent of BCG vaccination, and it is a favorable technology for qualitative detection of TB infection. However, it requires complicated equipment and operations by technicians, which increase its cost. In under-developed areas, its application is therefore limited. Many products based on IGRAs have been developed in China, with similar basic principles and detection procedures.

4.5 Other Detections

In 2017, American scholars successfully applied time-flight mass spectrometry (MALDI-TOF MS) to detect CFP10 and ESAT6 antigens in blood specimens, whose sensitivity and specificity for TB, extrapulmonary TB, and latent TB infection are clinically recognized. And its application has great clinical value. In addition, it has been reported that digital microparticle PCR amplification based on free DNA/RNA in blood/urine is capable of detecting the degraded nucleic acid fragments of Mtb for diagnosis of TB [19, 20]. The detection is independent of sputum specimen and has significance in the diagnosis of extrapulmonary TB and latent TB infection as well as quantitative differential diagnosis of latent TB infection and active TB. If its sensitivity can be further improved, the clinical value would be great.

5 Diagnostic Imaging of HIV/AIDS

AIDS is caused by HIV infection, and the HIV virus mainly attacks human CD4+ T lymphocytes, causing cellular immunodeficiency in the body. AIDS complicated with tuberculosis is related to the immune status of the body and the occurrence, development and manifestation of tuberculosis are related to the count of CD4+ T lymphocytes [21]. When CD4+ T- lymphocytes in HIV infected individuals are activated by M. tuberculosis, they can promote the replication of HIV virus. The relationship between both is very close. Clinically, CD4+ T lymphocyte counts are directly related to the clinical manifestations of tuberculosis. In the middle and late stages of HIV infection, the immune status of the body is severely inhibited, and the cellular immunity is severely damaged, which will result in greatly thriving of M. tuberculosis in the patient, the immune system being severely damaged, and being difficult to prevent the spread of M. tuberculosis in the body. The patients may present secondary pulmonary tuberculosis, hematogenous disseminated pulmonary tuberculosis, mediastinal and hilar lymphatic tuberculosis, as well as abdominal lymph node tuberculosis, liver and spleen tuberculosis, intracranial tuberculosis, and tuberculosis in other organs.

The imaging manifestations of AIDS complicated with pulmonary tuberculosis were significantly different from the manifestations in patients with common pulmonary tuberculosis. From the proportions of different types of pulmonary tuberculosis, the incidences of hematogenous disseminated tuberculosis and mediastinal lymph node tuberculosis were significantly increased. In a retrospective analysis of 235 cases of AIDS complicated with pulmonary tuberculosis confirmed or clinically defined by pathology and laboratory tests from January 2013 to December 2017 in Tian Tan Hospital (Beijing, China), the signs in CT imaging showed the incidence of secondary tuberculosis, hematogenous disseminated pulmonary tuberculosis, and mediastinal lymph node tuberculosis was 66.8%, 31.9%, and 63.8%, respectively. A review of 1415 cases of HIV-negative chest tuberculosis in 1 month's visits to Beijing Chest Hospital (Beijing, China) included 47 cases of hematogenous disseminated tuberculosis, accounting for 3.2%, and 81 cases of chest lymphatic tuberculosis, accounting for 5.7%. More literature reports that the imaging manifestations of AIDS complicated with tuberculosis mainly depend on the immune status of the body. It is generally believed that in the early stage of HIV infection, when there is no significant decrease in the counts of CD4+ T lymphocytes, the imaging manifestations are similar to that of pulmonary tuberculosis without immune function damage, and are often characterized by typical tuberculosis. In the middle and late stages of HIV infection, when CD4+ T lymphocytes are significantly reduced or extremely reduced, the patients are in a moderate and severe immunosuppressive state, where the pulmonary tuberculosis represents atypical tuberculosis and is highly prone to be complicated with multiple infections. In addition, not only the function of macrophages that inhibit the growth of tubercle bacillus is reduced, but also the functions of Langerhans cells that limit the development of lesions as well as other functions are also significantly inhibited, and it is difficult to form tuberculous granuloma, which also contributes to the formation of atypical changes in tuberculosis lesions.

5.1 The Imaging Findings of AIDS Complicated with Pulmonary Tuberculosis Are Related to the Degree of Immune Damage

At different infection stages of AIDS, the patient's immune level is different, and the location, nature, lesion morphology, and distribution range of the imaging manifestations are also different. When the immunity is mildly decreased, the imaging manifestations of secondary pulmonary tuberculosis are similar to those in patients with normal immunity. The predilection sites are still in the apical segments of superior lobes, the posterior segments of upper lobes, and the dorsal segments of the lower lobes of both lungs. When the patient's immunity is low, the number of cases with lesions distributed in non-predilection sites increases, and the exudative lesions increase. The lesions involve a wide range, and may be found in all the lobes and segments, often involving two or more lung segments or lobes and without obviously specific sites. As the decrease of immunity, the lesion sites become more atypical, with significantly increased incidences observed in the following atypical sites: right middle lobe and left tongue segment, basal segment of lower lobe, and anterior segment of upper lobe (Figs. 8.3, 8.4, and 8.5). This is due to the low immunity of AIDS patients, the tuberculosis cannot be limited, so there is no predilection site, often involving multiple lobes and multiple segments, and rarely involving single lobe. According to the imaging findings, the ratio of exudative consolidation of varying sizes is higher, accompanying with the density of the grinding glass, bronchial dissemination and multiple nodules, and less formation of fiber proliferation and calcification. The patients with AIDS complicated with secondary pulmonary tuberculosis have depletion of CD4+ T lymphocytes, which will lead to the hypofunctions of macrophages, cytotoxic T cells, natural killer cells, and B cells, and the decreased ability of limiting the spread of lesions. The lesions appear as patches or large sheets of lesions of inflammatory changes in lung lobes. AIDS complicated with tuberculosis may be accompanied with cavity formation, but the proportion of cavity formation reported in the literature is quite different. Liu et al. [22] reviewed the results of 66 cases of AIDS complicated with pulmonary tuberculosis and 72 cases of HIV-negative pulmonary tuberculosis, the proportion of AIDS complicated with tuberculous cavities was 3.03% and the proportion of tuberculous cavities in HIV-negative patients was 18.06%, and the proportion of cavitations in AIDS complicated with tuberculosis was significantly lower than that in the HIV-negative group, and the difference was significant. The imaging analysis of 235 patients with AIDS complicated with pulmonary tuberculosis in Beijing Ditan Hospital (Beijing, China) showed that the incidence of consolidation with cavitation in patients with AIDS complicated with secondary pulmonary

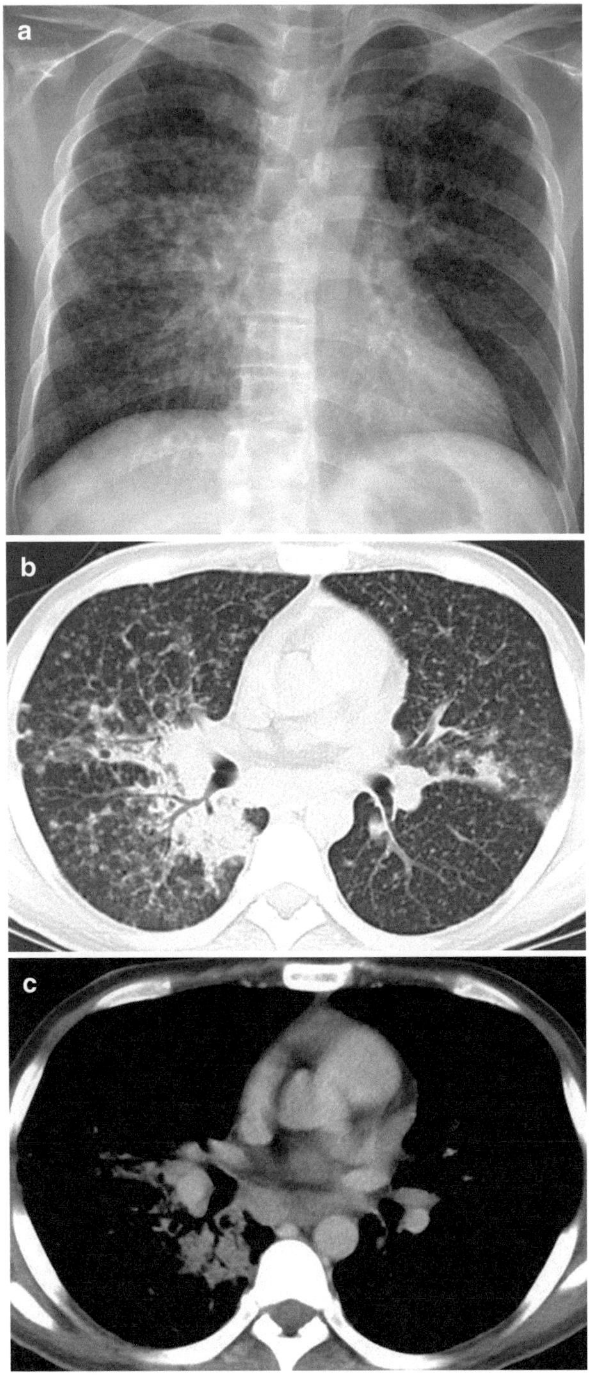

Fig. 8.3 AIDS complicated with secondary pulmonary tuberculosis, hematogenous disseminated pulmonary tuberculosis with lymphatic tuberculosis. Male, 36 years old, Han nationality. Laboratory examination: anti-HIV antibody positive, CD4+ T lymphocytes 60 cells/μL. The sputum smear was positive for acid-fast staining and positive for tuberculosis antibodies. Acid-fast bacilli were observed in the acid-fast staining of alveolar lavage fluid. (**a**) PA chest radiograph showing flocculent density in right lung hilar, with blurred boundary, and miliary nodules diffusely distributed in both lungs. (**b**, **c**) CT (lung window and mediastinal window), showing patchy and flocculent densities of the right hilar mid-lobe, back segment, and left tongue segment of right lower lobe, with blurred boundary, and miliary nodules diffusely distributed in both lungs. Lymph node enlargement in region 8 of the mediastinum. Intrapulmonary imaging showed synchronously typical imaging findings of pulmonary tuberculous infiltrates, hematogenous disseminated foci, and lymph node tuberculosis

tuberculosis was 31.6%, and cavities were formed in every lobe and segment of both lungs. When the CD4+ T lymphocyte count was less than $<100 \times 10^6$/L, the incidence of cavitation is significantly increased.

A small number of patients with AIDS complicated with secondary pulmonary tuberculosis represented atypical, mainly flaky, or patchy densities, and rarely showed disseminated lesions near the lung field (Figs. 8.6, 8.7, 8.8, 8.9, and 8.10). It is difficult to differentiate from non-specific inflammation based on simple images alone. It has been reported that when CD4+ T lymphocytes are depleted, especially when CD4+ T lymphocytes are less than 100 cells/μl, the functions of macrophages, natural killer cells, and B lymphocytes are extremely low, and some lesions easily presented as effusion changes.

5.2 The Incidence of AIDS Complicated with Hilar and Mediastinal Lymph Node Tuberculosis Is Significantly Increased, and Multiple Lymph Node Enlargement Is Easily to Be Complicated

The incidence of AIDS complicated with hilar and mediastinal lymph node tuberculosis is significantly increased, and multiple lymph node enlargement is easily to be complicated (Figs. 8.11, 8.12, and 8.13). CT plain scan showed uniform density or liquefaction area. After enhancement, a small number of enlarged lymph nodes presented uniform enhancement (suggesting proliferative lesions). Most of the lymph nodes showed annular enhancement or separated enhancement, and the central cheese-like necrosis was not enhanced. The enlarged lymph nodes were easy to fuse with each other. The proportion of AIDS complicated with mediastinal lymph node tuberculosis reported in each literature is slightly different. Li et al. [23] reported that 67 of 142 patients with AIDS complicated with tuberculosis had lymph node tuberculosis, accounting for 47.2%. In the enhanced scan, 50% of the enlarged lymph nodes showed uneven enhancement, 35.7% showed circular enhancement, and 14.3% showed uniform enhancement. Xue et al. [24] reported 235 cases of AIDS complicated with chest tuberculosis, including 150 cases of lymphatic tuberculosis, accounting for 63.8%, with lymph node enlargement in regions 4R, 7, and 2R being mostly seen; after enhanced scanning, 72.6% of the enlarged lymph nodes showed circular or separate enhancement, and the proportions of uniform enhancement and non-enhancement were 29.0% and 16.1%, respectively, of which the ratio of lymph node fusion was as high as 68.6%, the ratio of lymph node rupture was 24.6%, and the ratio of lymph node aeration was 16.0%. The study showed that AIDS complicated with mediastinal lymph node tuberculosis mainly represented circular or separated enhancement. The lesions mostly involved in

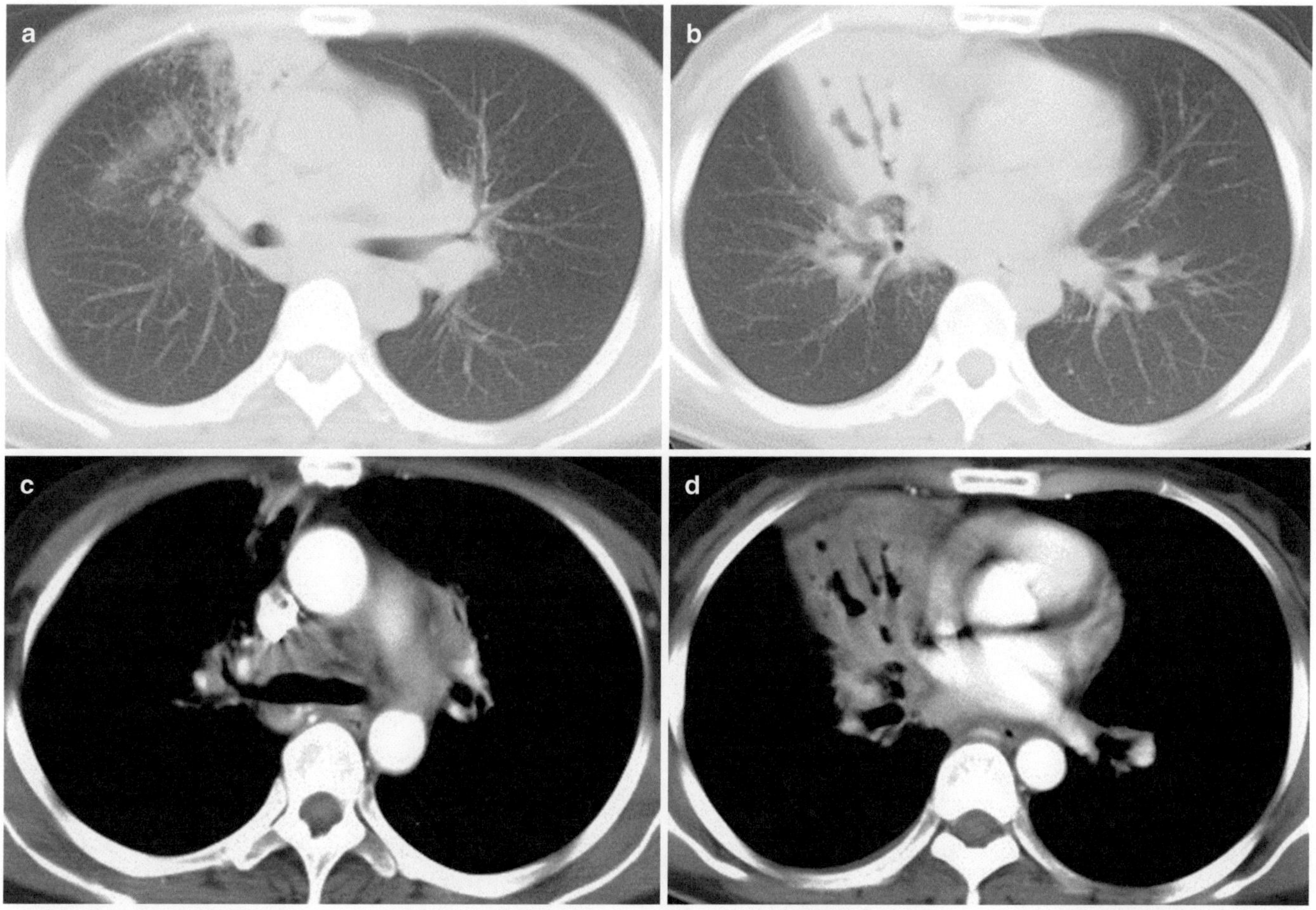

Fig. 8.4 AIDS complicated with tuberculosis and lymphatic tuberculosis. Female, 28 years old. Laboratory examination: anti-HIV antibody positive, CD4+ T lymphocytes 130 cells/μL. The sputum smear was positive for acid-fast staining and positive for tuberculosis antibodies. The sputum smear was positive for acid-fast staining of tubercle bacillus. (**a**, **b**) CT (lung window) showed lung consolidation in anterior and middle lobe, with air bronchogram, thickened bronchial wall in right upper and middle lobe with narrowed lumen; (**c**, **d**) enhanced CT scan (mediastinal window), showing soft tissue density of atelectasis, visible air bronchogram, multiple lymph nodes enlargement in the mediastinum

3 or more groups of lymph nodes, and the lymph nodes were easy to fuse or even be broken, with uneven density. However, when CD4 < 100×10^6/L, the incidence of lymph node enlargement in regions 6, 8, and 10R areas increased significantly; the enlarged lymph nodes often showed fusion, or even rupture and invasion of adjacent lung tissue to form tuberculous consolidation, with fusion, rupture, and invasion to adjacent lung tissue of enlarged lymph nodes in regions 6, 8, and 10R observed more commonly; and air-containing lymph nodes more found in regions 7and 4R, suggesting that the patients with AIDS complicated with lymphatic tuberculosis easily have the trachea and bronchus invaded to form bronchial lymphatic fistula, and the evacuation of cheesy necrosis in parenchyma of lymph nodes results in gas contained in the lymph nodes. The literature also observed that the fusion and rupture of lymph nodes or gas contained in lymph nodes strongly suggest the diagnosis of lymph node tuberculosis.

5.3 The Incidence of Hematogenous Disseminated Tuberculosis Was Very High

The proportion of hematogenous disseminated tuberculosis was also slightly different in the literature. Of the 142 cases of tuberculosis reported by Li, 29 were hematogenous disseminated tuberculosis, accounting for 20.4%. Among the 235 cases of AIDS complicated with pulmonary tuberculosis reported by Xue et al., there were 75 cases of hematogenous disseminated pulmonary tuberculosis, accounting for 31.9%, with the highest incidence (65.3% (49/75)) of subacute miliary tuberculosis and HRCT showing miliary nodules with uneven size, density, and distribution (i.e., "three non-uniformities" sign) (Fig. 8.14), and with the incidence of acute miliary nodules of 34.7% (26/75) and these miliary nodules were mainly distributed randomly and HRCT showing miliary nodules with uniform size, density, and

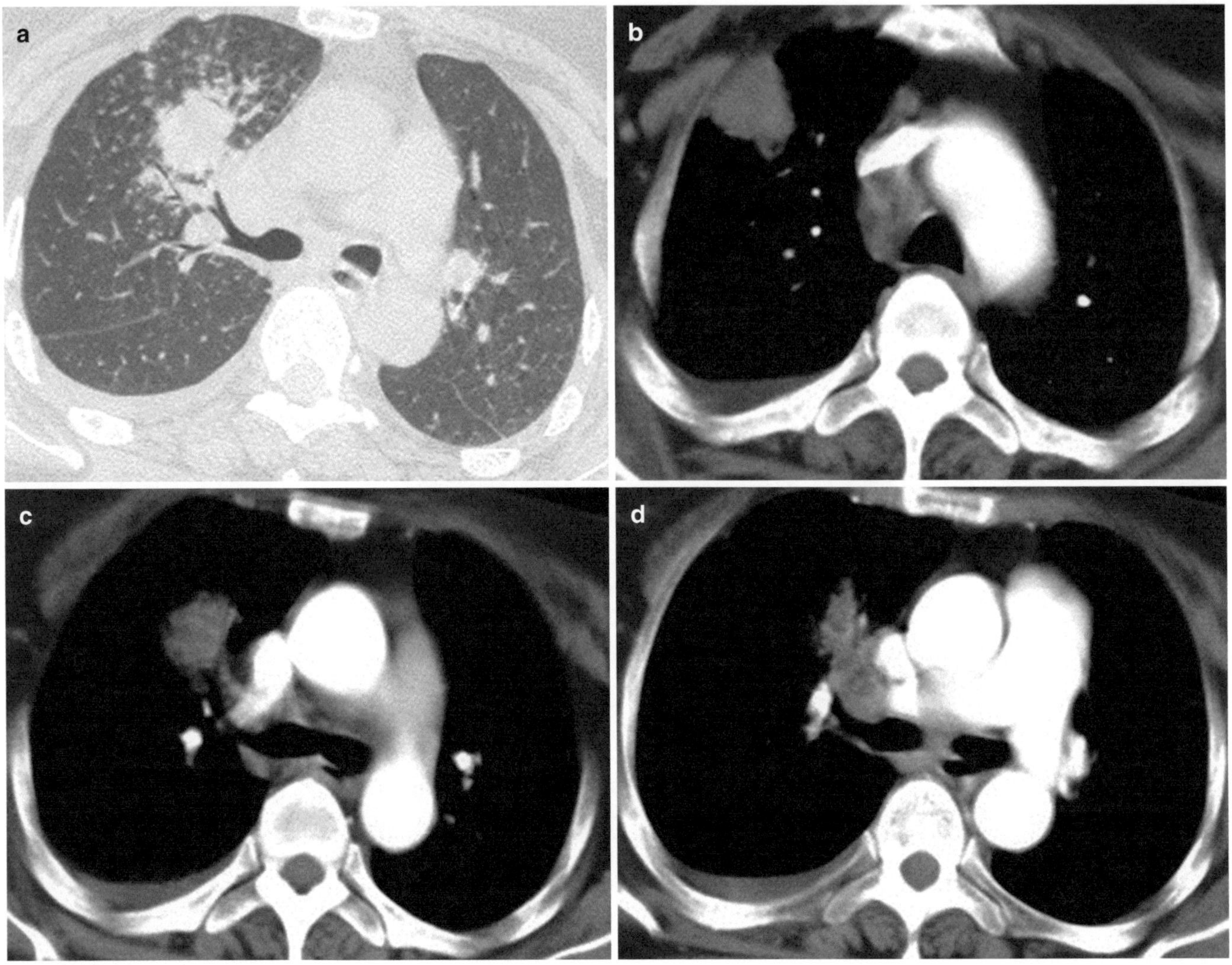

Fig. 8.5 AIDS complicated with tuberculosis and lymphatic tuberculosis. Female, 35 years old. Laboratory examination: anti-HIV antibody positive, CD4+ T lymphocytes 130 cells/μL. The sputum smear was positive for acid-fast staining of tubercle bacillus. (**a**) CT (lung window) showed a round-like high density in the anterior segment of right upper lobe, and a dotted patchy high density in the surrounding lung field. (**b**–**d**) CT (mediastinal window) showed multiple round-like soft tissue density in the anterior segment of right upper lobe, with slightly blurred boundary and enlarged lymph nodes in right lung hilar and mediastinum. There was a small amount of effusion in the right thoracic cavity, and enhanced scan showed enhancement of intrapulmonary lesions and mediastinal lymph nodes enlargement

distribution (i.e., "three uniformities" sign) (Fig. 8.15). With the decrease of CD4+ T lymphocytes, the hematogenous disseminated tuberculosis was uneven in distribution and size of lesion. The study showed that when CD4 < 100 × 106 cells/L, sub-acute hematogenous disseminated pulmonary tuberculosis was dominant, and the size, density, and distribution of miliary nodules were uneven, and the distribution in upper lung was more than that in the lower lung. It has been reported in the literature that with the decrease of CD4+ T cell count, the possibility of miliary tuberculosis is more likely to be found, and the extent of involvement is more extensive. The hematogenous disseminated pulmonary tuberculosis in the late stage of AIDS is characterized by uneven distribution of nodules and a fusion tendency. Some cases can be complicated with lymph node enlargement, easily companied with multiple-site dissemination.

5.4 Pleural Effusion and Pericardial Effusion Are Also Common in AIDS Complicated with Tuberculosis

The incidence of tuberculous pleural effusion and pericardial effusion in patients with AIDS complicated with chest tuberculosis was about 43% and 35%, respectively. It has been reported in the literature that pleural effusion is closely related to the diagnosis of AIDS complicated with M. tuberculosis infection, and it is believed that, when the chest imaging signs are not typical and the differential diagnosis is difficult, the diagnosis of tuberculosis should be considered first if the pleural effusion or pericardial effusion is found. The results of literature reports are inconsistent for the correlation between the tuberculous pleural effusions and the CD4+ T lymphocytes. There is no correlation between

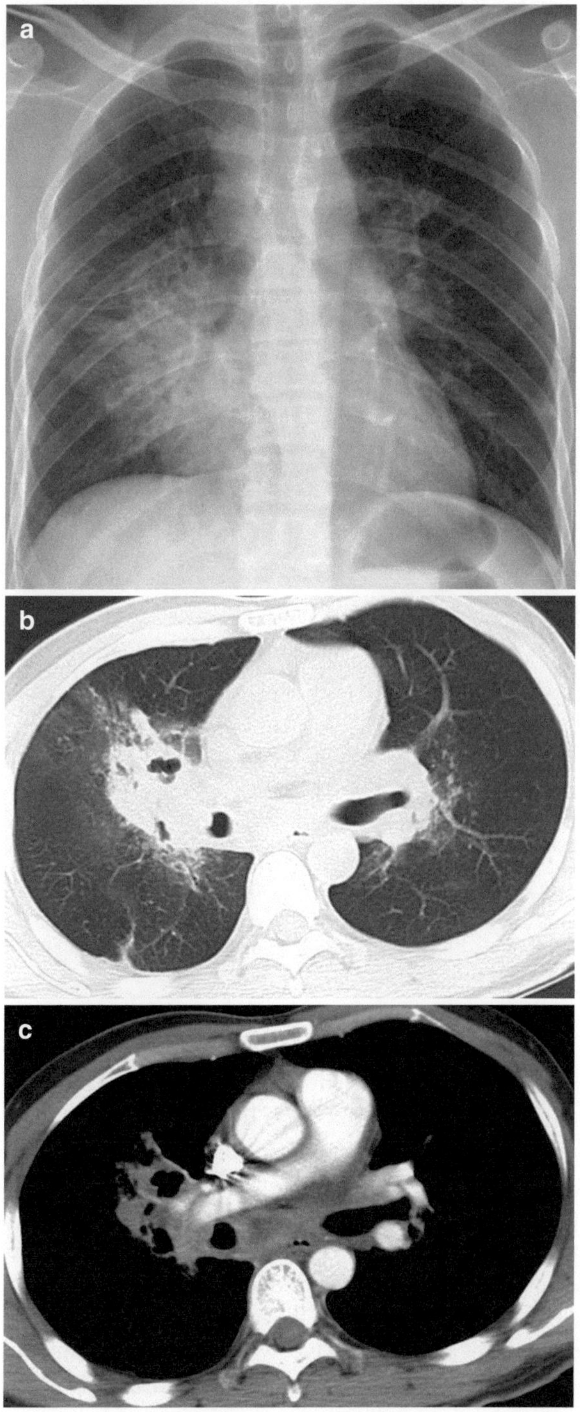

Fig. 8.6 AIDS complicated with tuberculosis and lymphatic tuberculosis. Male, 31 years old. Laboratory examination: anti-HIV antibody positive, CD4+ T lymphocytes 31 cells/μL. The sputum smear was positive for acid-fast staining of tubercle bacillus and positive for tuberculosis antibodies. (**a**) PA chest radiograph showing a patchy dense density in the middle, lower, middle and lower lung fields, with unclear outer edge from the lung tissue and uniform density of parenchyma. The right upper mediastinum widened and lobulated at the interface with the lungs. (**b**, **c**) CT (lung window and mediastinal window) showing patchy soft tissue density in the middle lobe of right lung with uniform parenchymal density, multiple gas-containing dissolved cavities, and light patchy density in the middle lobe lesions adjacent to the lung field and the lower right lobe. In the mediastinal window, enhanced scan showing enlarged lymph nodes in regions of 10R and 7, central liquefaction necrosis of lymph nodes in region 7, showing annular enhancement

pleural effusion and CD4+ T lymphocytes in literature; the results summarized by Ditan Hospital in Beijing, China showed that the incidence of pleural effusion and pericardial effusion is negatively correlated with CD4+ T lymphocyte count, which is inconsistent with the reported fact in other literatures. The authors believed that when the CD4+ T lymphocyte count is <200 × 106/L, the patient is prone to have bacteremia and invasion of the serosal cavity, so it causes pleuritis, pericarditis, and effusion generation (Fig. 8.16). It is believed that effusion represents an allergic reaction to tuberculosis proteins.

5.5 The Chest Tuberculosis in Patients with AIDS Often Presents Two or More Types of Tuberculosis

The incidence of secondary pulmonary tuberculosis complicated with mediastinal lymph node tuberculosis can reach 25%, often manifested as consolidation with grinding glass density, consolidation with cavities, bronchial dissemination, single or multiple-cavity formation, and mediastinal hilar lymph node enlargement and fusion. Two or more types among the secondary tuberculosis, hematogenous disseminated tuberculosis, mediastinal/hilar lymph node enlargement, and tuberculous pleurisy are commonly concurrent (Figs. 8.3, 8.4, 8.5, 8.6, 8.7, 8.8, 8.9, 8.10, 8.11, 8.12, 8.13, 8.14, and 8.16).

5.6 In Addition to Tuberculosis, the AIDS Patients Are Prone to Concurrent Extrapulmonary Tuberculosis, Often Showing Multiple Organ or Multi-System Tuberculosis

Li et al. [25] analyzed 97 cases of AIDS complicated with multi-organ tuberculosis infection confirmed in Beijing Ditan Hospital from January 2014 to December 2015, most of which were patients with tuberculosis, altogether 89 cases, accounting for 91.8%, followed by lymph node tuberculosis of 64 cases, accounting for 66.0%, central nervous system tuberculosis of 23 cases, accounting for 23.7%, multi-serosal effusion of 36 cases, accounting for 37.1%, liver and spleen tuberculosis of 15 cases, accounting for 15.5%, adrenal tuberculosis of 5 cases, accounting for 5.2%, intestinal tuberculosis of 5 cases, accounting for 5.2%, reproductive system tuberculosis of 3 cases, accounting for 3.1%, bone and joint tuberculosis of 2 cases, accounting for 2.1%, and soft tissue tuberculosis of 3 cases, accounting for 3.1%. The most common multi-organ tuberculosis infection is tuberculosis complicated with lymph node tuberculosis, a total of 59 cases, accounting for 60.8%. The lesion of AIDS complicated with lymph node tuberculosis has a wide range of involvement, and the diameter of lymph nodes is more than

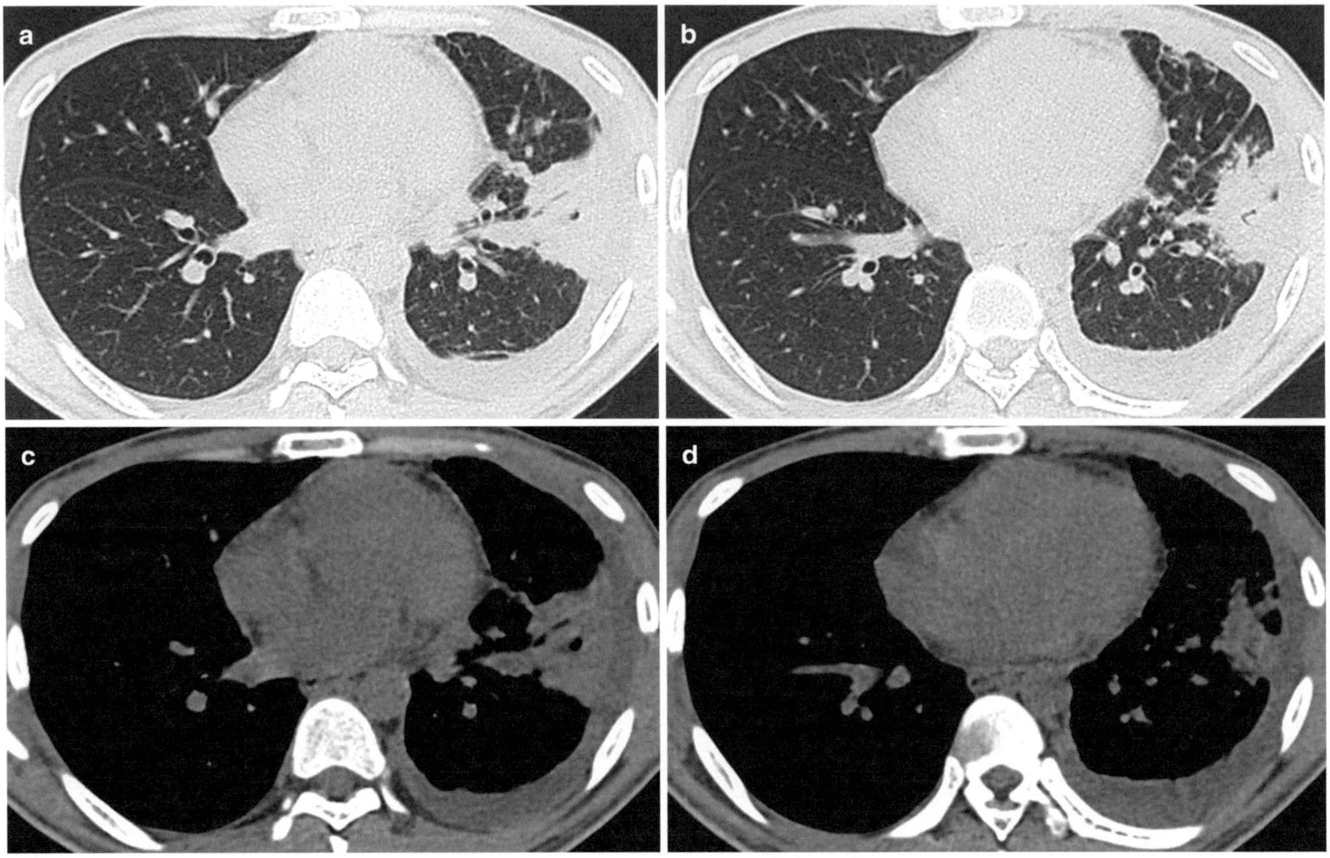

Fig. 8.7 (**a**–**d**) AIDS complicated with secondary pulmonary tuberculosis. Male, 28 years old. The patient showed positive for HIV upon PE 3 months ago, and confirmed as test positive, with the CD4+ T lymphocyte count of 27 cells/uL. The sputum smear was positive for acid-fast staining. The CT (lung window and the mediastinum window) showed fan-shaped consolidation density in the lower lobe of left lung, with clear boundary, and gas phase of gas-containing bronchial and the gas-containing dissolved small cavities in parenchyma. A small amount of effusion was found in the left chest

2 cm (56 cases). The enhanced scan showed circular or separated enhancement, and the lymph nodes have a tendency to fuse. The patients with AIDS complicated with central nervous system tuberculosis mainly represent skull base meninges and/or spinal dura mater thickening and nodular strengthening (12 cases), also represent multiple nodular and ring-shaped lesions in the brain parenchyma (7 cases) (Figs. 8.17, 8.18, and 8.19).

5.7 The Patients with AIDS May Have their Existed Tuberculosis Aggravated or Their Potential Tuberculosis Activated, thus to Develop New Tuberculosis, When Immune Restoration Inflammatory Syndrome (IRIS) Occurs during Highly Active Antiretroviral Therapy (HAART)

Immune restoration inflammatory syndrome (IRIS) occurs in patients with AIDS after highly active antiretroviral therapy (HARRT), resulting in a transient deterioration of tuberculosis infection. Tuberculosis with typical IRIS occurs within a few days or weeks after HARRT starts. Studies have shown that about 15.3% of patients develop IRIS from 3 days to 8 weeks after HAART, and get improved in 2–3 weeks after deterioration, with CD4+ T lymphocyte counts $<200 \times 10^6$ cells/L, suggesting that the lower the baseline level of CD4+ T lymphocytes, the more likely to develop IRIS; the imaging signs mainly present as intrapulmonary consolidation and mediastinal lymph node enlargement, of which the intrapulmonary lesions mainly present as segmental or lobe consolidation in right middle lobe and the left tongue segment, with peripheral exudation and micro-nodules, and the mediastinal lymph node enlargement mainly presents as necrosis and fusion, often accompanied by pleural effusion and pericardial effusion (Fig. 8.20).

6 Treatment of TB/HIV Coinfection

6.1 Overview on Treatment of TB/HIV Coinfection

According to the statistics reported by WHO in 2018, the global success rate of TB treatment is 82%, and its mortality rate is 4%. However, the success rate of treatment for HIV-

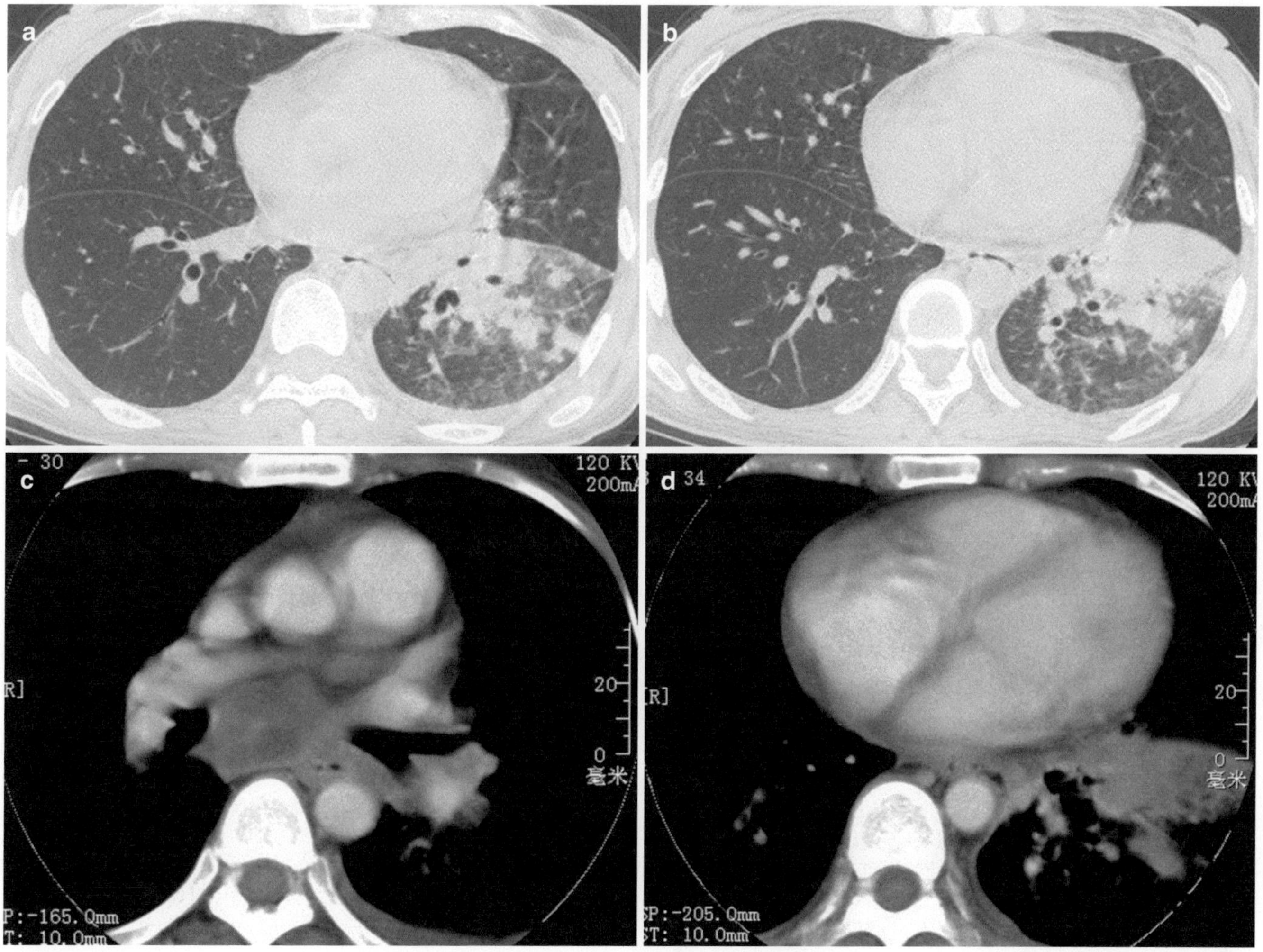

Fig. 8.8 (**a**–**d**) AIDS complicated with secondary pulmonary tuberculosis and lymphatic tuberculosis. Male, 35 years old. Laboratory examination: anti-HIV antibody positive, CD4+ T lymphocytes 15 cells/μL; sputum smear positive for acid-fast staining of tubercle bacillus. CT (lung window and mediastinal window) showed lung consolidation at the basal segment of left lower lobe, with slightly blurred boundary, and enlarged mediastinal lymph nodes. Enhanced scanning showed uneven enhancement of lymph nodes, and localized liquefaction zones

related TB is only 77%, and the mortality rate is as high as 11% [26]. The data indicates that the treatment of TB/HIV coinfection is still challenging. The further administration of antiretroviral therapy (ART) is beneficial to reduce the incidence of TB and improve the success rate of TB treatment.

Nowadays, the treatment of TB/HIV coinfection includes anti-tuberculosis and antiretroviral drugs. Due to many adverse reactions of anti-tuberculosis and antiretroviral drugs, in addition to overlapping of adverse reactions and antagonism of some drugs, the probabilities of adverse drug reactions and drug-resistant TB are increased. The treatment is more complex and the prognosis is poorer [27]. Therefore, in the treatment of TB/HIV coinfection, the timing of treatment, TB-associated immune reconstitution inflammatory syndrome (TB-IRIS), drug-induced liver injury (DILI), and drug interactions should be considered. Inappropriate management of these problems may cause sudden aggravation of the condition or even death. The treatment principle of TB in patients with HIV/AIDS is basically the same as that in non-HIV/AIDS patients. But the time and frequency in use of anti-tuberculosis drugs are different. In addition, the interaction and incompatibility between ART and anti-tuberculosis drugs should be paid close attention to prevent the occurrence of TB-IRIS.

In conclusion, for patients with TB/HIV coinfection, ART should generally be initiated as early as possible, but the timing of initiation depends on the CD4 cell count. Directly observed treatment and assessment on compliance of patient are also very important.

6.2 Anti-Tuberculosis Treatment for Patients with HIV/AIDS

Principles for Administration of Anti-Tuberculosis Treatment and ART

Anti-tuberculosis drugs should be firstly considered and following ART as long as the condition permits [28]. According

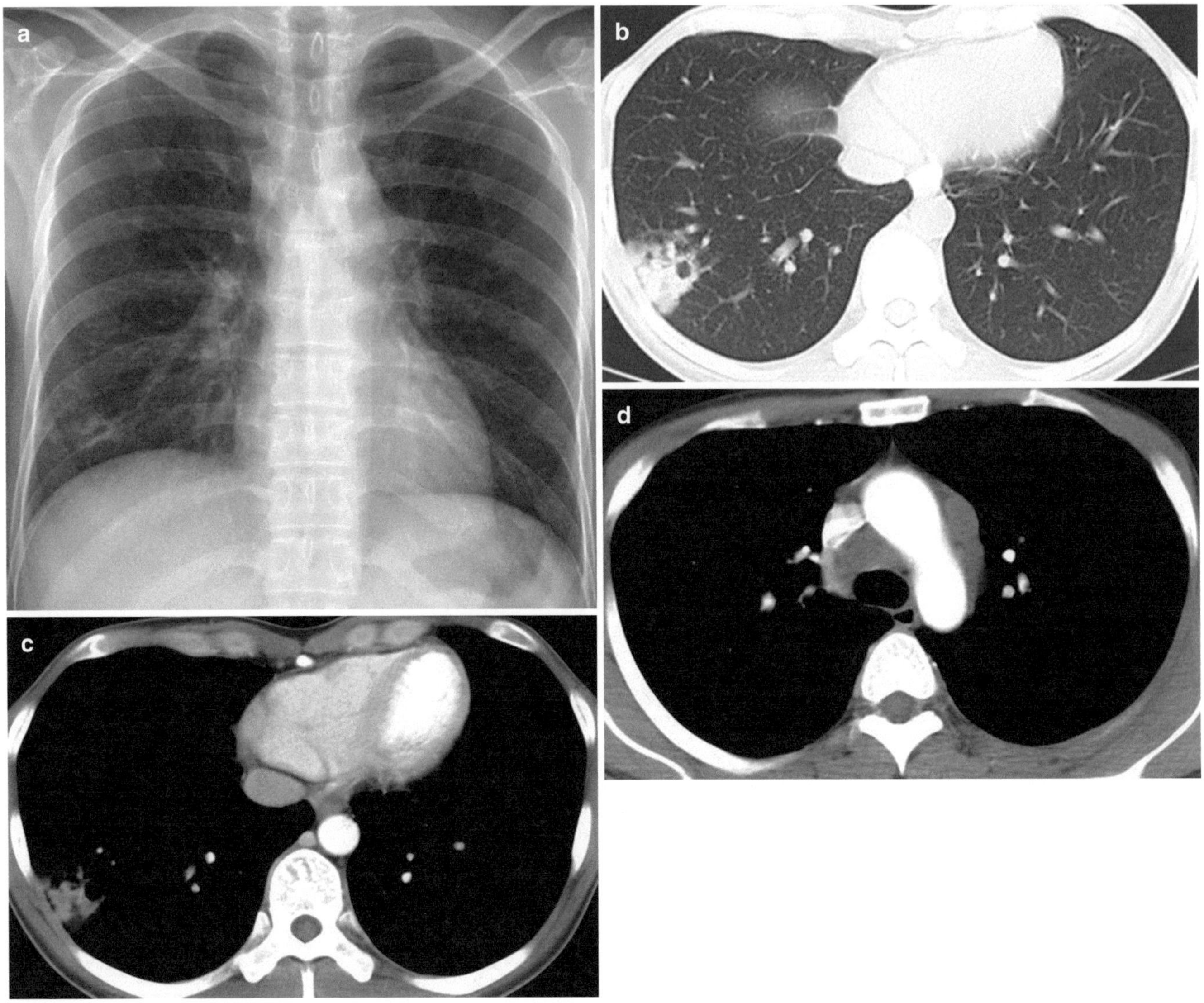

Fig. 8.9 AIDS complicated with tuberculosis and lymphatic tuberculosis. Male, 37 years old. Laboratory examination: anti-HIV positive, CD4+ T lymphocytes 2 cells/μL; sputum smear positive for acid-fast stained tuberculosis. (**a**) PA chest radiograph showed a high-density patchy shadow in the right lower lung field, with a slightly blurred boundary and enlarged both upper hilar, mainly in left hilum. (**b–d**) CT (lung window and mediastinal window) showed patchy soft tissue density on the lateral basal segment of the right lower lobe, and small gas-dissolving cavity visible in the parenchyma. Enhanced scan showed uneven lesion enhancement, and lymph node enlargement in mediastinal regions 4 and 6

to the condition of patient and CD4 T cell count, the timing of ART is selected.

(1) When CD4 T cell count is lower than 50/μL, the intensive phase of anti-tuberculosis drugs is firstly administered. If patients show favorable tolerance to anti-tuberculosis treatment, ART is initiated within 2 weeks if possible. For patients with central nervous system TB, ART can be delayed and administered as soon as possible after 4 weeks of anti-tuberculosis treatment.
(2) When CD4 T cell count is ≥50/μL, ART therapy can be initiated after 2 weeks of anti-tuberculosis treatment in mildly ill patients. For those with severe TB infection, such as low body mass index (BMI), hypoproteinemia, low level of hemoglobin, and multiple organ dysfunction, ART is initiated within 8 weeks after anti-tuberculosis treatment. For patients with central nervous system TB, ART is initiated after 2–4 weeks of anti-tuberculosis treatment.
(3) For pregnant women with TB/HIV coinfection, ART is administered as early as possible to block mother-to-infant transmission of HIV.

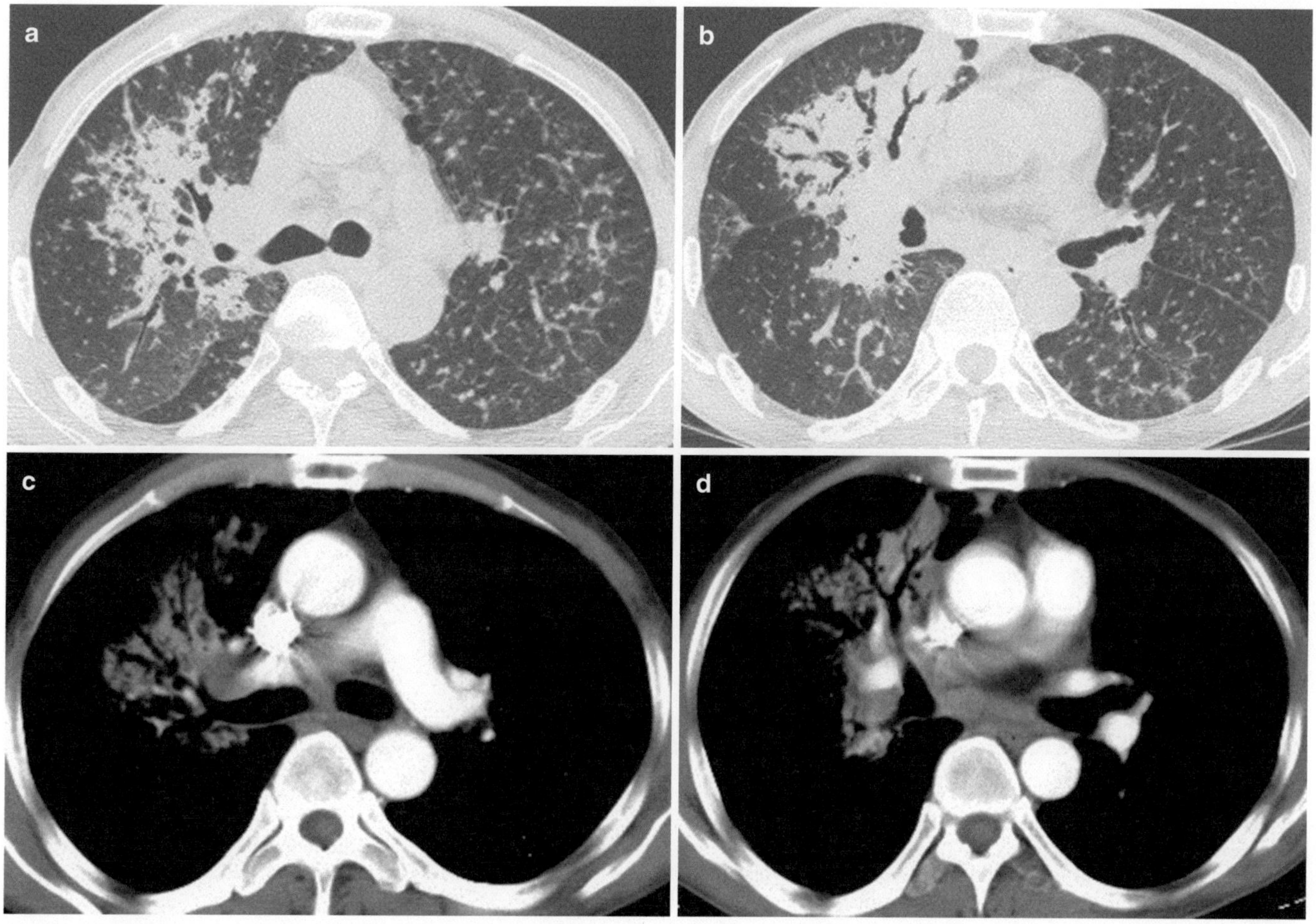

Fig. 8.10 (**a–d**) AIDS complicated with tuberculosis and lymphatic tuberculosis. Male, 33 years old. Laboratory examination: anti-HIV positive, CD4 + T lymphocytes 20 cells/μL; sputum smear positive for acid-fast stained tuberculosis. CT (lung window and mediastinum window) showed exudation and consolidation in the anterior segment of the right upper lobe, with blurred boundary and the bronchial aeration sign visible in the parenchyma of lesion. In the rest of the lung field, there were scattered micro-nodules, small patchy densities, and few streaked densities; the mediastinal and right hilar lymph nodes were enlarged

Selection of Anti-Tuberculosis Treatment Regimen

Clinical Treatment for TB in Patients with TB/HIV Coinfection

For patients with TB/HIV coinfection and a high CD4 cell count, the clinical manifestations resemble to those of simplex TB. However, patients with TB/HIV coinfection and a low CD4 cell count, especially those with a CD4 T cell count being lower than 200/μL, complication of extrapulmonary TB is common [29]. The most common extrapulmonary TB is central nervous system TB (such as tuberculous meningitis), followed by tuberculous pleurisy, lymph node TB (including peripheral lymph node, mediastinal lymph node, and abdominal lymph node TB), and abdominal TB (such as tuberculous peritonitis and intestinal TB). And extrapulmonary TB rarely involves liver, spleen, kidney, pericardium, bone and joint, and testicle. Therefore, in patients with TB/HIV coinfection, complication of extrapulmonary TB should be systematically excluded to avoid failed anti-tuberculosis treatment due to miss diagnosis of extrapulmonary TB.

Anti-Tuberculosis Treatment in Patients with TB/HIV Coinfection

Classification of Anti-Tuberculosis Drugs

The first-line anti-tuberculosis drugs include isoniazid (H), rifampicin (R), rifabutin (RFB), ethambutol (E), pyrazinamide (Z), streptomycin (Sm). And the second-line anti-tuberculosis drugs include sodium paraaminosalicylic acid (PAS), amikacin (Am), capreomycin (Cm), levofloxacin (LFX), moxifloxacin (MFX), gatifloxacin (GFX), ethionamide (ETO), prothionamide (PTO), meropenem (MPM), and imipenem–cilastatin (IPM/CIN).

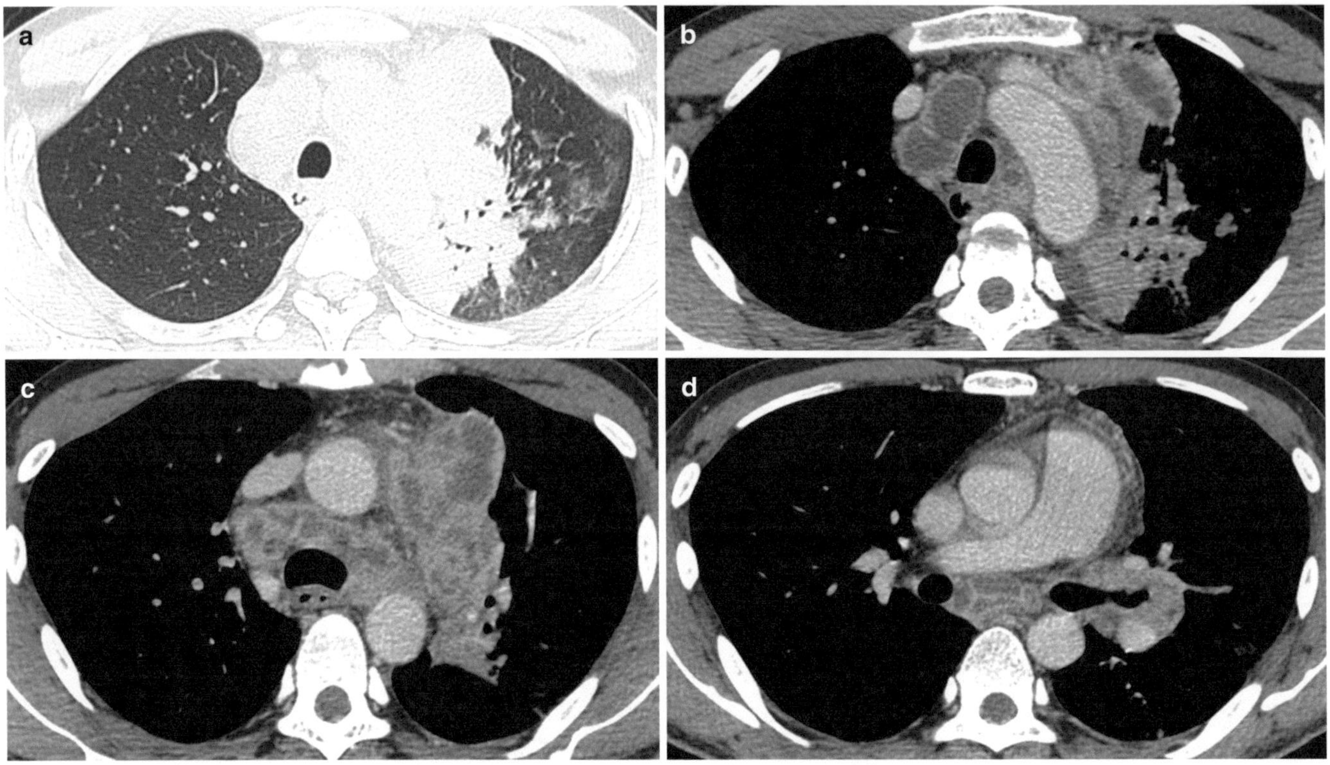

Fig. 8.11 (**a–d**) AIDS complicated with mediastinal lymphocyte tuberculosis and pulmonary tuberculosis. Male, 27 years old. Laboratory examination: anti-HIV positive, CD4+ T lymphocytes 15 cells/μL; sputum smear or bronchial brushing detection positive for acid-fast stained tuberculosis. CT (lung window and mediastinal window) showed enlargement of multiple groups of mediastinal lymph nodes, and the enhanced scan showed circular enhancement. Mutual fusion was found between the lymph nodes, and the pulmonary parenchyma adjacent to the left superior lobe was invaded and consolidated

For Patients with Initially Treated TB

For patients with initially treated TB and HIV/AIDS, the usage and dose of anti-tuberculosis treatment are the same as that for patients with simplex TB, namely administration of 2HRZE/4HR regimen. However, at the intensive phase of anti-tuberculosis treatment, it is strongly recommended to intake drugs each day instead of intermittent medication (such as twice or three times a week). Meanwhile, vitamin B6 (oral intake 25–30 mg daily during whole course of treatment) is simultaneously administered to reduce the occurrence of peripheral neuritis. If the sputum bacteriology test still shows positive after 2 months intensive phase of medication, the intensive phase is prolonged for 1 month, followed by the consolidation phase. During the consolidation phase, the anti-tuberculosis drugs can be taken daily or at least three times a week. During the whole course of anti-tuberculosis treatment, sputum specimen is collected each month for sputum smear with acid-fast staining and Mtb culture to assess the therapeutic efficacy of anti-tuberculosis treatment. And the anti-tuberculosis treatment is believed effective if two consecutive sputum cultures for Mtb are negative during the intensive phase. If one of the following conditions occurs, the initial treatment for TB fails: (1) The sputum smear test shows positive after 5 months treatment or at the end of the treatment course. (2) Any one of the sputum smear tests shows positive during the treatment for patients with newly detected smear-negative TB.

After the diagnosis of initially treated TB is defined, the drug sensitivity test of Mtb should be ordered for appropriate selection of anti-tuberculosis treatment regimen.

For Patients with Retreated TB

The commonly applied treatment regimen for retreated TB is 2SHRZE/6HRE. If streptomycin cannot be applied, an additional one-month intensive phase is necessary, and 3HRZE/6HRE regimen is administered. If patient treated with streptomycin included regimen still shows positive in sputum smear test with acid-fast staining after 2 months treatment, one additional month of intensive treatment regimen is necessary. If the sputum smear test still shows positive after 5 months of anti-tuberculosis treatment or at the end of the treatment course, the treatment for retreated TB fails. In areas that sputum culture for Mtb and drug sensitivity test can be performed, patients with failed treatment for retreated TB should receive sputum culture for Mtb and in vitro drug sensitivity test (DST) of Mtb. Based on the findings of DST, anti-tuberculosis treatment regimen is formulated. In the areas that routine drug sensitivity test cannot be

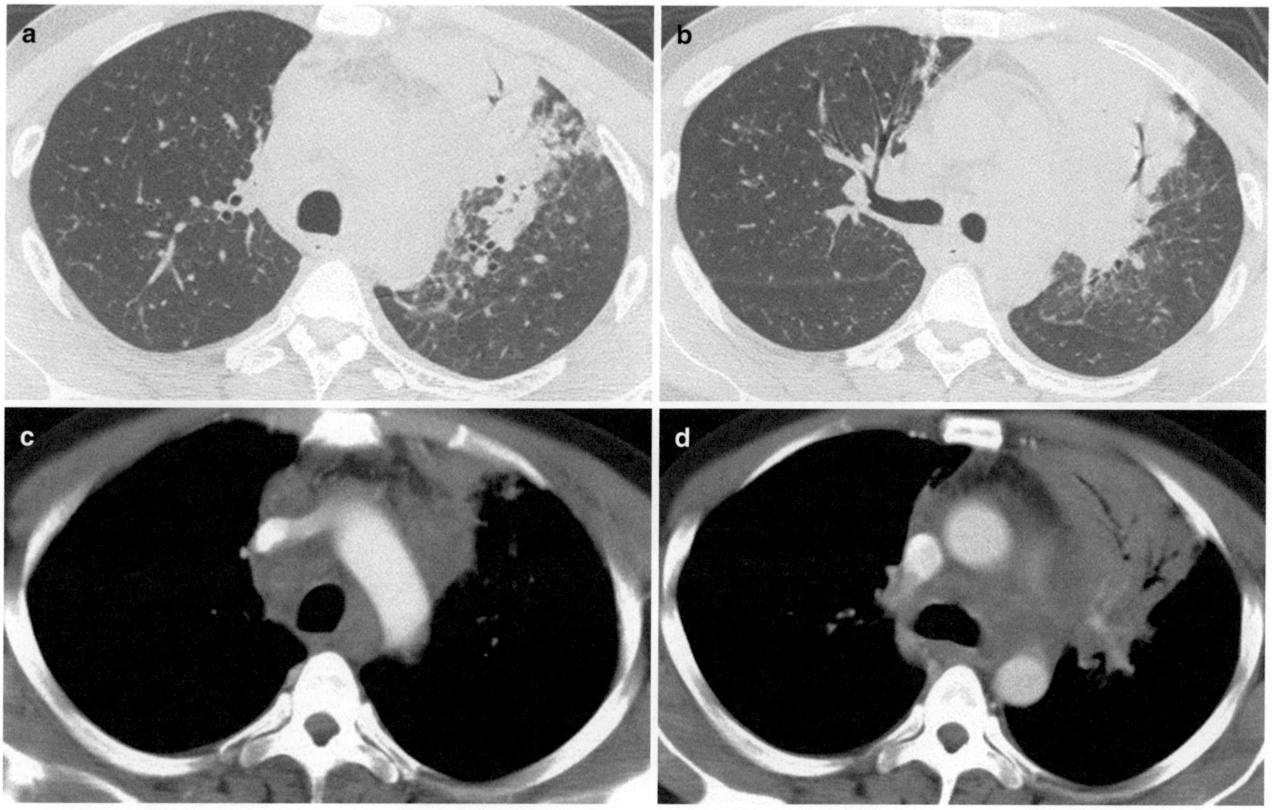

Fig. 8.12 (**a**–**d**) AIDS complicated with mediastinal lymphocyte tuberculosis and pulmonary tuberculosis. Male, 38 years old. Laboratory examination: anti-HIV positive, CD4+ T lymphocytes 25 cells/μL; sputum smear positive for acid-fast stained tuberculosis, and positive for tuberculosis antibodies. CT (lung window and mediastinal window) showed enlargement of multiple groups of mediastinal lymph nodes, and the enhanced scan showed necrosis and liquefaction of some enlarged lymph nodes, without significant enhancement; the adjacent anterior segment of the left upper lobe showed consolidation accompanied by flocculent densities, with blurred boundary and air bronchogram in consolidation area

performed, the treatment regimen is formulated according to the local epidemic of drug resistance of Mtb.

For Patients with HIV/AIDS and DR-TB

China is one of the countries with high incidence of DR-TB. The incidence of drug resistance in initially treated patients with TB in China is as high as 7.1%, and that in retreated patients with TB is as high as 24%. The incidences are much higher than the global average incidence of drug resistance in initially treated patients with TB and retreated patients with TB, being 3.5% and 18%, respectively [26]. Epidemic of HIV infection is always associated with epidemic of MDR-TB, and is an independent risk factor of XDR-TB. In an internationally published research report, it has been demonstrated that the incidences of single drug-resistant TB and multi-drug resistant TB in patients with HIV/AIDS are significantly higher than those in non-HIV/AIDS individuals [30]. Therefore, the treatment of DR-TB in patients with HIV/AIDS is very important in population with TB/HIV coinfection, and deserves focused attention.

DR-TB in patients with HIV/AIDS includes: (1) Mono-resistant TB (MR-TB), which is referred to as resistance of Mtb to one of the first-line anti-tuberculosis drugs that is detected by in vitro DST. (2) Polydrug-resistant TB (PR-TB), which is referred to as resistance of Mtb to more than one of the first-line anti-tuberculosis drugs (with simultaneous resistance to isoniazid and rifampicin excluded) detected by in vitro DST. (3) Multidrug-resistant TB (MDR-TB), which is referred to as resistance of Mtb to at least isoniazid and rifampicin detected by in vitro DST. (4) Extensively drug-resistant TB (XDR-TB), which is referred to as resistance of Mtb to isoniazid, rifampicin, any one of fluoroquinolones, and at least one of the three second-line injectable anti-tuberculosis drugs detected by in vitro DST. (5) Rifampicin-resistant TB (RR-TB), which is referred to as resistance of Mtb to rifampin detected by in vitro DST, including MR-TB, PR-TB, MDR-TB, and XDR-TB with rifampin resistance.

The treatment regimen for DR-TB contains at least 4 effective anti-tuberculosis drugs and pyrazinamide. If there are no 4 effective anti-tuberculosis drugs for selection or the effectiveness of one drug in the regimen is uncertain or questionable, the treatment regimen may include more than 5 anti-tuberculosis drugs, which are common in treatment of XDR-TB. The sequential drug selection is to select

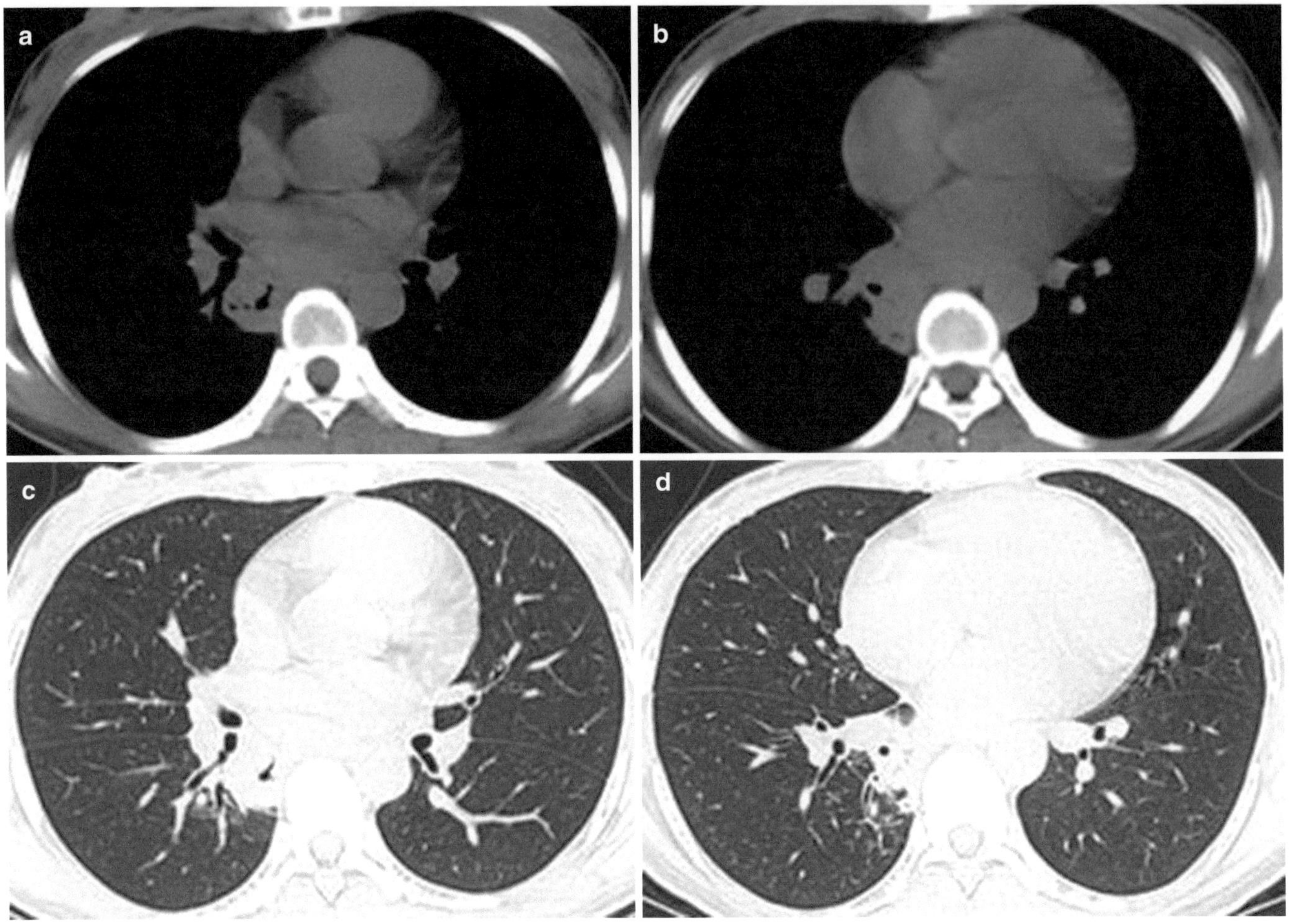

Fig. 8.13 (**a**–**d**) AIDS complicated with mediastinal lymphocyte tuberculosis and pulmonary tuberculosis. Female, 32 years old. Laboratory examination: anti-HIV positive, CD4+ T lymphocytes 96 cells/μL; sputum smear positive for acid-fast stained tuberculosis, and positive for tuberculosis antibodies. CT (lung window and mediastinal window) showed enlargement and fusion of multiple groups of mediastinal lymph nodes, and air-containing sign and local rupture of the enlarged lymph nodes; the adjacent medial basal segment of the right lower lobe showed consolidation accompanied by flocculent densities, with blurred boundary and air bronchogram in consolidation area

appropriate drug downward sequentially from the first group with reference to the five groups of drugs, which is applicable for MR-TB and PR-TB with no R resistance. The five-step drug selection is to firstly select second-line injections and fluoroquinolones. On the basis of 4 effective second-line anti-tuberculosis drugs, pyrazinamide is routinely added. This type of selection is applicable for RR-TB, MDR-TB, and XDR-TB.

According to the DST of Mtb, there are corresponding anti-tuberculosis treatment regimens, which are basically the same as that for patients with simplex TB.

For Pregnant Women with TB

For pregnant women with TB, anti-tuberculosis drugs may include isoniazid, ethambutol, and p-aminosalicylic acid, which are not teratogenic in animal or human studies. However, for pregnant women with TB receiving medication of isoniazid, liver damage is more likely to occur. Therefore, it is necessary to closely monitor the liver function during medication of isoniazid for pregnant women. During the second and third trimester of pregnancy, RFP can be selected, and its course of treatment is the same as that for common TB. Pyrazinamide shows no teratogenicity in animal experiments, but there is limited research data from pregnant women. Therefore, its application in pregnant women remains controversial. The neurotoxicity of aminoglycosides affects fetal hearing, and they are contraindicated for pregnant women. Due to the negative effects of quinolones on bone and joint, they are contraindicated to pregnant women and children aged under 18 years.

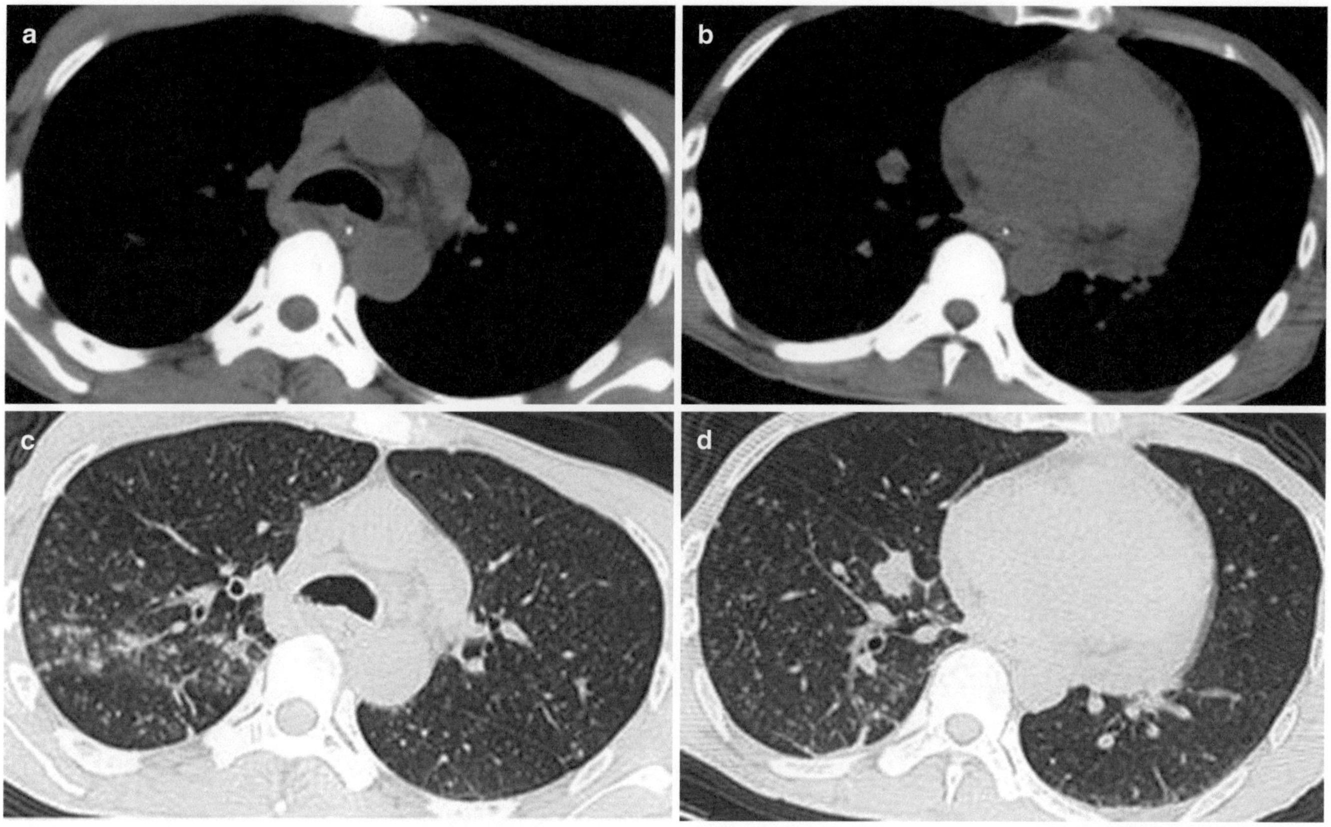

Fig. 8.14 AIDS complicated with subacute miliary tuberculosis, lymphatic tuberculosis, tuberculous pleurisy. Male, 41 years old. Laboratory tests: anti-HIV antibody positive, CD4+ T lymphocytes 16 cells/μL; bronchial brushing detection positive for acid-fast stained tuberculosis. (**a**, **b**) CT (mediastinal window) showed mediastinal lymph node enlargement, with uneven density and a small amount of effusion in the left thoracic cavity; (**c**, **d**) CT (lung window) showed diffuse distribution of miliary nodules in both lungs, with uneven size, density, and distribution (i.e., "three non-uniformity" characteristics), and the distribution in upper lung was more than that in the lower lung

For Patients with Bone/Joint TB or with Delayed Response to Anti-Tuberculosis Drugs

For patients with bone/joint TB or with delayed response to anti-tuberculosis drugs (showing TB toxic symptoms or sputum culture positive after intensive treatment for 2 months), the anti-tuberculosis treatment regimen should be administered for additional 9 months.

For Patients with Central Nervous System TB

For patients with central nervous system TB, the course of treatment is recommended to last for 9–12 months or even longer.

Application of Hormone for Anti-Tuberculosis Treatment in Patients with TB/HIV Coinfection

For patients with HIV positive and central nervous system TB or pericardial TB, hormone therapy can be appropriately administered, which increases the survival of such patients. The use of dexamethasone is recommended for patients with HIV positive and central nervous system TB. The administration of dexamethasone is started at a dose of 0.3–0.4 mg/kg body weight per day for 2–4 weeks and gradually decreased to 0.1 mg/kg body weight per day. The dose is further decreased by 1 mg/week. And the whole course of treatment lasts for 12 weeks. The administration of prednisone is recommended for patients with HIV positive and pericardial TB. The administration of prednisone is started at a dose of 60 mg/day, which is then gradually decreased by 10 mg/week. And the whole course of treatment lasts for 6 weeks.

6.3 Antiretroviral Therapy (ART) for Patients with TB/HIV Coinfection

Principles and Timing of ART

For all patients with TB/HIV coinfection, ART should be initiated as early as possible, regardless of their CD4 T cell

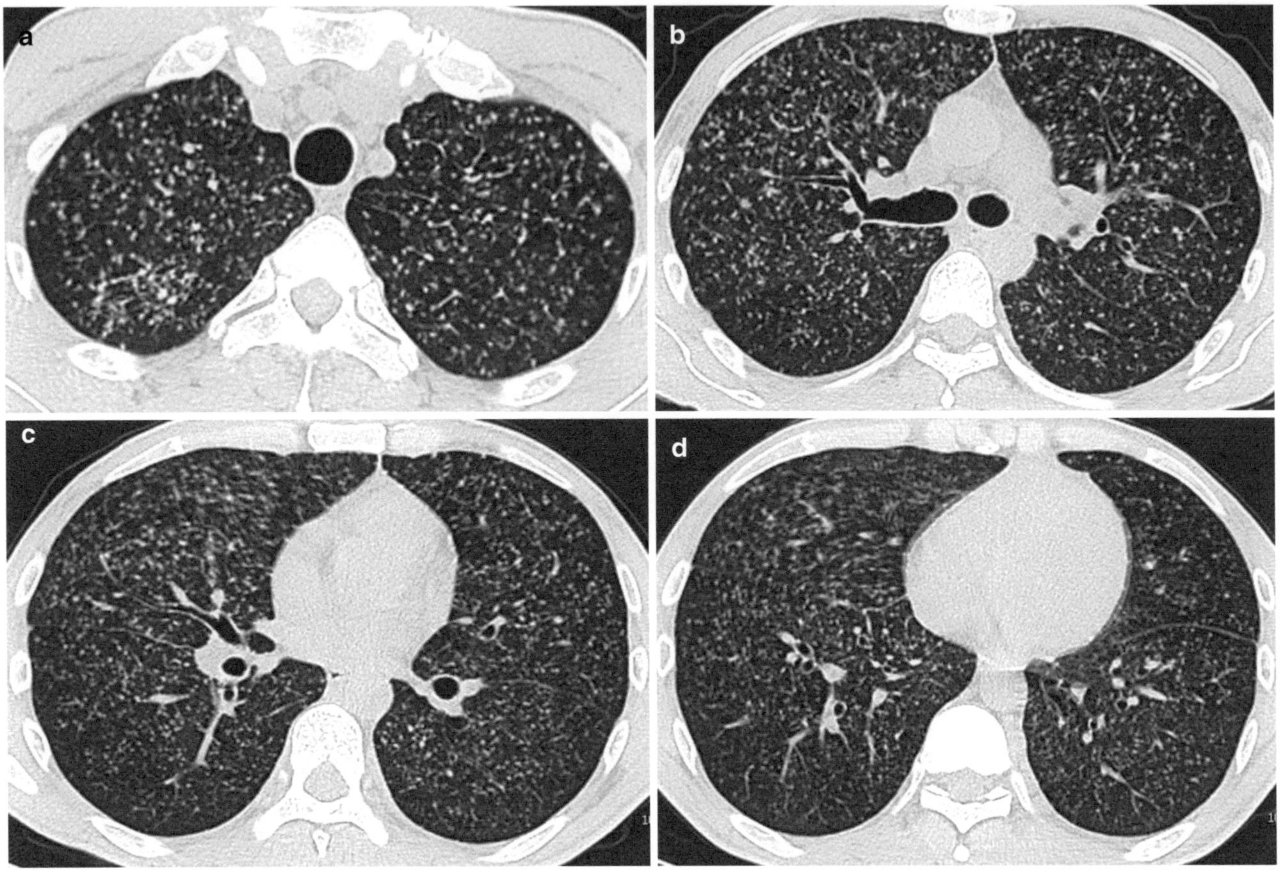

Fig. 8.15 (**a**–**d**) AIDS complicated with acute miliary pulmonary tuberculosis. Male, 36 years old. Laboratory tests: anti-HIV antibody positive, CD4+ T lymphocytes 40 cells/μL; bronchial brushing detection positive for acid-fast stained tuberculosis. The CT (lung window) showed diffuse distribution of miliary nodules in both lungs, showing a "three uniformity" feature

count. The initiation of ART depends on the condition of coinfection and CD4 T cell count of patient. And assessment on treatment compliance and following up surveillance are also very important [31].

ART Regimen

First-Line ART Regimen

Tenofovir/Emtricitabine (Lamivudine) + Latiravir (Dotiravir); Tenofovir/Entravir (Lamivudine)/Efavirenz (EFV).

Alternative ART Regimen

If the patient cannot be administered with ART regimen, special ART regimens can be applied as alternative.

Tenofovir/Entretabine (Lamivudine) + Ritonavir protease inhibitor. Rifabutin should be applied to replace rifampicin. If rifampicin is included in the anti-tuberculosis treatment regimen, tenofovir/Entretabine + Dotiravir can be administered, twice a day.

When raltegravir (RAL), dolutegravir (DTG), or rifampicin is not applicable in some patients, the following treatment regimen can be applied for short-term treatment until anti-tuberculosis treatment is completed. (1) For patients receiving rifampicin-containing anti-tuberculosis treatment regimen, when ART regimen is combined and their HIV viral load is less than 100,000 copies per μL, the following regimen can be applied: fixed dose of Abacavir/Lamivudine/Zidovudine (300/150/300 mg), twice a day; + tenofovir (600 mg), once a day. (2) For patients receiving rifampicin-containing anti-tuberculosis treatment regimen, when ART regimen containing protease inhibitor is combined, double dose of ritonavir (500 mg, twice a day) or ritonavir (400 mg, twice a day) + lopinavir (400 mg, twice a day) can be administered. (3) Other treatment regimens are based on two nucleoside reverse transcriptase inhibitors (NRTI) plus one non-nucleoside reverse transcriptase inhibitor (NNRTI), nevirapine (NVP), rilpivirine (RPV), evirtraine (ETV), or chemokine receptor-5 inhibitors on cell membrane surface, and maraviroc (MVC).

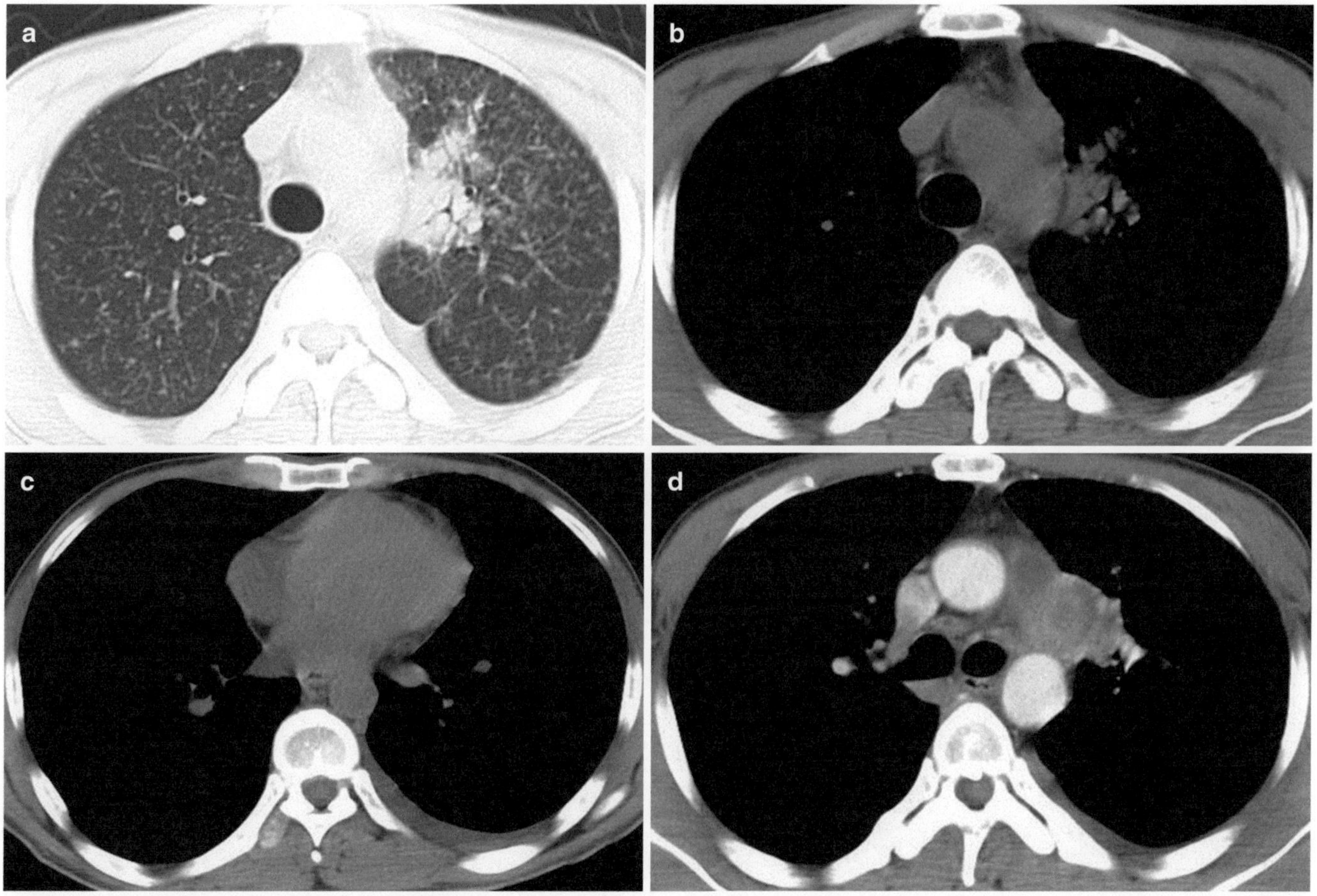

Fig. 8.16 (**a–d**) AIDS complicated with hematogenous disseminated tuberculosis, lymphatic tuberculosis, tuberculous pleurisy. Male, 35 years old. Laboratory tests: anti-HIV antibody positive, CD4+ T cells 1 cell/μL, acid-fast bacilli seen on acid-fast staining of alveolar lavage fluid. CT (lung window and mediastinal window) showed diffuse miliary lesions in both lungs, high density shadows projecting to the lung field in left upper hilar; the CT (mediastinal window) showed left pleural effusion, mediastinal, and left upper hilar lymph node enlargement; enhanced scan showed obviously unevenly enhanced mediastinal lymph nodes, localized liquefaction and necrosis, and circularly enhanced edge

Precautions in Administration of ART

Drug Interaction Between Tenofovir Alafenamide Fumarate (TAF) and Rifampicin

Drug interaction between TAF and rifampicin has not been assessed in detail. Because TAF may be induced by enzymes, patients taking TAF should avoid application of rifampicin-containing regimen in anti-tuberculosis treatment.

Combination with Ritonavir Protease Inhibitor

When combined with ritonavir protease inhibitor, the concentration of rifabutin and its active metabolites greatly increase. Pharmacokinetic data obtained from patients with TB/HIV coinfection showed that the combined use of ritonavir or ritonavir azanavir with rifabutin (150 mg, once every other day) causes a lower concentration of rifabutin than those subjects who take rifabutin (300 mg per day) but do not take ritonavir protease inhibitor. The data indicated insufficient dose of rifabutin. Therefore, in the guidelines for treatment of HIV/AIDS treatment, rifabutin is recommended to be administered at a dose of 150 mg, once a day, when ritonavir protease inhibitor is combined. Due to the limited data on safety of this dose and combination regimen, patients taking rifabutin (150 mg, once a day) should be closely monitored to assess the toxicity associated with rifabutin (such as uveitis and neutropenia).

Treatment for TB/HIV Coinfection Complicated by Viral Hepatitis B and C

Patients with TB/HIV coinfection should be routinely screened for hepatitis B and C. If patients are exposed to

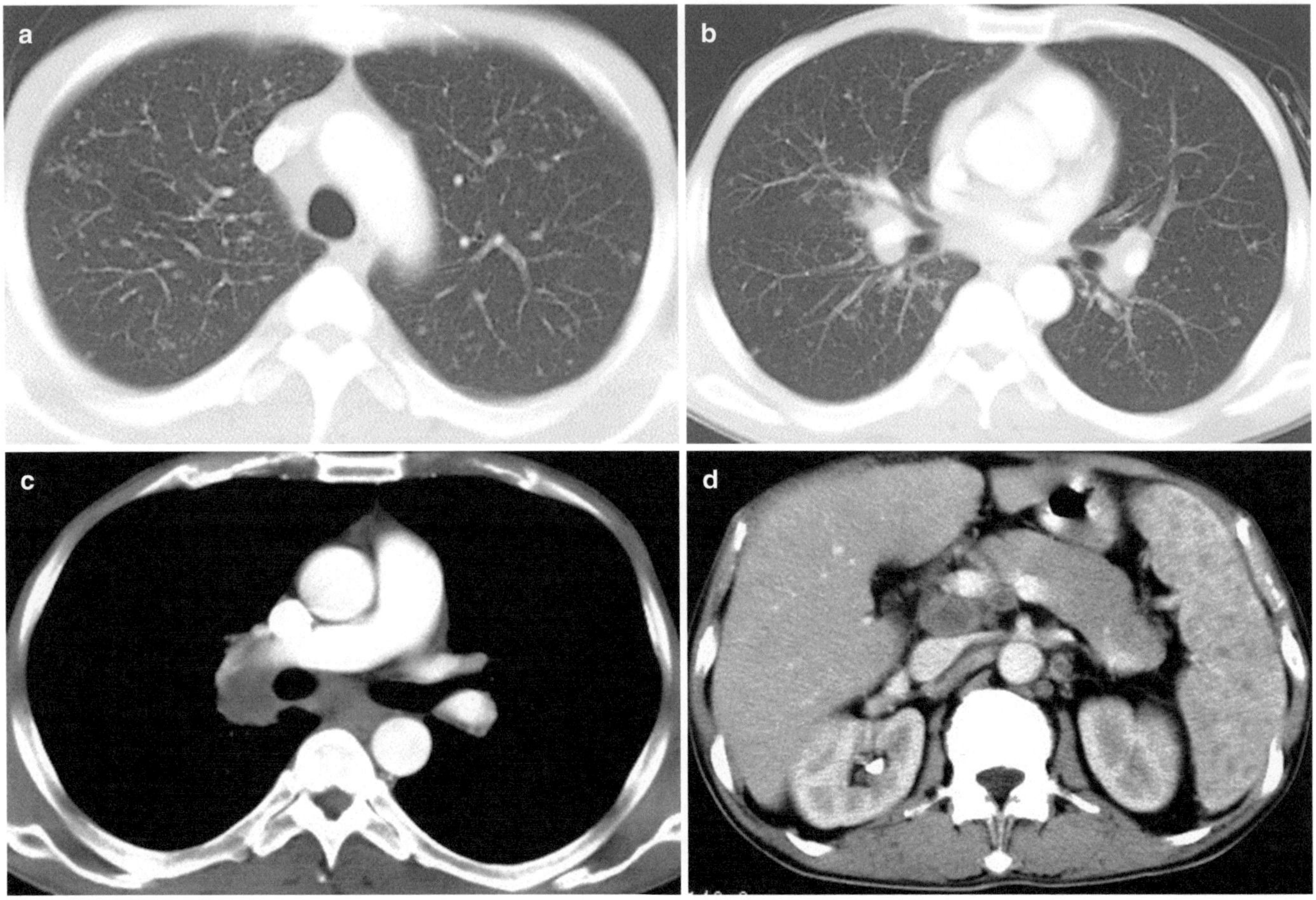

Fig. 8.17 AIDS with subacute hematogenous disseminated tuberculosis, lymphatic tuberculosis, and splenic tuberculosis. Male, 35 years old. Laboratory tests: anti-HIV antibody positive, CD4+ T cells 60 cells/μL, acid-fast bacilli seen on acid-fast staining of alveolar lavage fluid. (**a**, **b**) shows micro-nodules and miliary lesions unevenly distributed in both two lungs, (**c**) in mediastinal window, right hilar and subcarinal lymph nodes enlargement were found, (**d**) abdominal enhanced CT showed multiple low-density miliary foci and small nodules with varied sizes, and multiple lymph nodes enlargements found in the abdomen

the following risk factors, HCV-RNA detection should be performed for early HCV infection. The risk factors include persistently positive intravenous drug use, chemical sexual behaviors (sexual behaviors before and/or during the affected period by intravenous recreational drug abuse) with mucosal trauma, persistent unprotected anal intercourse, and recently diagnosed sexually transmitted disease with unexplained elevation of aminotransferase but HCV antibody negative. For patients with hepatitis B core antibody positive but surface antigen of hepatitis B virus negative, especially those with elevated aminotransferase, test for surface antigen of hepatitis B virus and hepatitis B virus DNA screening should be performed to exclude potential hepatitis B virus infection. For patients with HBsAg positive, screening for hepatitis D antibody is recommended. For patients with hepatitis C or hepatitis B cirrhosis, screening for primary liver cancer is recommended.

All patients with HCV/TB/HIV coinfection must receive direct acting anti-viral agent (DAA) treatment to eradicate hepatitis C, regardless of the severity of liver fibrosis and the availability of DAA drugs. In patients with HCV/TB/HIV coinfection, the progression of liver fibrosis is more rapid. Due to active HCV during anti-tuberculosis treatment and ART in patients with HCV/TB/HIV coinfection, it aggravates the damages to liver [32]. Therefore, the condition of a patient should be comprehensively assessed for administration of anti-tuberculosis treatment, anti-hepatitis C treatment, and ART. If the damages to liver are more serious in patients with HIV/AIDS and DAA drugs are available, anti-HCV treatment can be prioritized to achieve early SVR rapid response and decreased liver damage. By this way, anti-tuberculosis treatment and ART can be further implemented. If pulmonary TB infection is more serious in patients with HIV/AIDS, anti-tuberculosis treatment is prioritized. After the condition of TB is stabilized, anti-hepatitis C treatment and ART can be accordingly administered. In patients with HCV/HIV coinfection, the tolerance to and cure rate of DAA treatment are almost the same as those in patients with hepatitis C alone. Therefore, the indications of treatment regimens for patients with HCV/HIV coinfection are the same as those for patients with hepatitis C alone.

All patients with HBV/TB/HIV coinfection, if tolerant, are required to receive combined ART with tenofovir (TDF) or tenofovir-alaphenolamine (TAF). (1) If anti-HBV nucleosides are part of the antiretroviral combination therapy, lifelong treatment is recommended. In combination antiretroviral therapy (including lamivudine) for patients with inactive HBsAg positive, TDF or TAF should be added as

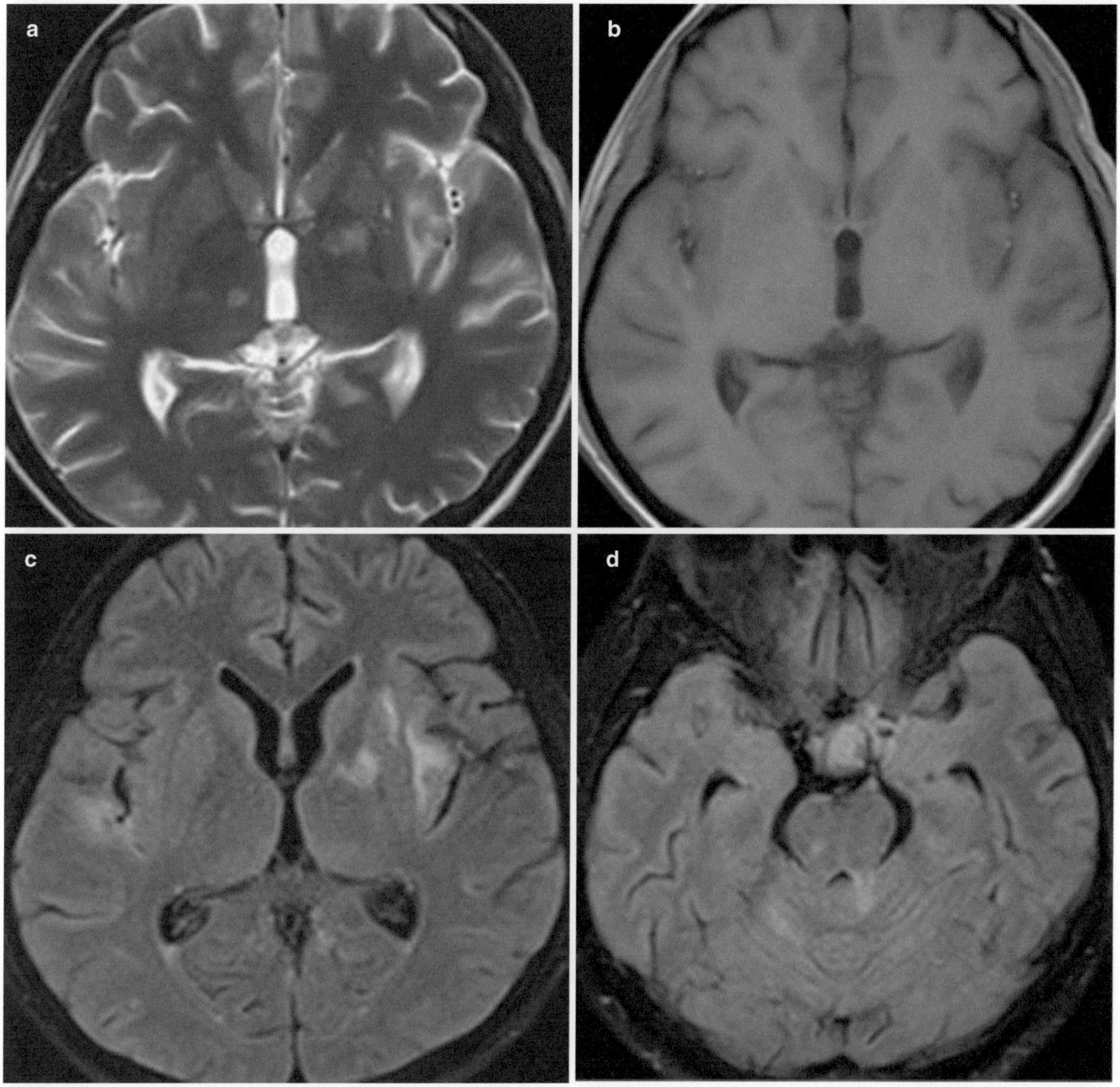

Fig. 8.18 AIDS with subacute hematogenous disseminated tuberculosis, lymphatic tuberculosis, and intracranial tuberculosis. Male, 28 years old. Clinical laboratory tests: anti-HIV antibody positive, CD4+ T cells 156 cells/μl, cerebrospinal fluid total cell count 376 cells/uL, white blood cells 176, monocytes 30%, polykaryocytes 70%, cerebrospinal fluid protein 87.1 mg/dL, glucose 0.44 mmol/L, and chlorides 112.6 mmol/L. It met the diagnosis of intracranial tuberculosis. (**a**–**g**) Brain MR plain scan and enhanced scan showed low signal of brain parenchyma on T1 W1, patchy and nodule high signal on T2 W1, FLAIR sequence showed more lesions with high signal located in the brain parenchyma and the right lateral fissure and cistern, high signal of cerebellar leptomeninges, and enhanced scan showed multiple circular, miliary enhanced lesions scattered in brain parenchyma, and skull base meningeal thickening and nodules. (**h**) CT (lung window) showed scattered and evenly distributed micro-nodules and miliary lesions in both lungs

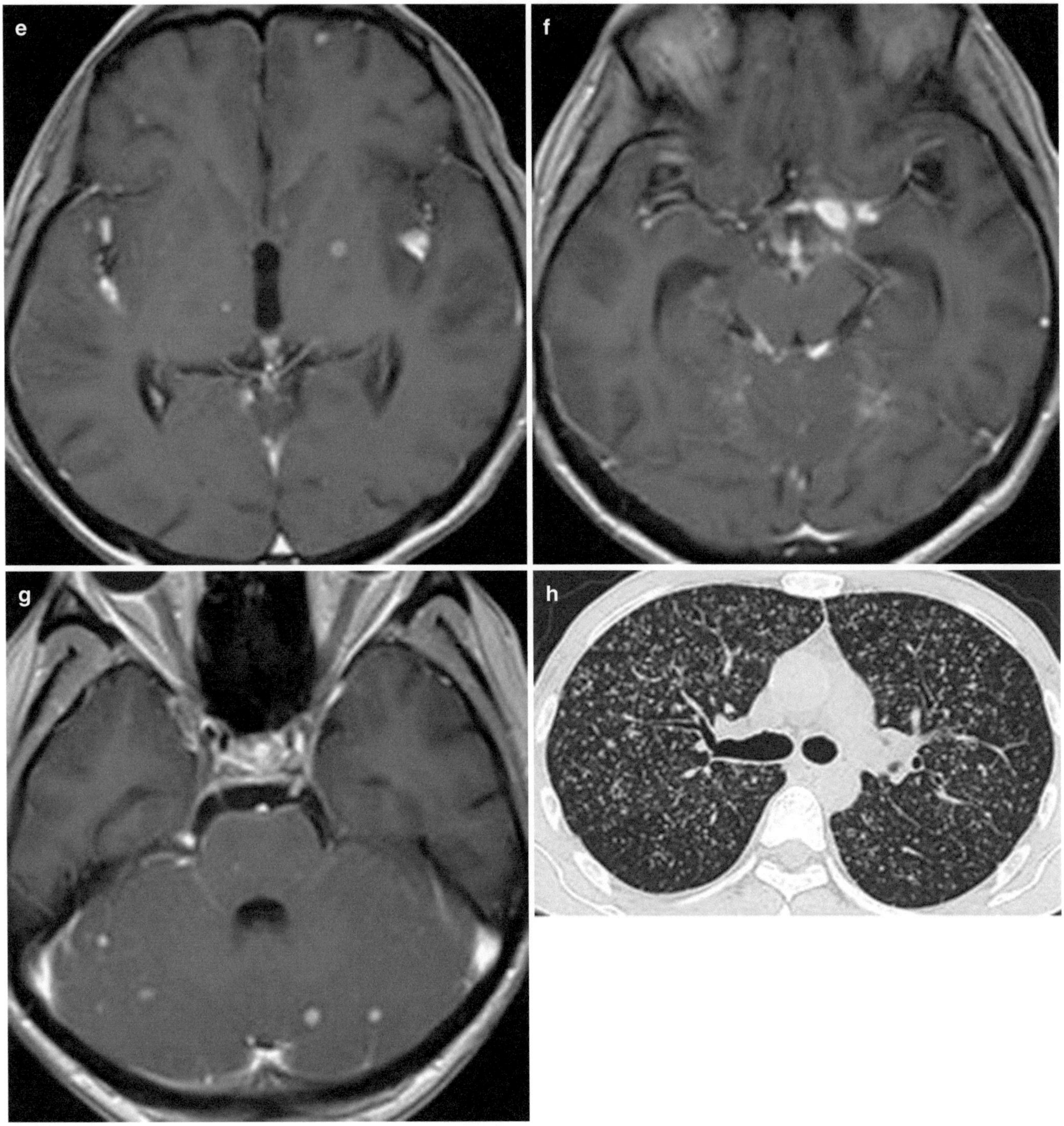

Fig. 8.18 (continued)

a prophylactic treatment. (2) If TDF or TAF are contraindicated, patients who have never received lamivudine should be treated with entecavir and adequately effective ART. (3) For patients receiving antiretroviral combination therapy including TDF or TAF, the bone mineral density and renal function should be monitored. Patients with hepatocirrhosis and low CD4 T cell count should be closely observed in the first month of ART for immune reconstruction syndrome and subsequent decompensation of liver function caused by sudden elevation of hepatic aminotransferase [33]. (4) Patients with HBV/TB/HIV coinfection should avoid retrieval of antiretroviral combination therapy, because it greatly increases the risk of sudden severe hepatitis, and causes decompensation after hepatitis induced by hepatitis B virus reactivation.

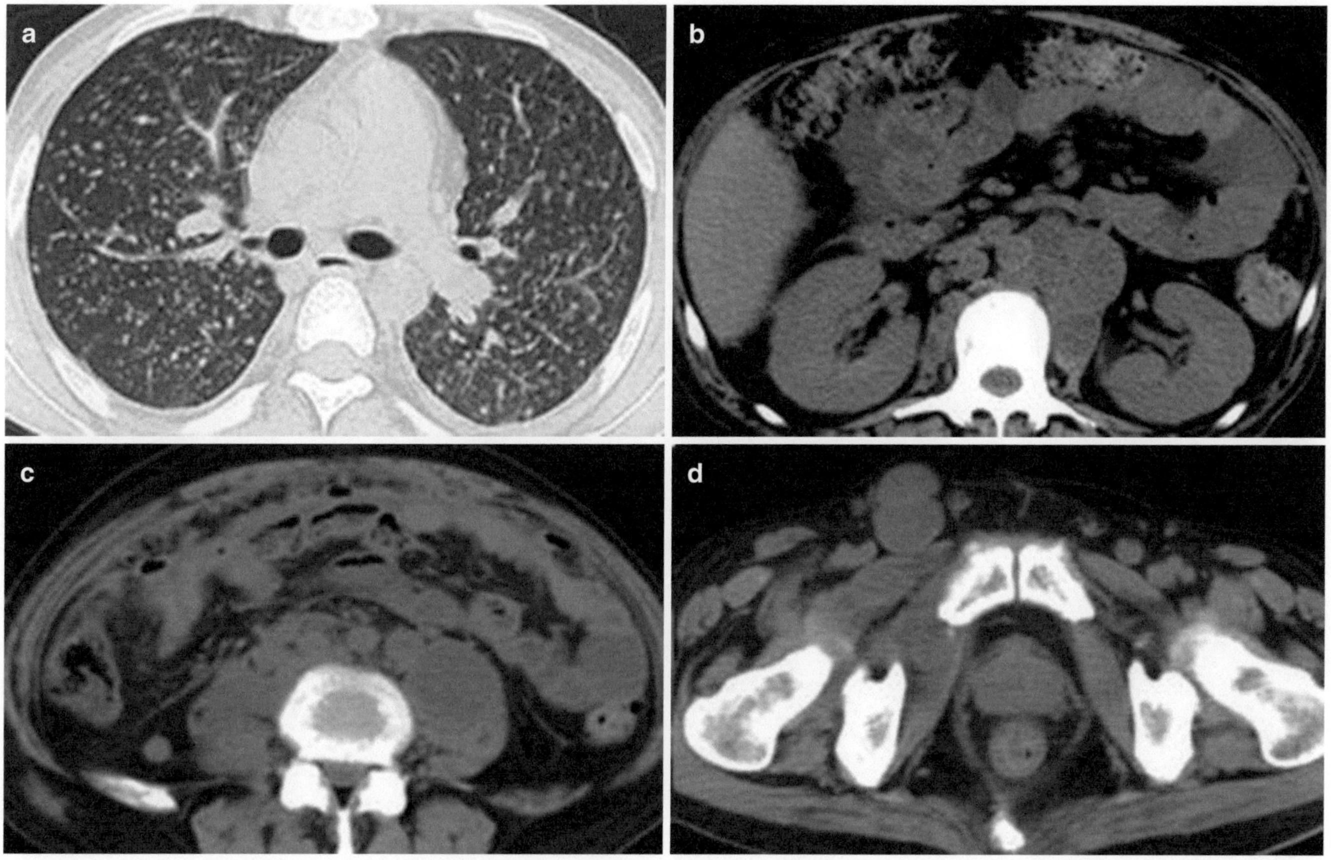

Fig. 8.19 AIDS complicated with subacute hematogenous disseminated tuberculosis, lymphatic tuberculosis, and intracranial tuberculous abscess. Male, 33 years old. Laboratory tests: anti-HIV antibody positive, CD4+ T cells 157 cells/μl, acid-fast bacilli seen on acid-fast staining of alveolar lavage fluid, tubercle bacillus found upon right inguinal lymph node puncture. (**a**) shows micro-nodules and miliary lesions evenly distributed in both lungs, (**b–d**) abdominal CT showed multiple lymph node enlargement and necrosis, and left psoas abscess formation with blurred, multiple nodules in peritoneum, with uneven density, and enlargement and necrosis of lymph nodes in the right inguinal region

6.4 Tuberculosis-Associated Immune Reconstruction Inflammatory Syndrome (TB-IRIS)

TB-IRIS is the most important and the most common early complication in patients with TB/HIV coinfection during the anti-tuberculosis treatment and efficient ART. TB-IRIS does not occur in patients with TB alone. The global incidence of TB-IRIS is 11.0–68.8% in patients with TB/HIV coinfection [34]. The mechanism of TB-IRIS is generally believed to be the destruction of cellular immune balance and excessive inflammatory responses. And it is suspected to be related to the imbalanced Th1/Th2 and Th17/Treg immune ratio, but the detailed mechanism has still been elusive. TB-IRIS occurs most frequently within 2 weeks to 3 months after initiation of ART. The common clinical manifestations include fever, cough, expectoration, enlarged primary lung lesions, and enlarged lymph nodes. The systemic toxic symptoms are not obvious, and TB-IRIS hardly affects the spiritual status and appetite of patient. Laboratory tests show elevated lactate dehydrogenase, elevated CD4 T cell count, and decreased HIV RNA load. All of these laboratory findings support the diagnosis of TB-IRIS. Clinically, TB-IRIS is classified into two types, self-contradictory TB-IRIS and exposed TB-IRIS [28].

Self-Contradictory TB-IRIS

Definition

Self-contradictory TB-IRIS occurs when ART is initiated after anti-tuberculosis treatment. The incidence is 48–54%, and the mortality rate is 2%. It usually lasts for 2–3 months. During anti-tuberculosis treatment, the clinical symptoms of patient are improved. However, within 1–4 weeks after ART, patient develops new symptoms or the condition deteriorates, with enlarged opacity by chest radiography.

Typical Clinical Manifestations

The typical clinical manifestations include repeated high fever, new enlarged lymph nodes or further enlarged lymph

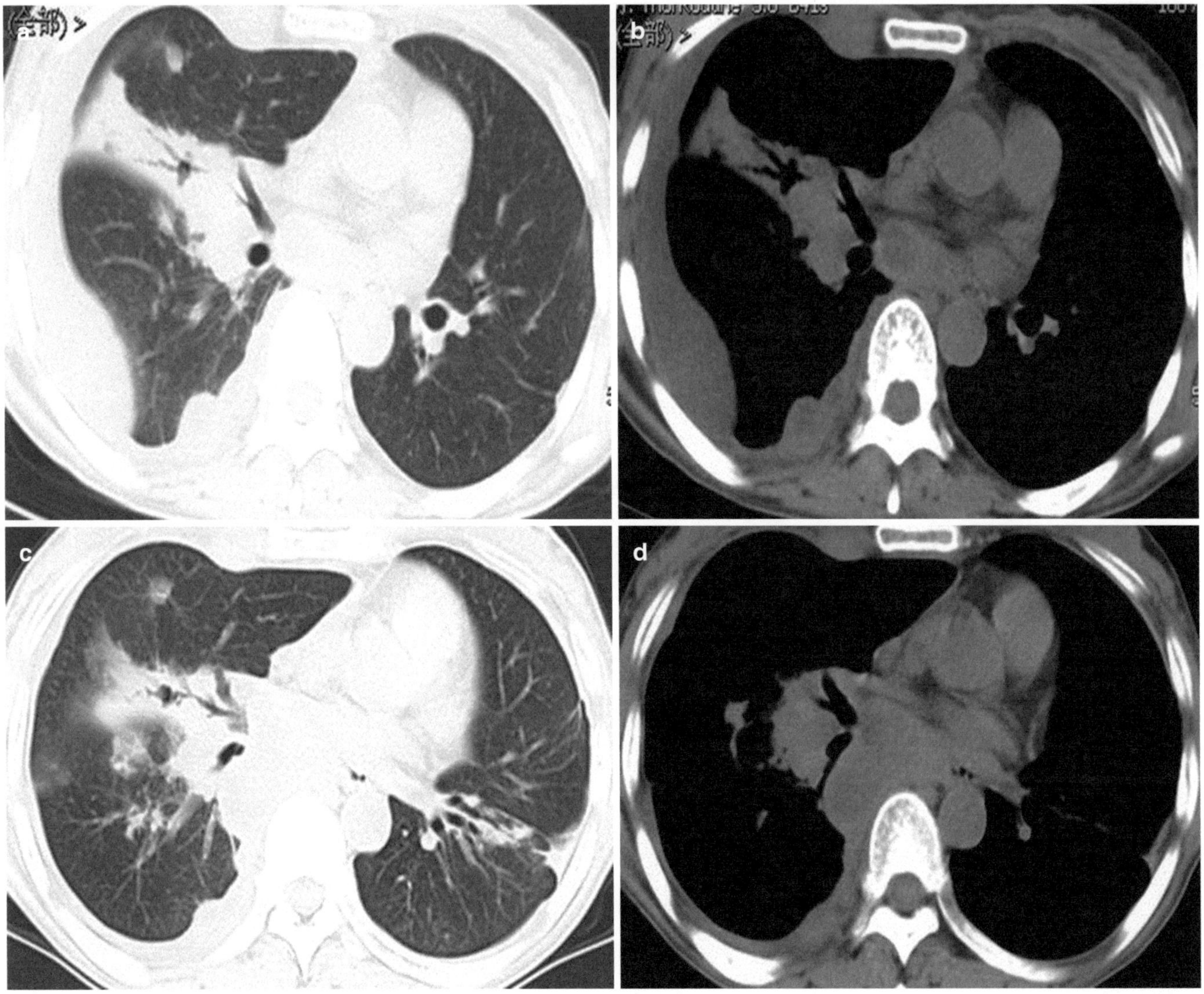

Fig. 8.20 AIDS complicated with IRIS response during tuberculosis. Female, 46 years old. (**a**, **b**) CT (2014-01-06) showed secondary pulmonary tuberculosis in right lung, mediastinal and hilar lymphatic tuberculosis, tuberculous pleuritis, and pleural effusion. CD4+ T cells: 43 cells/μL. (**c**, **d**) CT (2014-03-19, 2 months after HAART therapy) showed aggravation and progression of pulmonary tuberculosis and mediastinal and hilar lymphatic tuberculosis. It is immune restoration inflammatory syndromes

nodes, new pulmonary infiltration lesions or enlarged original pulmonary lesions. In addition, hepatic TB-IRIS is also common in patients with disseminated TB. Patients with hepatic TB-IRIS present nausea, vomiting, abnormal aminotransferase, jaundice, and hepatomegaly. Puncture for pathological biopsy demonstrates granulomatous inflammatory change. Clinically, hepatic TB-IRIS can hardly be distinguished from drug-induced hepatitis induced by anti-tuberculosis drugs.

High-Risk Factors of Self-Contradictory TB-IRIS

The high-risk factors of self-contradictory TB-IRIS include low CD4 T cell count, especially when CD4 T cell count is lower than $100/mm^3$, high HIV RNA quantification, disseminated TB or extrapulmonary TB, and short interval between anti-tuberculosis treatment and ART (being less than 1–2 months).

Diagnosis of Self-Contradictory TB-IRIS

Patients with TB/HIV coinfection show improved condition after initiation of anti-tuberculosis treatment before ART. After initiation of ART, the condition deteriorates with obvious inflammatory response. Along with the increase of CD4 T cell count, HIV RNA copies decrease. And the diagnosis can be made after other possible causes for deterioration of condition are excluded.

Treatment of Self-Contradictory TB-IRIS

For mild TB-IRIS, antipyretic and analgesic drugs can be administered to alleviate clinical symptoms. Hormones (dexamethasone or prednisone) are recommended for severe TB-IRIS, especially those with the central nervous system involved. The course of hormone therapy commonly lasts for about 4 weeks. Prednisone is started at a dose of 1.5 mg/kg body weight per day, which is then changed to 0.75 mg/kg body weight per day after 2 weeks. For some patients, administration of hormones needs to be maintained in gradually reducing dose, and the administration may be prolonged to more than 1 month. Exclusion of Kaposi's sarcoma or other serious infections is necessary before hormone therapy.

Prognosis

Self-contradictory TB-IRIS is commonly non-fatal. However, if brain TB or meningeal TB, pericardial tamponade induced by tuberculous pericarditis, respiratory failure induced by increased TB lesions, and other serious clinical symptoms occur, the life of patient is threatened.

Exposed TB-IRIS

If patient fails to be detected with TB due to mild symptoms of TB and ART is initiated, inflammatory responses appear in the earliest weeks of ART, which resemble to bacterial pneumonia. The inflammatory responses include high fever, respiratory distress, sepsis, and consolidation opacity in lungs. Exposed TB-IRIS may also present as progressive focal inflammatory responses, such as abscesses or lymphadenitis. The standard anti-tuberculosis regimen and hormones are recommended for the treatment of exposed TB-IRIS on the basis of ART.

6.5 Interaction and Adjustment of Anti-HIV Drugs and Anti-Tuberculosis Drugs

Rifampicin is a potentially potent inducer of cytochrome enzyme CYP450, especially CYP450 isoenzyme CYP3A4 [28]. Rifampicin can induce the activity of CYP3A4. When combined with other anti-HIV drugs, it can accelerate the metabolism of these anti-HIV drugs (NNRTIs and protease inhibitors, PIs), and reduce the blood concentrations of NNRTIs and PIs. Therefore, combination of rifampicin with PIs is forbidden in anti-tuberculosis and anti-HIV treatment. When combined with EFV, the dosage of rifampicin remains the same, but the intake of both drugs should be at an interval of 8–12 h. It has also been reported that when rifabutin (RFB) is combined with PIs [31], the drug concentration of RFB increases by 45%. Therefore, the dosage of RFB should be reduced by half for oral intake of 0.15 g/day when combined with PIs. When combined with EFV, the concentration of RFB decreases by about 38%, so the dosage of RFB should be increased to 0.45 g/day for oral intake. The combination of nevirapine tablets (NVP) and RFB may cause serious or even fatal liver necrosis. The blood concentration of NVP decreases significantly when combined with RFP, which also increased the chance of failed ART. Therefore, when anti-tuberculosis treatment is combined with NVP-based anti-HIV treatment, the regimen should be changed. In addition, due to the imbalanced immunity induced by anti-HIV and anti-tuberculosis treatment, the risk of hepatic immune impairment during the treatment is higher than in patients with TB alone. Especially in the treatment of patients with chronic hepatitis B or hepatitis C, active HCV or HBV aggravates liver damage. Therefore, the liver function should be more closely monitored to avoid the occurrence of liver dysfunction and even liver failure.

6.6 Side Effects of Anti-HIV Drugs and Anti-Tuberculosis Drugs and Their Management

General Principles

Side effects of anti-tuberculosis drugs in patients with HIV positive are almost the same as those in non-HIV-infected individuals, which are mainly drug-induced hepatitis and drug-induced dermatitis. Drug toxic and side effects of anti-tuberculosis drugs in patients with HIV positive are related to its combination with ART. Since the change of first-line anti-tuberculosis drugs may lead to reduced efficacy of anti-tuberculosis treatment, the retrieval of any anti-tuberculosis drug should be tried to avoid without definitive evidence supporting the correlationship between the toxic and side effects with the anti-tuberculosis drugs (isoniazid, rifampicin, and rifabutin).

Definition of Drug-Induced Hepatitis

Drug-induced hepatitis is a condition which the level of aminotransferase is 3 times as high as its normal level with accompanying fever, skin rash, fatigue, anorexia, jaundice, and other symptoms, or the level of aminotransferase is 5 times as high as its normal level with no clinical symptoms. Isoniazid, rifampicin, pyrazinamide, sulfamethoxazole, and many anti-HIV drugs may induce hepatitis. In general, the aminotransferase in patients with HIV positive during anti-tuberculosis treatment and ART is transiently and mildly increases. In such cases, treatment to reduce the level of aminotransferase and protect the liver is administered. Once drug-induced hepatitis occurs, all drugs that may impair liver function should be discontinued. At the same time, the liver function should be assessed, laboratory tests for various hepatophilic viruses (hepatitis A, B, and C viruses) should be performed, and histories of biliary diseases and alcoholism should be assessed. After retrieval of drugs that may affect liver function, the anti-tuberculosis regimen with ethambutol, aminoglycosides, moxifloxacin, or levofloxacin should be temporarily applied. Meanwhile, the causes of liver dysfunction should be explored. Once the cause of liver dysfunction is detected, the first-line anti-tuberculosis drugs are gradually applied, followed by reuse of anti-HIV drugs and sulfamethoxazole. The liver function should be closely monitored, once a week as recommended, during the course of re-administration.

Drug-Induced Dermatitis

All first-line anti-tuberculosis drugs (especially isoniazid and rifampicin), all anti-HIV drugs (especially non-nucleoside antiretroviral drugs), and sulfamethoxazole may cause drug-induced dermatitis. If skin rash is scattered and itchy, antihistamines, such as loratadine or desloratadine, can be administered. Meanwhile, antiallergic treatment can applied to alleviate symptoms, with continuation of all anti-tuberculosis drugs. If skin rash is severe, with accompanying fever, drug-induced hepatitis, or mucosal involvement, all anti-tuberculosis drugs, related anti-HIV drugs and sulfamethoxazole should be immediately discontinued. After the skin rash subsides, the anti-tuberculosis drugs, anti-HIV drugs, and sulfamethoxazole are gradually re-used.

6.7 Prophylactic Treatment of TB in Patients with HIV/AIDS

For HIV-infected patients, routine surveillance of latent TB infection is conducted, including tuberculin skin test and/or interferon γ release assay (IGRA) (IGRA is recommended) [35].

Prophylactic Treatment of Latent TB Infection

Patients with tuberculin skin test and/or IGRA positive and HIV infection without evidence of active TB should receive prophylactic treatment for latent TB infection. And patients with HIV infection and close contact to patients with active TB should also receive prophylactic treatment for latent TB infection.

Prophylactic Treatment Regimen for Latent TB Infection [36]

Regimen of First Choice

Isoniazid tablets 300 mg orally once a day for 9 months (AII) or isoniazid tablets 900 mg orally twice a week for 9 months (BII); its combination with vitamin B6 to prevent peripheral neuritis (oral intake of 25–30 mg daily till the end of prophylactic treatment).

Alternative Regimen

Rifampicin 600 mg orally once a day for 4 months (BIII); rifabutin 300 mg orally once a day (BIII) (with corresponding adjustment of rifabutin dosage according to different ART regimens, see the chapter of interaction between anti-tuberculosis drugs and ART for reference). Isoniazid 300 mg orally, once a day + Rifampicin 600 mg orally, once a day, combination of isoniazid and rifampicin for 3 months.

Precautions and Notes

Before administration of prophylactic treatment, it is necessary to exclude active TB.

Notes: The recommendation level and evidence level (A: strongly recommended; B: moderately recommended; C: recommended as an option. I: with evidence from one or more randomized clinical trials; II: with evidence from one or more well-designed non-randomized cohort clinical trials; III: expert opinion.)

There are many interventions to reduce the relapse of TB in patients with HIV/AIDS, such as prolonged treatment for TB, increased frequency of medication, prolonged administration of isoniazid, and prolonged administration of ART. However, no randomized clinical trial has been conducted to demonstrate the effectiveness of these interventions in reducing incidence of TB. In areas with high incidence of TB, such as Africa, it is possible to reduce the relapse of TB in patients with TB/HIV coinfection by continuing oral intake of isoniazid for 6–9 months for prophylactic treatment of TB after the completion of standard combined anti-tuberculosis treatment. But in areas with low incidence of TB, such as the USA, isoniazid for prophylactic treatment is not recommended.

6.8 Recent Progress in Treatment of TB/HIV Coinfection

At present, there are many advances in treatment of TB/HIV coinfection, which mainly focus on shorter and more effective anti-tuberculosis regimens, and new ART drugs and regimens with less impact on anti-tuberculosis drugs.

Studies on Interaction Between Anti-Tuberculosis Drugs and the Latest ART Drugs

In a 24-week study applying rifampicin and dotiravir for TB/HIV coinfection, the safety and efficacy of dotiravir were observed during the treatment. It has been demonstrated that the safety and efficacy of dotiravir-based ART are close to those of EFV-based ART. But the group receiving dotiravir-based ART showed lower incidence of TB-IRIS [37].

Studies on Shorter Course of Anti-Tuberculosis Treatment

In the intensive phase of anti-tuberculosis treatment, three groups receiving rifampicin at different doses, 10, 15, or 20 mg/kg body weight per day, were observed for the efficacy and side effects of rifampicin. It was demonstrated that the safety of rifampicin at different doses is similar in the three groups, but high dose of rifampicin at 20 mg/kg body weight per day helps to shorten the course of anti-tuberculosis treatment [38].

In a study on prophylactic treatment for latent TB infection in patients with HIV infection, one-month administration of isoniazid at 300 mg/day plus rifampicin 450–600 mg/day was compared to nine-month administration of isoniazid alone. It was found that the efficacy is similar in the two groups, but the combination of isoniazid with rifampicin has less toxic and side effects [39].

7 Management of Patients with TB/HIV Coinfection

7.1 Registry and Reporting of Patients with TB/HIV Coinfection

TB control agencies and HIV/AIDS control agencies are responsible for information registration and inter-agency exchanges about TB/HIV coinfection. The collected data should be input into the TB management information system and the HIV/AIDS control information system. And a mechanism for registry, reporting, statistics of patients with TB/HIV coinfection should be established and gradually improved [40].

Agency Responsible for Registry

Local TB control agency and HIV/AIDS control agency are responsible for registry and management of patients with TB/HIV coinfection whose residence is within the localized management.

Subjects of Registry

Patients with TB/HIV coinfection.

Agency and Staff Responsible for Reporting

All health-care institutions, TB control agencies, and HIV/AIDS control agencies are responsible for reporting the patients with TB/HIV coinfection. The executive staff and physicians are responsible for reporting patients with TB/HIV coinfection.

Procedures of Reporting

Before confirmation by TB control agency, the patients with HIV/AIDS who are suspected with TB referred from HIV/AIDS control agency should be reported as suspected cases of TB/HIV coinfection. Before confirmation by HIV/AIDS control agency, the patients with TB who show HIV antibody positive should be reported as suspected cases of TB/HIV coinfection.

The first consulted physician or other consecutive staff is responsible for filling in the reporting card of TB/HIV coinfection. Within the time limit, the suspected cases of TB/HIV coinfection should be reported on-line, and the relevant information should be feedback to the local TB control agency or HIV/AIDS control agency. After receiving the information feedback, the TB control agency or HIV/AIDS control agency should register the information timely [41].

Preservation of Registry Data

A specific staff should be responsible for preserving the registry and reporting data and keeping the data about patients with TB/HIV coinfection confidential.

7.2 Management of Patients with TB/HIV Coinfection

According to the requirements in the Technical Guideline for Implementation of Tuberculosis Control Planning in China and the Handbook for Free-in-charge Anti-HIV Treatment in China, anti-tuberculosis and anti-HIV treatment, management, and follow-ups are performed for patients with TB/HIV coinfection. The relevant information registry and reporting on the treatment, management, and outcome of patients are also conducted. For patients with TB/HIV coinfection, the relevant hospitals are responsible for anti-HIV and anti-tuberculosis treatment, management, and information feedback to TB and HIV/AIDS control agencies for registry and reporting [42].

References

1. World Health Organization. 2016 TB-HIV fact. http://who.int/tb/areas-of-work/tb-hiv/tbhiv_factsheet_2016_web.pdf?ua=1.
2. World Health Organization. Global tuberculosis report 2016. Geneva: World Health Organization; 2016.
3. WHO policy on collaborative TB/HIV activities guidelines for national programmes and other stakeholders; 2012.
4. Wang XW, Dong BQ. Research developments on TB/HIV coinfection. China Trop Med. 2005;2005(06):1331–2, 1324.
5. Peng H, Xu WG, Wang F, et al. Prevalence of TB/HIV coinfection and measures for its management. Chin J Antituberculosis. 2011;33(11):769–72.
6. Han GL, Zhang FJ. Prevalence of TB/HIV coinfection and its diagnosis and treatment. Chin J AIDS STD. 2008;2008(01):87–9, 92.
7. Shen JY, Lu HZ. Research developments on prevention and treatment of TB/HIV coinfection. Chin J AIDS STD. 2015;21(06):543–6.

8. Lin DW, Cui ZZ, Liu FY, et al. Screening and management of TB/HIV coinfection in Guangxi Zhuang autonomous region of China. Chongqing Med. 2017;46(35):4987–90.
9. Yang R, Qiu YB, Su WW, et al. Survival analysis in patients with TB/HIV coinfection receiving anti-tuberculosis treatment in Yunnan province of China. Chin J Dis Control. 2016;20(12):1212–5, 1226.
10. Fang XH, Ma DC, Zou Z, et al. Correlation between social support and psychological health in patients with TB/HIV coinfection in Anhui province of China. Chin Rural Health Serv Adm. 2016;36(2):228–31.
11. Moore D, Liechty C, Ekwaru P, et al. Prevalence, incidence and mortality associated with tuberculosis in HIV-infected patients initiating antiretroviral therapy in rural Uganda. AIDS. 2007;21(6): 713–9.
12. Prakash S, Katiyar SK, Purwar S, et al. Clinical evaluation of the mycobacteriophage-based assay in rapid detection of Mycobacterium tuberculosis in respiratory specimens. Indian J Med Microbiol. 2009;27(2):134–8.
13. Shinu P, Nair A, Singh V, et al. Evaluation of rapid techniques for the detection of mycobacteria in sputum with scanty bacilli or clinically evident, smear negative cases of pulmonary and extra-pulmonary tuberculosis. Mem Inst Oswaldo Cruz. 2011;106(5):620–4.
14. Gul Yurtsever S, Bicmen C, Gunduz AT, et al. Comparison of proportion method in Lowenstein-Jensen medium with the BACTEC 460 TB system for antimycobacterial susceptibility testing of Mycobacterium tuberculosis isolates. Mikrobiyol Bul. 2011;45(4):623–31.
15. Dave P, Patel P, Modi B, et al. Evaluation of use of line probe assay on smear-positive direct specimen from extra-pulmonary tuberculosis site. Indian J Tuberc. 2015;62(4):218–21.
16. Matabane MM, Ismail F, Strydom KA, et al. Performance evaluation of three commercial molecular assays for the detection of Mycobacterium tuberculosis from clinical specimens in a high TB-HIV-burden setting. BMC Infect Dis. 2015;15:508.
17. Shah M, Hanrahan C, Wang ZY, et al. Lateral flow urine lipoarabinomannan assay for detecting active tuberculosis in HIV-positive adults. Cochrane Database Syst Rev. 2016;(5):CD011420.
18. Kerkhoff AD, Kranzer K, Samandari T, et al. Systematic review of TST responses in people living with HIV in under-resourced settings: implications for isoniazid preventive therapy. PLoS One. 2012;7(11):e49928.
19. Yamamoto M, Ushio R, Watanabe H, et al. Detection of Mycobacterium tuberculosis-derived DNA in circulating cell-free DNA from a patient with disseminated infection using digital PCR. Int J Infect Dis. 2018;66:80–2.
20. Yang J, Han X, Liu A, et al. Use of digital droplet PCR to detect Mycobacterium tuberculosis DNA in whole blood-derived DNA samples from patients with pulmonary and extrapulmonary tuberculosis. Front Cell Infect Microbiol. 2017;7:369.
21. Lu P, Yu W, Zhu W, et al. Imaging characteristics of AIDS complicated with tuberculosis and its correlation with CD4+ T lymphocytes. Chin J Tuberc Respir Dis. 2005;28(01):16–9.
22. Liu J, Wang M, Pang H. Clinical comparison analysis of 66 cases of AIDS complicated with pulmonary tuberculosis and simple pulmonary tuberculosis. Jilin Med J. 2012;33(31):6745–7.
23. Li C, Lv S, Shu W, et al. CT findings of acquired immunodeficiency syndrome complicated with pulmonary tuberculosis and normal immune tuberculosis. Chin J Med Imaging. 2015;2015(12):924–8.
24. Xue M, Li J, Xie Y, et al. HRCT imaging signs of AIDS complicated with chest tuberculosis and analysis of its correlation with CD4+ T lymphocyte count. Chin J Antitubercul. 2018;40(7): 682–8.
25. Li J, Xue M, Xie Y, et al. Correlation of MR imaging features with CD4 technology for acquired immunodeficiency syndrome complicated with brain tuberculosis. Chin J Antituberculosis. 2018;40(7):689–95.
26. Global tuberculosis report 2018 [DB/OL]. World Health Organization; 2018. http://www.who.int/tb/publications/global_report/en/. 18 Sep 2018.
27. Van der Werf MJ, Ködmön C, Zucs P, et al. Tuberculosis and HIV coinfection in Europe: looking at one reality from two angles. AIDS. 2016;30(18):2845–53.
28. National Institutes of Health, Centers for Disease Control and Prevention, HIV Medicine Association of the Infectious Diseases Society of America. Guidelines for prevention and treatment of opportunistic infections in HIV-infected adults and adolescents. AIDS info [DB/OL]; 2017, pp. 1–17. https://aidsinfo.nih.gov/contentfiles/lvguidelines/adult_oi.pdf. 23 Feb 2017.
29. Manosuthi W, Wiboonchutikul S, Sungkanuparph S. Integrated therapy for HIV and tuberculosis. AIDS Res Ther. 2016;13:22.
30. Katz IT, Essien T, Marinda ET, et al. Antiretroviral therapy refusal among newly diagnosed HIV-infected adults. AIDS. 2011;25(17):2177–81.
31. European AIDS Clinical Society. EACS treatment guidelines 9.0. Belgium: European AIDS Clinical Society [DB/OL]; 2017, p. 16. http://www.eacsociety.org/files/guidelines_9.0-english.pdf. 1 Oct 2017.
32. Nino L, Lali K, Archil S, et al. Hepatitis C virus co-infection increases the risk of anti-tuberculosis drug-induced hepatotoxicity among patients with pulmonary tuberculosis [DB/OL]. PLoS One. 2013;8(12):e83892.
33. Mo P, Zhu Q, Teter C, et al. Prevalence, drug-induced hepatotoxicity, and mortality among patients multi-infected with HIV, tuberculosis, and hepatitis virus. Int J Infect Dis. 2014;28:95–100.
34. Zhou Y, Wang H, Li SX, et al. Analysis of tuberculosis-associated immune reconstitution inflammatory syndrome in HIV/TB co-infected patients during HAART. Inf Int. 2014;3(3):122–8.
35. National Institute for Health and Care Excellence. NICE guideline [NG33] tuberculosis [DB/OL]; [2016-113]. https://www.nice.org.uk/guidance/ng33.
36. Group of AIDS, Branch of Infectious Diseases, Chinese Medical Society and Center for Disease Control and Prevention of China. Guideline for diagnosis and treatment of HIV/AIDS in China (edition 2018). Chin J Intern Med. 2018;57(12):1–18.
37. Kelly D, Richard K, Noluthando M, et al. Safety and efficacy of dolutegravir-based art in TB/HIV coinfected adults at week 24. 25th conference on retroviruses and opportunistic infections; 2018, p. 14 [201834]. http://www.croiconference.org/sites/default/files/uploads/croi2018-abstract-ebook.pdf.
38. Gustavo EV, Meredith BB, Julia MC, et al. Randomized controlled trial of high-dose rifampin for pulmonary tuberculosis. 25th conference on retroviruses and opportunistic infections; 2018, p. 17 [2018-34]. http://www.croiconference.org/sites/default/files/uploads/croi2018-abstract-ebook.pdf.
39. Susan S, Ritesh R, Amita G, et al. One month of rifapentine/isoniazid to prevent TB in People with HIV: brief-TB/A5279. 25th conference on retroviruses and opportunistic infections; 2018, p. 16 [2018-34]. http://www.croiconference.org/sites/default/files/uploads/croi2018-abstract-ebook.pdf.
40. Xiao WL, Hu TQ, Hu Y. Employment of supervisors for management of patients with TB/HIV coinfection. Mod Prev Med. 2013;40(12):2262–4.
41. Xu J, Zheng QQ, Zhang TH, et al. Bidirectional screening of TB and HIV/AIDS and prognosis of patients with TB/HIV coinfection after anti-tuberculosis treatment. China Trop Med. 2018;18(6): 619–23.
42. Technical guideline for implementation of tuberculosis control planning in China. Peking Union Medical College Press; 2009.

New Technologies for TB Control in Migrating Population

9

Pu-Xuan Lu, Ya-rui Yang, Sheng-yuan Liu, Li Xie, Fleming Lure, and Mu-Lan Li

1 Overview

1.1 Background and Challenges of TB Control in Migrating Population

According to the 2017 Development Report of migrating Population in China, the migrating population in China reached 245 million in 2016, accounting for 18% of the total population. In the next decade or two, China is still in the rapid development stage of urbanization. According to the implementation of the National New Urbanization Planning, there are still more than 200 million migrating population in China by 2020. During the 13th Five-Year Plan period, the population continues to aggregate in the large delta areas, coastal areas, and major transportation areas, and the population of mega-cities and metropolis continues to grow. The migrating population is characterized by high mobility, poor awareness about health, high incidence of TB, and difficult treatment and management after the occurrence of TB. Therefore, the migrating population is vulnerable to TB epidemic. Since 2006, TB epidemic in migrating population has gained focused attention from Chinese government. Previous surveys have found that the new registry rates of TB and smear-positive TB in the migrating population in large cities of China are higher than those in the local population [1]. In Shenzhen, Guangzhou, Zhuhai, Shanghai, Suzhou, Wuxi, Nanjing, and other large cities, surveys found that the increase of patients with TB in the migrating population is the main reason for the high number of TB in these large cities [2]. There are also studies showing that the estimated incidence of active TB in China in 2014 is 64 per 0.1 million, while the estimated incidence of TB in the migrating population is 85 per 0.1 million. The proportion of trans-regionally managed patients with TB in the migrating population is much higher than that in the non-migrating population. Meanwhile, the percentage of unknown prognosis in patients with TB is 8–9% nationwide, and most of these patients are trans-regionally managed patients [3]. Migrating patients with TB have been a bridge for the spread of TB from high-prevalence areas to low-prevalence areas. The TB control in migrating population is one of the three challenges in TB control in China.

In 2002, in the Technical Guidelines for Implementation of Tuberculosis Control Plan in China and the Implementation Plan of the National Tuberculosis Control Plan (2006–2010) issued by the Disease Prevention and Control Bureau of the Ministry of Health, the tasks of TB control in the migrating population have been clearly defined. In addition, it has been required that the same policies be implemented for the migrating population and the local residents [4]. To solve difficulties of TB control in the migrating population in China, the Global Funding Program for Tuberculosis Control in migrating Population of China has been initiated in some provinces (municipalities) since 2006. In the Notice on the 13th Five-Year Plan for Tuberculosis Control issued by the General Office of the State Council, it has been clearly pointed out that TB control in the migrating population should be strengthened. According to the principle of territorial management, the diagnosis, reporting, referral and trace, information registry, treatment, and follow-ups of migrating patients with TB should be well performed. For trans-regional patients with TB, information of the patients

P.-X. Lu (✉)
Department of Radiology, The Shenzhen Center for Chronic Disease Control, Shenzhen, Guangdong, China

Y.-r. Yang · S.-y. Liu
Shenzhen Nanshan Center for Chronic Disease Control, Shenzhen, Guangdong, China

L. Xie
Shenzhen Center for Chronic Disease Control, Shenzhen, Guangdong, China

F. Lure
College of Engineering, University of Texas, El Paso, TX, USA

M.-L. Li
Shenzhen Smart Imaging Healthcare Co. Ltd., Shenzhen, Guangdong, China

W.-y. Yu et al. (eds.), *Tuberculosis Control in Migrating Population*, https://doi.org/10.1007/978-981-32-9763-0_9

should be well exchanged. Direct settlement of basic medical insurance in different places should be well performed. And health education at aggregating places of migrating population should be strengthened to improve their awareness and capability about TB control.

Significant progress has been made in TB control in the migrating population nationwide. In Guangzhou, Shanghai, Shenzhen, Dongguan, and Wenzhou, the migrating patients with TB have successively incorporated into the TB control plan, and the cure rate of the initially treated patients with smear-positive TB has increased to between 86% and 98%. However, most areas of China are still facing challenges in TB control in the migrating population.

1.2 Difficulty in Detecting Patients with TB in the Migrating Population

The low detection rate of patients with TB is an important reason restricting the effective implementation of TB control plan in China. In the migrating population, the difficulty is particularly prominent.

High Diagnostic Delay Rate

Due to the high mobility of the migrating population, their poor accessibility to health-care service, and low awareness rate about core knowledge of TB, they commonly do not know about the symptoms of TB and the places providing relevant health-care service.

Multiple surveys show that a high percentage of migrating population tends to delay their presentation to health-care institutions for diagnosis and treatment. In an analysis on the intension of the migrating population to present to health-care institutions for diagnosis and treatment of TB in six provinces and municipalities in China, the analysis indicated that the rate of delayed presentation to health-care institutions for suspected mild and moderate symptoms of TB in the migrating population is 22.8% and 14.9%, respectively. The rates of delayed presentation to health-care institutions for suspected symptoms of TB in the migrating population of Shandong province and Xiamen city are 56.2% and 37.1%, respectively. The obstacles perceived by the migrating population with the intention of delaying presentation to health-care institutions include “need to ask for leave,” “too much time is needed for presentation to health-care institutions,” and “an economic burden.” The time cost and the economic cost are the important reasons for their delayed presentation. Li et al. have found that the total delay in migrating patients with TB in China is mainly attributed to the delayed presentation to health-care institutions [5].

Meanwhile, most migrating patients with suspected symptoms of TB choose private clinics, district/county-level small general hospitals, or drug store for diagnosis and treatment, and the proportion of presentation to designated health-care institutions for TB is relatively low.

In addition, less than 50% of patients with suspected symptoms of TB detected in general health-care institutions voluntarily present to designated health-care institutions for TB. Most of the suspected TB patients are traced by TB control agency. However, some patients with TB detected by employment health examination are more difficult to be traced, treated, and managed due to its negative impact on their employment. Some patients migrate to other places, which makes it more difficult for TB control agency to trace. Otherwise, some stay at the original place and conceal their illness during the other employment health examination as hidden patients. And the others are afraid of discrimination by colleagues and the surrounding population, and refuse to be followed up, treated, and managed. These factors lead to delayed detection, diagnosis, and treatment of TB in the migrating population [6], and even constitute the reason for the occurrence of DR-TB and its epidemic.

Different Level of Imaging Diagnosis

Patients with TB in the migrating population are mainly detected in health examination. Direct digital radiography (DR) is the first choice for detection, diagnosis, treatment, and reexamination of TB. CT scan is ordered for suspected cases of TB. The two radiological examinations are important diagnostic measures for TB [7]. However, due to imbalanced medical resources, chest X-ray fails to be effectively and rapidly provided for high-risk populations of TB.

No Rapid and Effective Etiological Diagnostic Technique for TB

Due to high mobility of the migrating population, rapid diagnosis of TB plays an important role in appropriate treatment and management of detected patients with TB, and reducing the spread of Mtb.

In 2010, the national epidemiological sampling survey on TB found that the morbidity of active pulmonary TB is 459 per 0.1 million in population aged 15 years and above, that of smear-positive pulmonary TB is 66 per 0.1 million, and that of bacteriologically positive pulmonary TB is 119 per 0.1 million. It has been estimated that about 70% of all patients with TB are bacteriologically negative in China. Due to no specific clinical manifestations in patients with bacteriologically negative pulmonary TB, its misdiagnosis, overdiagnosis, and miss diagnosis based on clinical experience are common.

1.3 Difficult Treatment and Management of Patients with TB in Migrating Population

After patients with TB in migrating population are detected, it is very important to implement treatment and management. Most of the patients with TB in the migrating population have low family economic status and high mobility, which causes difficulty for observed treatment and management.

Unfavorable Compliance of Patient

Nowadays, management of TB in the migrating population has been incorporated into the regional TB control plan. The same TB control policies are implemented in the migrating population and local residents, with free-in-charge diagnostic examination, treatment, and management. However, due to many factors such as low income, no medical insurance, and unstable residence, the patients with TB in the migrating population show unfavorable compliance to treatment and high missing rate. Many patients in the migrating population return to their permanent registered residence and are missed [8] due to their insufficient confidence in future expense on health-care service, fear of discrimination by the surrounding population, and unemployment. They fail to receive standardized management. Meanwhile, the symptoms and psychological anxiety of initially treated patients with smear-positive TB in the migrating population are more serious than those in the local residents, while their knowledge about diagnosis and treatment of TB and social support are relatively insufficient [9]. A survey conducted in Shenzhen found that the overall drug resistance rate and multi-drug resistance rate of TB in the migrating population in Shenzhen are relatively high. And the main factors influencing occurrence of DR-TB in the migrating population include females, interruption of initial treatment, and history of chemical retreatment [10].

Currently, DOTs strategy is adopted in China for management of patients with TB. It is necessary for patients with TB to present to a basic health-care institution every day for directly observed medication. In such a way, the patients are under the psychological and transportation pressure for medication. For instance, the average transportation time of a patient with TB to local TB control agency in Donglan County of Guangxi is 4.4 h, and the average travelling time to the village clinic is 1.4 h [11]. Due to the increasing awareness of privacy protection, patients are strongly resistant to taking medicine under the direct observation. A survey conducted in Shenzhen showed that 85.9% of the patients with TB are unwilling to inform their workplace about their illness, and 9.9% of the patients with TB are unwilling to inform their family member about their illness. Only 28.8% of the patients with TB are willing to take medicine under direct observation of the physician, 7.3% are willing to take medicine under direct observation of their family member, and 20.0% are willing to take medicine under supervision by telephone. In addition, 43.9% of the patients are willing to take medicine by themselves without any observation and supervision, and 88.4% of the patients believe direct observation by a physician for medication is unnecessary [12]. In basic health-care institutions, irregular medication is common, and irregular medication is more serious in patients who take medicine by themselves. Frequent missed medication and inappropriately managed adverse reactions commonly cause low cure rate, relapse, and even drug resistance [13].

At present, the policy of free-in-charge diagnosis and treatment for TB implemented in China is limited to some essential drugs, while some necessary auxiliary drugs (such as drugs for hepatotoxicity and adverse reactions) and auxiliary examinations are expensive and at their own expense. It negatively affects the compliance of patients to treatment in the migrating population with relatively low socioeconomic status.

Inefficient System and Performance for TB Control

The national basic public health service is an important part of the public health system in China, in which the health management of patients with TB is one of the 12 basic public health services. The public health service for TB control mainly includes screening and referral, housing condition assessment, health education, directly observed treatment, surveillance for adverse reactions and complications, follow-up assessment, and case closure assessment, which are implemented in community-based health-care institutions. Professional institutions for TB control are mainly responsible for the follow-ups, diagnosis, treatment, reexamination, and management of patients with TB. In addition, prevention, surveillance, screening, and control of TB in common populations and special groups, such as personnel in schools and places of detention, the elderly, patients with diabetes, populations at workplaces, and individuals of close contacts, are also implemented in professional institutions for TB control.

In addition, nationwide study conducted by CDC of China showed that the human resources in some county/district-level TB control agencies are not sufficient as required [18]. At present, the local TB control system and its performance for population with present residence can hardly meet the demands of the patients with TB in the migrating population. The coverage of DOTs is not wide enough, and the effect of TB control in migrating population is not satisfying [6].

Concerning the trans-regional referral management of migrating patients with TB, many cases are re-registered to increase the number of managed patients, and the procedures of standardized management are complex. Meanwhile, the entrusted treatment and management of referrals are insufficiently assessed. Trans-regional referral management of patients with TB in migrating population may fail due to any break of the chain procedures.

1.4 Prospects of TB Control in Migrating Population

"Early detection, early quarantine and early treatment" is a basic consensus on the measures for optimal TB control. The measures to reduce the delayed diagnosis and interrupted treatment are keys for TB control and patient management in migrating population in China.

To Improve the Diagnostic Technology for TB

First of all, the etiological diagnosis of TB should be paid focused attention, and detection of patients with TB should be strengthened to control the spread of TB in communities. Therefore, it is urgent to develop rapid, accurate, and inexpensive diagnostic techniques for laboratory evidence of TB. In recent years, with the rapid development of molecular biology, a number of rapid diagnostic techniques for early diagnosis of TB have been developed [14]. The results of multi-center and large-scale clinical trial showed that many molecular biological techniques have a high detection rate for bacteriologically positive TB, and a certain detection rate for bacteriologically negative TB. The trial expands the application prospects of molecular biological technology in the diagnosis of bacteriologically negative TB. Especially in 2013, the diagnostic criteria for TB was revisited by WHO, and WHO recommended molecular biology positive is equivalent to bacteriologically positive as the diagnostic basis for etiologically positive TB [15]. In China, the diagnostic criteria for TB was also revisited in 2017, the positive finding by molecular biological technology is the diagnostic basis for etiologically positive TB. Therefore, traditional bacteriological detection of TB is greatly complemented, and the advantages of molecular biological technology for the diagnosis of bacteriologically negative TB are fully exerted to serve clinical practice. The new diagnostic technologies, such as Hain and GeneXpert, shorten the time for diagnosis and improve the diagnostic accuracy, which are helpful for timely treatment of TB and control of its spread.

In order to solve the problem of large demand for imaging diagnosis, artificial intelligence-based CAD automation system applies advanced artificial intelligence algorithm in digital diagnostic imaging for accurate diagnosis of TB. The technology is applied for efficient and accurate imaging diagnosis of TB, which opens up a new way for accurate imaging diagnosis of TB.

To Explore Innovative Observed Treatment

It is necessary to strengthen the management of migrating patients with TB and improve the effectiveness of DOTs strategy. With the continuous innovation and widespread application of Internet technology, information technology-based eDOT and vDOT should be developed to save human resources and to assist the implementation of DOTs strategy, which is also actively advocated by WHO.

2 Innovations of Traditional Technologies

2.1 Directly Observed Treatment for TB

Since the advent of effective anti-tuberculosis drugs, the treatment of TB steps into the era of chemotherapy, and effective treatment and management are the key for successful treatment. Treatment and management of patients with TB is a very important part in the end TB strategy. However, due to difficulty in implementing treatment and management after diagnosis, poor compliance to treatment, occurrence of drug resistance, and difficult implementation of trans-regional collaborative management policies, TB control in migrating population has been the difficulty and emphasis worldwide for many years. In the Tuberculosis Control Plan in China (2011–2015), TB control in migrating population is one of the important works. And the target rates of successful treatment and trans-regional patient information feedback are defined. Due to different levels of technology development in different periods, the TB control strategies and measures are also different, so are the ways of patient management.

Early Direct Observation of Medication

Before 1940, the treatment of pulmonary TB was mainly rest and nutritional food. Since chemical treatment began to be applied for TB, the course of early chemical treatment lasted mostly for 12–18 months and the patients took medicine at home. The compliance was unfavorable, with low cure rate and unfavorable treatment effect. Since 1979, non-hospitalized chemical treatment under direct observation (also known as direct face-to-face treatment) was implemented in Beijing for patients with TB. By 1992, the coverage rate of directly observed treatment reached 98%. The rate of regular medication in patients with TB increased from 40% to above 95%. Another mode of treatment and management for patients with TB has also been improved in Shanghai, whole-course chemical treatment and management. The implementation procedures included first health education in the clinic before chemical treatment, regular follow-ups in the clinic, and regular family visits by physician in TB control agency to ensure regular medication of patient [16].

DOTs Strategy

In 1992, the Chinese government for the first time initiated the World Bank Funding Program for TB control in China in 13 provinces, municipalities, and autonomous regions. In 1993, the Ministry of Health in China initiated the TB Control Promotion Program in 15 provinces, municipalities, and autonomous regions, with self-pooled funds. DOTs by physician have been fully implemented and applied in these two program covered areas, and remarkable success has been achieved. Since then, DOTs have gradually been incorporated as the main measure for TB control in China. In the Technical Guidelines for Implementation of Tuberculosis Control Planning in China (edition 2002) the Technical Guidelines for Implementation of Tuberculosis Control Planning in China (edition 2008), the management of TB patients, especially implementation of DOTs strategy, was stipulated and required in detail [16]. DOTs are implemented on the premise that the physician, health-care staff, volunteers, or family members are well trained for direct observation of intake of anti-tuberculosis drugs by patient

[17]. DOTs have been, so far, the most effective strategy for management of TB patients in TB control.

DOT Strategy in Basic Health-Care Institution

In daily management, patients need to present in basic health-care institutions every day for regular medication under direct observation by physician. The patients commonly complain of the frequent travelling to and back from the basic health-care institutions. In addition, inquiring, drugs dispensing, information input, and other tedious paperwork have also been a heavy burden for physicians in basic health-care institutions. Due to limited health-care resources and the shortage of professionals working in TB control, the proportion of patients receiving DOT is much lower than the reported data. In most cases, DOT is only implemented formally and favorable effects can be hardly achieved [18]. According to a survey on the demand for treatment and management of TB in the migrating population in Shenzhen, only 28.8% of the patients are willing to take medicine at the basic health-care institution, 7.3% are willing to take medicine at home under direct observation by family member, 20.0% are willing to take medicine at home under urge of physician by telephone, 43.9% of the patients are willing to take medicine by themselves without any observation, and 88.4% believe that direct observation by physician is unnecessary [19]. Hu et al. conducted a study in 401 patients with smear-positive TB in Chongqing and found that only 15.96% of the patients receive DOT management, and the proportion of patients with no observed medication is as high as 72.07% [20]. Irregular medication is common in patients managed by basic health-care institutions, but it is more common in patients who take medicine by themselves. Often, missed medication is frequently, and adverse reactions are inappropriately treated and managed, which result in low cure rate, relapse, and even drug resistance. Even for patients with favorable compliance, DOT strategy can hardly be implemented due to short-term travelling for business, hospital transfer, and change of treatment regimen [21].

In addition, in Yixing city of Jiangsu province, the following measures have been adopted for management of migrating population communities. In the management mode, community-based health-care service center (station) is mainly responsible for management of patients with TB in the migrating population.

(1) Regular follow-ups via telephone and family visits are performed. And health education on TB control is performed about the importance of the "ten-word guidelines" for chemical treatment of TB. The family members of patients are selected and trained for directly observed treatment and reporting of adverse reactions.
(2) Patients with TB are followed up monthly for regular medication and sputum reexaminations. The patients who delay their sputum reexamination for above 3 days are urged to receive sputum reexamination.
(3) Sputum reexamination at designated health-care institutions is ensured after anti-tuberculosis treatment for 2, 5, and 6 months (8 months for re-treated patients).
(4) Regular appointments with patients for follow-up are made to establish a communication mechanism between patients to improve their compliance with treatment, and the patients with unfavorable compliance are emphasized and guided.

DOT Strategy Implemented by Volunteers

As early as 1999, Li et al. selected and trained volunteers to implement DOTs strategy for patients with active TB in the migrating population because the original adaptive anti-tuberculosis system fails to simultaneously manage a large number of patients in the migrating population [22]. It was found that the volunteers implemented DOTs strategy is feasible and can effectively improve the compliance to treatment. Zhao et al. investigated the attitude, demand, and factors influencing the management of patients with TB in central urban area of Wuhan. It was found that the proportion of patients with TB who choose volunteer implemented DOTs management is high. And the main factors influencing the choice of management mode include the distance to basic health-care institution and employment status [23].

Family Member Implemented DOTs

Due to limited health-care resources, it is difficult for health-care professionals to implement whole-course DOTs. Family member implemented DOTs then emerged. In Zhuhai and Shijiazhuang [24, 25], family member implemented DOTs has been tried for management of patients with TB in the migrating population, which effectively improves the compliance to anti-tuberculosis treatment in migrating population. In Foshan [26] and other places, DOTs jointly implemented by family member and health-care professional has been tried and it was found that the joint implementation is more effective in management of patients, compared to family member implemented DOTs.

Relatively highly educated immediate relatives (such as parents, spouses, and offsprings) are selected to receive training on DOTs. Health-care professionals from TB control clinic are responsible for the training.

The training of family member on DOTs includes the basic knowledge about TB control, the hazards of TB, the importance of regular medication, the hazards of irregular or interrupted medication, direct observation on regular drugs taking at TB control clinic, regular sputum reexamination, regular liver and kidney function test and chest X-ray, basic knowledge about anti-tuberculosis drugs and their doses, notes taking about medication, observation of adverse reactions, households disinfection and quarantine, and screening of close family contacts to patients with smear-positive TB.

The selected family members are trained by means of centralized training, in combination with "one-to-one" guidance. Centralized training is performed via one 60-min lecture per month. And "one-to-one" guidance is performed via telephone or family visits for 15–20 min. Responses to adverse reactions and other special conditions are also trained. The initial training lasts for no less than 10 min.

Long-Distance Follow-Up

In Zhuhai and other places [27], the following mode has been adopting for management of patients with TB in the migrating population, which greatly improves the compliance of the initially treated patients with TB in the migrating population.

First of all, the nurses with sufficient expertise in TB control and humanistic quality are selected for the long-distance follow-up. A hierarchical management mechanism is then established, and the responsible nurse conducts the follow-ups based on the requirements. And the head nurse assesses the completion and quality of follow-ups.

Health record of each patient is established. The recorded information includes basic personal information of the patient, diagnosis and treatment, follow-up management, sputum reexaminations, and other information.

The follow-ups are performed via text message communication, brochures on TB control, websites and QQ on-line doctors, telephone calls, and letters. During follow-ups, medications, adverse reactions, causes of treatment interruption, regular reexaminations, liver function test and chest X-ray, diets, psychological support, rest and exercise, and changes of symptoms are communicated.

Telephone follow-up begins in 3 days after treatment. During the intensive phase of medication, follow-ups are conducted once a week, and during the continuation phase of treatment, follow-ups are conducted twice a month. For special patients, follow-ups are appropriately increased according to the needs of patient to ensure that the condition of patient is known and managed by health-care professionals.

Management Model of Trans-Regional Referral and Tracking

In Guangzhou, Shenzhen, and other places, the following model has been adopted for management of trans-regional referral in the migrating population [28, 29].

Based on the diagnosis and treatment before and after referral, the compliance of patient after referral is assessed. For patients with poor compliance, individualized management measures are adopted in advance. Meanwhile, the family members of patients with TB are educated about TB control.

When the diagnosis is defined before and after referral, the intention of trans-regional referral is inquired. And the name of patient, present residence, emergency contact, permanent registered residence, mobile phone number, and telephone number should be correctly recorded to ensure tracking of patient after referral-out.

When patients are referred out, the referral-out form is filled and the referral-in TB control agency is informed in advance about the referral. And the patients are instructed to contact the referral-in TB control agency, and the contact number of referral-out TB control agency is informed to the patients. If contacts to the referral-in TB control agency fail, the patients should contact to the referral-out TB control agency within 7 days. And the referral-out TB control agency should try the best to help the patients to contact the referral-in TB control agency for following treatment and management.

After referral, the referral-out TB control agency is responsible for tracking the patients about their presentation in the referral-in TB control agency within 3 days. If the patients fail to present in the referral-in TB control agency, the referral-out TB control agency is responsible for contacting the referral-in TB control agency. Joint tracking is performed if necessary. Health education is performed within 1 month after trans-regional referral. The high-risk groups, vulnerable groups, special groups, and patients with poor compliance should be paid close attention.

An incentive mechanism for referral-in TB control agency is established to provide patient management fees according to the criteria stipulated by the Global Funding Program for TB Control in migrating Population.

The TB Information Management System (TBIMS) has been developed by CDC of China. It is an effective platform for trans-regional management of patients with TB in migrating population [3].

Precaution System

Lin DW et al. conducted a prospective nested case-control study to collect data of the physical factors of patients, treatment factors, sociological factors, and psychological factors. Logistic regression was applied to screen the significant factors as indicators for predicting regular medication of patients. The system predicts the compliance of patients and provides basis for individualized treatment and management for TB [30]. Guo et al. established a "real-time surveillance of medication and reminding module in on-line DOTs system, which improves the prompt management of medication and quality of patient management" [31].

Electronic Direct Observed Treatment (eDOT)

In recent years, the application of information technology in health-care system has been rapidly developed. Video telephone technology, computer and internet-based video technology, website platform, mobile phone text message and voice message technology, application program (APP), electronic medicine box technology, clinical laboratory information system (LIS), and hospital information system (HIS) have been applied in prevention, management, and treatment of TB. These technologies have played active roles in rational allocation of health-care resources, improving efficiency of health-care professionals, and optimizing diagnosis and treatment of diseases. Internet-based video technology and electronic network based on mobile phones and computer terminals have been gradually applied in medication management of patients with TB. And eDOT has gradually been developed.

The migrating population in Shenzhen is characterized by high mobility and unstable residence. To facilitate medication in patients with TB, the application of Tuberculosis Electronic Direct Observed Treatment System (TBEDOTS) has been promoted in the city since April 2012. The TBEDOTS is firstly developed and applied in China, which replaces the paper medication record card by electronic information system. In Shenzhen, there is a well-established network for TB control, which can meet the demands in managing patients with TB across the city. When the residence of patient is changed, the patient can be referred to any TB control agency for DOTS. However, due to insufficient awareness of the hazards of TB, the patients show unfavorable compliance to anti-tuberculosis treatment. In addition, transportation and nutrition subsidies are provided for patients with TB in the migrating population in Shenzhen, which improves their compliance to the treatment and the success rate of TB treatment in initially treated patients with smear-positive TB has reached 73.6% [32].

In recent years, in order to improve the compliance to treatment, researchers have explored other models of DOTs, such as telephone-based supervision and Wechat-based supervision [33]. In 1970, electronic medicine box with the functions of containing drugs, reminding medication, and monitoring doses has been firstly developed in the USA [34, 35]. In 2009, the Ministry of Health-Gates Foundation Joint TB Control Program was initiated in Inner Mongolia, Heilongjiang, Jiangsu, Henan, Chongqing, and Hunan provinces of China. In the program, electronic medicine box was applied in pilot work for TB patients management [36]. The attempts have achieved success. But due to the limitations of technology and its dependence on human resources, it is difficult to achieve a fundamental breakthrough. In addition, various new electronic devices are constantly available, but their application is limited within generating medication reminder and patient self-management. The physicians cannot be real-time informed about the medication of patient and the adverse reactions. The on-line communication about the condition of patient, on-line housing assessment, on-line health education, and on-line treatment regimen adjustment can hardly be realized. And the effects are limited.

Video-Based Direct Observed Treatment (vDOT)

China has been the country with the largest number of mobile Internet users and the largest number of smartphone users in the world. Along with the advent of network era and the widespread use of mobile terminals, communication is more flexible and convenient, and the corresponding hardware basis is provided for better management of TB patients. In addition, the wide application of free instant communication software (such as Wechat and QQ) provides the corresponding software and platform for real-time communication between health-care professionals in TB control and patients. At present, vDOT has been explored and developed, such as TV-based vDOT, telephone-based vDOT, mobile phone-based vDOT, social software-based vDOT, and APP-based vDOT [37, 38]. The application of vDOT can improve the compliance of patients to the treatment, reduce the time and transportation costs consumed in taking medicine, and improve the efficiency of health-care professionals in TB control. And it has favorable cost-effectiveness ratio [39, 40]. A survey has been conducted in 113 TB control agencies in the USA in 2017. And it has been found that vDOT has been adopted in 47 TB control agencies, with synchronous vDOT in 31 TB control agencies and asynchronous vDOT in 4 TB control agencies. In addition, there are 41 TB control agencies with intention to try vDOT in the next year [41].

New Technology for Space Epidemiology of TB

Epidemiologically, the spread of disease is closely related to spatial social activities of patients [42]. With the improvement of attributes database of global positioning system (GPS) and geographic information system (GIS), researchers in the field of TB control have applied GPS technology, GIS, and SaTScan spatiotemporal scanning analysis to detect the hot spots of TB [43, 44]. In 2017, Liu et al. applied GPS technology for family quarantine of smear-positive TB patients [45]. However, there has been no study based on integration of GPS activity track with GIS. Systematic analysis of the transmission trajectory of communicable pulmonary TB (especially MDR-TB) plays an active role in tracing the source of infection, identifying close contacts individuals, defining key areas of public health, and preventing the spread of TB.

2.2 Traditional Detection of TB Patients

Since Robert Koch discovered the pathogen of TB in 1882, the diagnosis and treatment technologies for TB have been developed rapidly. The sputum smear test and bacteria culture have been rapidly developed as its diagnostic technology. Application of X-ray technology has made diagnostic imaging as the main way for detection of TB. In recent years, the development of TB immunology and molecular biology technology has made it possible to predict outbreak of TB.

Bacteriological Diagnosis

Sputum Smear for Microscopy

After Koch applied alkaline methylene blue staining to detect Mtb from sputum of tuberculosis patient in his laboratory in 1882, Mtb biology-based sputum smear has been the main bacteriological diagnosis of TB for a long period of time, and it has been the main way to detect TB patients. In 1883, Neelsen improved the Mycobacterium Carbonate staining to develop the Ziehl–Neelsen acid-fast staining. Since then, the Ziehl–Neelsen acid-fast staining has been explored and developed. Yan et al. increased the thickness of sputum smear by 3–5 times and prolonged the staining time by 5–10 min, which increased the positive rate of sputum smear by 44.4% [46]. After the introduction of fluorescent staining, many studies have shown that the sensitivity and specificity of fluorescent staining are improved compared to Ziehl–Neelsen acid-fast staining [47].

In 2016, the positive detection rate of Mtb in nano-silica membrane sandwich cup system established by Peng et al. was much higher than that of direct sputum smear (10.9% vs 6.2%, $P < 0.05$). The sensitivity of nano-silicon sandwich cup system was higher than that of direct smear method, compared sputum culture as standard (97.3% vs 55.2%) [48]. In the same year, Huang et al. [49] coupled specific polyclonal antibodies to magnetic beads for Mtb isolation and enrichment, and then streptavidin labeled QD was applied to detect Mtb with monoclonal antibodies to heparin hemagglutinin labeled with biotin, which also effectively improves the detection rate of acid-fast bacilli.

Sputum Culture

In 1925, Sumitomo in Japan successfully isolated and cultured Mtb from sputum of patients. In 1930, Roche culture medium was developed. And in 1949, Ogawa's culture medium was successfully prepared. These developments render Mtb culture to be the golden standard for diagnosis of TB. In addition, the Mtb culture is not limited to the diagnosis, and subsequent strain identification and drug sensitivity test have been playing an important role in the diagnosis of TB. In 1955, Zhu et al. introduced and improved the Pryce slide culture in 1941. Zheng et al. found that the positive rate of isolation and culture of modified Roche medium with sodium glutamate (40.8%) was slightly higher than that with asparagine (35.1%) in Japan. In 1980, Zheng et al. introduced the 1% hemolytic half-stream culture medium, which was developed in China. Shan JS, et al. found that the medium containing sodium pyruvate promotes the growth of Mtb. The two-way medium with both solid and liquid culture medium properties shortens the culture time, increases the positive rate of culture, and provides direction observation on the properties of colonies.

In 1990, Bactec 460, an automatic liquid culture medium labeled with 14C for metabolites of Mtb, was introduced in China. It has the advantages of short culture time, high culture positive rate, and low contamination rate, but it may cause radioactive pollution to the environment.

In 2000, Bactec MGIT 960 began to replace Bactec 460. Bactec MGIT 960 applies fluorescent indicators that are very sensitive to the concentration of oxygen molecules. When Mycobacterium grows, oxygen molecules are consumed in the test tube and the inhibited fluorescent indicators collect to be emitted. Bact/ALERT-3D applies a special color sensor sensitive to CO_2. With the growth of Mtb, CO_2 in the test tube increases and pH value decreases. The color sensor changes irreversibly from blue-green to yellow.

Imaging Diagnosis

In 1895, W. K. Roentgen, a German physicist, discovered X-ray in his research on cathode ray. Based on the penetration, differential absorption, sensitization, and fluorescence of X-ray, it has rapidly been the main way to detect the internal human body.

In 1920, X-ray began to be widely applied to detect thoracic diseases. When X-ray passes through human body, it receives different degrees of absorption (the amount of X-ray absorbed by bone is more than that absorbed by muscle). By this way, X-ray carries the information of density distribution in various parts of human body whose magnitude of fluorescence or sensitization on the screen or photographic film varies greatly. In this way, even small lesions can be clearly shown, as one of the main ways for diagnosis of TB. Based on comparison of pathology of TB to imaging diagnosis of TB, the imaging characteristics of primary pulmonary TB and secondary pulmonary TB have been described. Due to facilities and other reasons, radiography has been the main way for detection of TB in China for a long period of time after the founding of People's Republic of China.

In 1972, computed tomography (CT) was applied in clinical practice. In the late 1970s, CT technology was introduced into China. In the 1990s, CT technology began to be widely applied for the diagnosis of TB. Since then, the imaging diagnosis of tuberculosis stepped into a new era. In 1978, Damadian first applied nuclear magnetic resonance (MRI) technology into clinical practice. Based on the MRI technology, many very small lesions in the human body can be detected.

In recent years, the application of digital subtraction X-ray camera (DR) has been rapidly promoted, with faster imaging speed, higher resolution, lower radiation, and digital storage, which greatly reduces the times of radiography for diagnosis.

Molecular Biology

In 1983, Mullis successfully developed Polymerase Chain Reaction (PCR) technology, which is simple, rapid, and specific with low purity requirements. It has soon attracted much scholarly attention for detection of Mtb. In PCR, a pair of specific oligonucleotide primers is applied to mediate in vitro enzymatic action of specific sequence fragments of Mtb nucleic acid in the examined specimen. Target sequences are repeated dozens of times through denaturation, renaturation, and extension, resulting in millions of times amplification of the detected nucleic acid. The sensitivity of DNA detection is as high as 1 fg-10 pg, 1–10 bacterial cells (bacterial fluid) and 10–100 bacterial cells (sputum specimen). However, contamination has been one of the problems to be solved in PCR technology. At present, the main research directions of molecular biological detection of Mtb include PCR sequencing, qualitative detection of PCR, and various probe technologies.

Immunological Assay

Tuberculin Skin Test

In tuberculin skin test for diagnosis of TB, tuberculin is applied for skin test and its effect on skin delayed hypersensitivity is observed, based on which the immunity to Mtb and previous infection of Mtb are determined.

In 1890, Koch successfully prepared old tuberculin (OT) from Mtb solution cultured in glycerol broth after heating and filtering. In 1907, Clemens F von Pirquet established a skin scratch test. In 1908, the Mantoux method was established. In 1928, P. B. Seibert successfully prepared tuberculin pure protein derivatives (PPDs) with only immunologically active tuberculoprotein but no other non-specific substances. Compared with OT, PPD has more stable titer and higher specificity. At present, the diagnosis of TB is mainly based on the result of tuberculin skin test worldwide. However, by PPD, the immune response produced by BCG vaccination cannot be distinguished from that caused by pathogenic Mtb infection.

TB-IGRA

After Mtb infection, antigen-specific sensitized T cells are produced in human body. When stimulated again by Mtb antigen, the sensitized T cells can be rapidly activated to proliferate and release interferon γ. The principle of TB-IGRA is to detect interferon γ released by sensitized T lymphocytes in vivo by using RD1-encoded TB specific antigen as stimulator. Being different from PPD in tuberculin skin test, these proteins are specifically expressed in all Mtb and pathogenic Mycobacterium bovis, but not expressed in BCG and most non-Mtb. TB-IGRA assay has high specificity for the diagnosis of Mtb infection, especially for differentiation of natural infection from BCG vaccination. And it can be applied to diagnose latent TB infection.

Bronchoscopy and Other Endoscopies

The trachea, bronchus, lobes, segmental bronchus, and their openings can be observed directly under bronchoscope. In addition, it can be applied for secretions, brushing, biopsy, and bronchoalveolar lavage fluid for bacteriological, pathological, cytological, immunological, and biochemical examinations. In 1949, Auerbach summarized autopsy data from 1000 TB patients and discovered that 42% suffers from complications of tracheal and bronchial TB. In subsequent clinical trial, it was found that the detection rate of bronchial TB by bronchoscopy is 20–85% [50]. With the development of fiber optics, bronchoscope has developed from rigid bronchoscope to flexible bronchoscope, and electronic fiberoptic bronchoscope with additional video and computer control has emerged. In recent years, electromagnetic navigating bronchoscopy, transbronchoscopic needle aspiration biopsy technology, and virtual navigation combined with bronchial ultrasound have developed rapidly, which is of great significance for auxiliary diagnosis of TB.

3 Application of Internet Technology

New Internet technologies have been gradually applied to health promotion, diagnosis, surveillance, and patient management of TB. It plays an active role in rationally allocating health care resources, improving the efficiency of health care professionals, and optimizing services for diagnosis and treatment [51]. Meanwhile, highly informationized TB prevention and control system can timely and accurately report the epidemic of infectious diseases, improve the emergency response to epidemic of TB, and conduct in-depth data mining to improve the quality of medical treatment [52]. At the same time, internet technology-based eDOT and vDOT help to save a lot of manpower and improve the quality of treatment, which are actively advocated by WHO [53]. The development of Internet technology has presented more opportunities and challenges to TB prevention and control.

3.1 Telephone-Based Video Technology

In the USA, Australia, and Canada [54], telephone-based video technology has been developed for supervision and management of patients with TB. It has been found that it can greatly save the cost of health-care service for supervision and management of patients with TB, effectively improve the completion rate of treatment, and shorten the time consumed in direct observation. However, there are still some problems. It requires appointment of patients and health-care professionals on a fixed time for telephone follow-up, which limits the space and time for activities of patients. Meanwhile, telephone has small bandwidth, if widely applied, blockage of telephone follow-ups tends to occur.

3.2 Mobile Phone Text/Voice Message Technology

In recent years, DOT management via mobile phone text/voice message system and its supporting platforms is developed in many regions in China for medication reminder, reexamination reminder, and health education. A number of studies [55–57] showed that the model has favorable effects on compliance to treatment in patients with TB. However, there are some limitations. For instance, medication based on text/voice messages is unreliable, and frequent phone calls and messages interfere and constitute economic burden to health care professionals [58].

3.3 Internet-Based Video Technology

In 2010, in Huizhou of Guangdong province [59], computer- and internet-based video technology is applied for DOT management of TB patients. The technology effectively reduces the time cost and transportation cost for DOT management, and greatly improves the efficiency of DOT management.

3.4 Mobile Terminal Application Technology (APP)

APP of mobile health care is a third-party application software based on mobile smartphone for health care service. It is a technology for implementation of mobile health care service. It incorporates various functions to provide services for both patients and health care professionals, including data collection, physician–patient communication, health care services, and health education. While providing intellectualized health care services for patients, it also greatly improves the service efficiency of health care professionals. In 2016, there were more than 100,000 health-related APPs worldwide and more than 2000 mobile health care APPs in China [60]. Researchers firstly apply social APP for DOT management of TB patients, then gradually try to develop specialized APP for DOT management of TB patients.

Social Software

Tencent QQ

In Xinjiang Autonomous Region, Xuchang city, Huainan city, and other places in China, Tencent QQ, via single-line contact or QQ groups, is applied for extended TB care services. The services mainly include consultation and management of PPD strong positive population, patients information collection, health care demands of the patients, and health education about TB core knowledge [61]. The QQ-based management effectively improves compliance of patients to diagnosis and treatment, and increases the awareness rate of TB core knowledge.

Wechat

In 2013, Wechat is applied for medication management and health education in patients with MDR-TB in Foshan City and Quanzhou City of China. The Wechat-based management effectively improves the compliance of patients to treatment. In 2014, China TB Prevention and Control Wechat platform was officially launched by the Health Commission of China. And TB-related Wechat subscription number or public number [62] was established successively throughout the country for health education about TB prevention and control, which greatly improves the public awareness about TB prevention and control and patients' compliance to diagnosis and treatment of TB. In 2015, health education for TB patients in migrating population was conducted via Wechat by the Guangdong TB Control Center, which effectively improves the treatment compliance and health care experience in migrating TB patients [63]. By applying Wechat, Nanshan Health Care Easy was established in Nanshan district of Shenzhen, which realized on-line registration, payment, report viewing, health care consultation, Wechat payment, and mobile medical insurance payment. The specialized Wechat platform facilitates health care services provided by the hospitals.

Other Social Software

Many websites-based reports in the USA showed that Skype, FaceTime, and other software have been tried for their application in the management of TB patients. In 2013, a study in the USA pointed out that application of Skype in the DOT management of TB patients, on-line communication, and surveillance of adverse drug reactions can effectively save the time and expenses of the patients and health care professionals [64].

Specialized APP for DOT Management of TB

The mobile APP for management of TB has been developed jointly by CDC Clinical Center for Tuberculosis Prevention and Control and Beijing Thoracic Hospital. There are two client terminals, TB Assistant APP and TB Physician

APP. TB Assistant APP is a mobile application for TB patients and their families, including medication reminder, reexamination reminder, Q & A in TB prevention and control, and patient-to-patient communication. TB Physician APP is a mobile application for health care professionals and scientific researchers, including information, activities, Q & A, cases, and management, for information exchange in health care professionals, and convenient management of patients. In 2016, the APP was tested in Tongzhou district of Beijing [65], with 264 patients included, and all the patients appraised the APP. However, there are still some limitations. APP functional plate and content are insufficient, and the applying activity of APP needs to be improved. In 2017, in Longhua district of Shenzhen, a joint platform of APP + Wechat Public Number was established for TB patient management, and the effects showed that the management mode is feasible. However, it is necessary to increase its acceptance by male patients aged under 20 and above 39 years. In 2016, in Nanshan district of Shenzhen, Health-enjoying Internet APP was independently developed for video-based DOT management of TB, adverse reactions management, and GPS-based family quarantine of TB [66]. In addition, a number of companies in the USA have developed specialized APPs for TB management, such as AICure [67] and Sure Adhere. A comparative study of vDOT and DOT in the USA has demonstrated that vDOT is more feasible and acceptable, with more favorable treatment compliance and lower cost than DOT.

3.5 Electronic Medication Box Technology

In actual management of TB, the reason for the low rate of regular medication in some patients is that they often forget to take medication, and even some forgetful patients have repeated medication. Based on these facts, the development of intelligent electronic medication box has been explored all over the world.

In 1970, electronic medicine box began to be developed in the USA, which can remind patients to take medicine and monitor the drugs dispensing in addition to container of medicines [35]. In 2009, the joint program of the Ministry of Health and Gates Foundation on TB control was implemented in Inner Mongolia, Heilongjiang, Jiangsu, Henan, Chongqing, and Hunan provinces and municipalities, and pilot work for application of electronic medicine box in management of TB was initiated [68]. In 2011, a research team of CDC and Peking University of China conducted a study on consistency between electronic medicine box records and urine test results as gold standard for intake of medicine by patients. And a high consistency was found [69]. Another study, with 104 patients with latent TB infection included in the study, has demonstrated that electronic medicine box for TB patient management can improve treatment compliance [70]. The electronic medicine box is promising to be an assistant tool for monitoring and promoting medication of TB patients.

3.6 Wirelessly Observed Therapy (WOT)

To ensure the medication by TB patients, WOT is also an alternative to replace traditional DOT. Patients receive anti-tuberculosis treatment by taking tablets with absorbable sensors, while wearing a wearable sensor to collect data about their compliance. And then the data is transmitted from the wearable sensor to the patient's mobile phone and central server, while the responsible physician can monitor and confirm the medication via the management platform. The system is capable of recording the type, dosage, and time of medication by patients. It also supports the responsible physician to confirm the medication objectively at any time and at any place [71]. A study conducted in the USA has shown that the direct cost of WOT for TB treatment is lower than that of traditional DOT. However, within a short period of time, due to its implementation based on wireless/mobile network, the system is not feasible in underdeveloped regions [17].

3.7 Internet Website Platform

Internet On-line Direct Reporting and Internet On-line Special Reporting System

In January 2004, the infectious disease internet on-line reporting system (IDRS) was launched in China, which is also known as the internet on-line direct reporting system and can be accessed by all the health care institutions in China to report and monitor the incidence of TB. It has been the best information platform for the detection and surveillance of TB patients. With the help of the internet on-line direct reporting system and the supporting intervention measures, the overall arrival rate of suspected TB patients has been greatly increased [72]. In 2005, TB Information Management System (TBIMS), also known as the internet on-line special reporting system, was developed by CDC of China, through which designated health care institutions for TB can know about the diagnosis, treatment, management, and prognosis of TB patients. And it provides a fast and more comprehensive information platform for the detection, diagnosis, and treatment of TB patients [73]. Based on the system, trans-regional management of TB patients in migrating population can be performed.

TB Epidemic Surveillance System

In practice, health care institutions are responsible for reporting the original data via the internet on-line direct reporting system. The timeliness and accuracy of reported data directly affect the data quality in the internet on-line direct reporting system and the decision-making in TB prevention and control. In many regions of China, various measures have been actively attempted or systems have been built to assess the data and to reduce the missed report rate and missed registry rate. A real-time monitoring and warning system for infectious diseases has been developed by the PLA General Hospital of China, which greatly improves the data quality for surveillance of infectious diseases. In 2016, with the help of the information platform, the Large-scale Data Research Base for Chronic Diseases, it has been found in Zhijiang city that the overall missed report rate of 13 health care institutions is 1.01%, the missed registry rate of suspected TB patients in designated health care institutions for TB is 6.96%, and the missed registry rate of defined TB patients is 0.36%. The main factors influencing the rates include insufficient training of working staffs and insufficient data quality control [74].

Internet-Based Health Care Resources

Currently, large quantities of health care information resources, including electronic health care journals, internet-based health care academic exchanges, professional news reports, various health care databases, on-line continuing education services in health care, and information search engines, are running on the internet. Such electronic resources as the National Library of America Medical Retrieval System, Wanfang Data Resource System, China Knowledge Information Resource System, WHO TB Control Program, and website of China Anti-tuberculosis Association can be applied for knowledge, experience, and policy in TB control [75].

Informatization Platform on TB

In 2011, Shenzhen took the lead in developing TBEDOTS by applying Internet technology, which was incorporated into the management system of Shenzhen community-based health care service center. The system is based on computer terminal and IC card reader, providing health care services of supervising medication, follow-up records, adverse reactions, drug dispensing, follow-up reminder, and system management. The patients with an IC card can obtain anti-tuberculosis drugs at any health care institution with TBEDOTS. And the information about drug dispensing and follow-up is shared in the system. Meanwhile, there is a real-time monitoring and warning reminder to supervise the medication of patients [76].

In 2011, a TB information system was established in Beijing, which incorporated hospital information system (HIS), clinical laboratory information system (LIS), and regional health care resource management platform. Via the system, the information about diagnosis and treatment of TB and community-based management are shared, which promotes the construction of TB outpatient management [77].

Student Health Surveillance Information System

To improve the surveillance for symptoms of common diseases and absence due to illness in students and to provide early warning information for TB epidemic, a student health surveillance information system [78] was developed in Shenzhen in 2012. The system supports real-time recording of morning health examination and absence due to illness. And by applying the system, surveillance gateway for suspected symptoms of TB in schools is shifted forward, and information is provided to ensure prevention of TB clustering epidemics and sudden public health events of TB.

3.8 Public Information Resource Base in the Network Project

By using government public information resources, identification of TB patients, follow-up services for TB patients, real-time surveillance and dynamic management of TB epidemic are performed. The TB control across the whole city has been more efficient. Shenzhen is a mega-city with permanent residents of more than ten million and the highest proportion of migrating population in China. The population structure is complex with high mobility and incomplete basic data, and information collection is challenging. For a long period of time, due to the information exchange barriers between different departments, it is impossible to obtain clear and accurate data about population and to understand all the subjects of service management. In order to solve the problem of "Information Island," social management has been innovated to improve public services. In 2012, the Network Project was creatively implemented in Shenzhen [78]. Based on cloud computing and large-scale data technology, the only public information resource database in the city has been established for the four-level vertical information connection of city, district, neighborhood committee office, and community. Thirty-six departments, such as the Municipal Public Security Bureau, the Civil Affairs Bureau, and the Municipal Education Bureau, have access to the public basic resources database, which promotes the dynamic management, interconnection, and sharing of information resources across districts, levels, and departments. By using the resource database, 3-dimensional surveillance system and 3-dimensional relationship network are established by correlating the distribution of public information such as population, legal person, building (urban component) with the location of electronic map. The epidemic features, spatial distribution, and hot spots of TB are obtained by visualization analysis, which provides a scientific basis for TB risk surveillance, TB epidemic early warning, its transmission chain analysis, and emergency response to TB epidemic.

3.9 Global Positioning System (GPS) and Geographic Information System (GIS)

GPS is a mid-range circular orbit satellite navigation system, which can provide accurate positioning, speed measurement, and high-precision time standard in more areas across the world. Studies have reported that the GPS technology is applied to locate the family address of patients, and GIS and SaTScan space-time scanning analysis are applied to explore the hot spots of TB cases. There are also studies concerning application of GPS technology to analyze the transmission of Mycobacterium bovis between badgers and cattle [79]. In recent years, GPS positioning data of TB patients has been continuously collected in Nanshan district of Shenzhen city to acquire the trajectories of quarantined TB patients, which provides a basis for accurate and effective family quarantine of TB patients and control of TB transmission.

With the support of computer hardware, GIS is a computer system to collect, store, manage, retrieve, analyze, and describe the location distribution of space objects and the corresponding attribute data, so as to realize the requirement of information management [80]. In many studies, GIS technology was applied to map the spatial distribution for tendency analysis and spatial autocorrelation analysis to explore the spatial distribution and the hot spots of case or strain. Moran's I and Getis-Ord G spatial autocorrelation analysis and SaTScan space-time scanning analysis technology were also applied to analyze the spatial, temporal, and space-time clustering characteristics of TB. In addition, high-risk place and scope of TB clustering epidemic are detected accurately and the risks are assessed. Moran's I spatial autocorrelation analysis and spatial cross-sectional regression model, F test, Hausman test, error Moran's I test, and Lagrange multiplier (LM) test have been applied to explore the sociological and meteorological factors affecting the incidence of TB. Moran's I, Getis-Ord G spatial statistics, and Poisson multiple regression model have also been applied to explore the impact of migrating population on TB epidemic. A Canadian study attempted to apply GIS technology, related laboratories, clinical and demographic databases to track individuals with close contacts and monitor outbreak of TB [81].

3.10 Hospital Information System (HIS) and Laboratory Information System (LIS)

HIS is an information management system that covers all the processes within a hospital. HIS can be applied to manage the clinical diagnosis and treatment information of TB and the economic activities in a hospital involved in the process of its diagnosis and treatment.

Concerning clinical information management of TB, HIS system is mainly applied to collect and process clinical diagnosis and treatment information of TB, to assist decision-making for physicians, and to improve the efficiency and quality in TB diagnosis and treatment. In addition to participating in the diagnosis and treatment of TB, HIS is also applied in the management of economic activities in hospitals, such as drug management, charge management, and ward management. The diagnostic imaging information system in HIS, namely the picture archiving and communication system (PACS), is an important way to diagnose or exclude TB, especially in patients with bacteriologically negative TB. After diagnostic imaging of lungs is performed in TB patients in a hospital, the radiologist uploads the imaging data to the cloud. The physician can obtain the imaging data at any time and any place via computer or mobile phone. In such a way, the imaging data can be shared among different hospitals, which realizes TB consultation and case reporting at different hospitals.

LIS is one of the important components of HIS. During prevention and treatment of TB, the computer technology and computer network are applied to collect, store, process, transmit, query, and provide clinical laboratory data for analysis and diagnosis of TB. Its main functions are to assist the laboratory staff to pre-treat the laboratory test application form and specimen, to automatically collect or directly input the laboratory data, to process the laboratory data, to examine and review the laboratory report, and to inquire and print the laboratory report. Via LIS, various laboratory equipment are connected to the local network of the hospital. After the orders from physicians are obtained via HIS, LIS manages the laboratory tests based on the bar code on the test tube, and the electronic report is then generated and feedback to HIS. The clinicians have convenient access to the relevant information.

Compared to the traditional laboratory test procedures, LIS reduces the error rate and improves the accuracy and timeliness of laboratory reports. And the laboratory report is convenient for inquiries. Via internet, TB patients can even view the laboratory test results at home. The possibility of nosocomial infection of Mtb has been further reduced due to the reduced exposure to Mtb during the laboratory test procedures.

3.11 Application of Internet Technology in Other Fields

The development and application of Internet technology continuously promote the progress in early detection of TB and subsequent patient management. For instance, large-scale data analysis is applied to screen and identify DNA molecular markers responsible for TB susceptibility. The risk of TB in individuals is thus assessed to provide a basis for prophylactic treatment of latent TB infection. Intelligent video analysis and digital image processing analysis are applied to detect, isolate, track, and identify moving targets in dynamic scene video, which helps to track and manage entry–exit TB patients as well as patients with MDR-TB and EDR-TB. The network analysis platform for whole genome sequencing of Mtb has been established to analyze the evolution and genetic map of DR-TB for rapid prediction of drug resistance spectrum, description of the transmission path, optimization of treatment regimen, and guidance of clinical precise treatment. In the diagnostic technology of TB based on sputum microimaging, via integration of high accuracy automatic sputum loading control platform, the sputum smear test can be performed via automatic loading, continuous automatic scanning, and computer-aided artificial intelligence detection. Thus, automatic identification of Mtb and its strains in sputum smear is achieved.

The challenges of Internet information security, insufficient subsidies, uneven levels of technological development, and asynchronization of Internet standards in health care industry limit the development of Internet+ health care [82]. However, the policies, the development of Internet technology, and the demand for health care services bring unprecedented opportunities for development of Internet+ TB prevention and control. These factors will greatly promote the early detection and intervention, rapid diagnosis, teleconsultation, precise treatment, and health management of TB. In the era of mobile internet, more network data should be run for TB prevention and control but less transportation of patients. The technologies will help to improve the detection, diagnosis, treatment, and management of TB in basic TB control agencies, and provide more timely and accurate scientific basis for effective policy-making by government officials.

4 Application of New Technologies in Molecular Biology

The diagnosis of TB has stepped into the era of molecular biology for rapid diagnosis and identification of TB and DR-TB with optimal cost-effective ratio. By molecular biology, the diagnosis of TB saves the time of several weeks compared to conventional culture for its diagnosis. Recent advances in molecular biology for TB detection include more rapid and simpler nucleic acid amplification test (NAAT) and whole genome sequencing (WGS), both of which can shorten the time for diagnosis.

Rapid and accurate detection of pathogens and their drug sensitivity is essential for early treatment and control of diseases. These new technologies can be applied to optimize the culture medium, optimize the culture system, detect early proliferation, strictly control oxygen partial pressure, and identify the matrix-assisted laser desorption ionization time-of-flight mass spectrometry (MALDI-TOF-MS) [83]. Advances in Mtb molecular assays have shortened the diagnostic time to several days, whereas conventional culture systems usually take several weeks to diagnose. Most molecular technologies aim to detect specific nucleic acids in Mtb DNA and RNA by amplification technologies such as polymerase chain reaction (PCR), or to detect drug resistance related mutants by sequencing and nucleic acid hybridization. In addition, WHO has announced that sputum smear-based microscopy for TB diagnosis needs to be replaced by new diagnostic technologies. In general-level laboratories, non-sputum-based biomarkers can be applied for simple exclusion tests and rapid drug sensitivity tests in suspected patients. Innovative microscopes (e.g., light emitting diode [LED] microscopes), Mtb culture systems (e.g., Becton Dickinson MGIT 960), linear probe analysis, and automation systems for nucleic acid amplification (e.g., Cepheid Xpert MTB/RIF systems) are constantly being developed in developing and developed countries [84].

4.1 Fully Automated Nucleic Acid Amplification Test (NAAT)

Because of the limitations in traditional bacteriological diagnosis of TB, NAAT has gradually been a new choice. The fast turnover time of NAAT system is convenient for patients to complete detection and treatment within once presentation, which thus improves the follow-up rate of patients. Most NAATs are applied to identify insertion element IS6110 in Mtb, and NAAT has been applied to detect Mtb ribosomal RNA or DNA in sputum specimen from patients with acid-fast bacilli (AFB) smear positive and AFB smear negative, respectively. NAAT shows a very high sensitivity in patients with sputum smear-positive TB, while its sensitivity in patients with sputum smear-negative is about 61–76%. Currently, the WHO approved NAAT detection is Xpert/RIF MTB. And the other two NAAT detections are Mtb Rapid Detector (Gen-Probe, Inc) and Amplicor Mtb Detection System (Roche Molecular Systems, Inc). Both have been approved by the Food and Drug Administration (FDA) to detect specimen of respiratory AFB smear positive. Other commercially available NAATs include RING-mediated isothermal amplification-based MTB detection system, cross-primer amplification-based TB diagnosis system, and Mtb gene-driven technology [85].

Among various bacterial diseases with high Mycobacterium load, NAAT positive and AFB smear-positive indicate active TB. And AFB smear positive and NAAT negative with no inhibitors indicate non-Mtb (NTM) infection. If the culture shows positive in the above cases, TB is bacteriologically defined. NAAT can be applied to detect TB in patients with AFB smear-positive. In addition, for the cases of NAAT positive and AFB smear negative, anti-tuberculosis treatment is performed based on clinical manifestations before the culture results are available. According to the requirements of CDC, if both sputum smear and NAAT are negative, NAAT should be applied to detect other specimens [86]. However, if Mtb growth is detected by culture, the patient is bacteriologically defined with TB. Finally, if all of AFB smear, NAAT, and Mtb culture show negative, the condition can be categorized into clinically diagnosed TB or other diseases.

In the regions with low positive rate of Mtb culture, the promotion of NAAT in patients with sputum smear positive may be more effective. On the other hand, in the regions with more TB cases, NAAT should also be applied in patients with sputum smear negative. A meta-analysis showed that commercially available NAAT alone should not replace the traditional diagnostic tests for TB [87].

4.2 Xpert MTB/RIF Detection Technology

Xpert MTB/RIF detection is a nucleic acid amplification detection based on GeneXpert instrument system. Xpert MTB/RIF detection technology is based on the principle of full-automatic real-time fluorescence quantitative PCR, which can be applied to detect Mtb specific DNA sequence in sputum specimen. Direct sputum detection by Xpert MTB/RIF can detect 99% smear-positive patients and more than 80% smear-negative patients. According to the WHO report in 2013, Xpert MTB/RIF can be applied for additional test after TB microscopy, alternative of AFB smear microscopy, detection of Mtb in AFB smear positive or negative and culture positive, detection of Mtb in pleural effusion, detection of Mtb in lymph node specimen harvested by biopsy or fine needle aspiration, detection of Mtb in gastric juice, detection of Mtb in cerebrospinal fluid specimen, and detection of Mtb in tissue specimen. In 2014, WHO indicated that Xpert MTB/RIF technology can be applied as a preliminary diagnostic test for all suspected patients of pulmonary TB [88].

Xpert MTB/RIF has been applied to detect rifampicin resistance by PCR amplification of 81 bp fragment of rpoB gene of MTB specific sequence and subsequent detection of rifampicin resistance-related mutations in the region. And the results can be obtained within 2 h [89]. Xpert MTB/RIF is recommended by WHO to detect sputum from high-risk population of MDR-TB. Xpert MTB/RIF can be applied as initial detection and additional detection after AFB smear negative. By using Xpert MTB/RIF, the time for detection is shortened, and the average time to treat AFB smear-negative TB has been shortened from 56 days (range: 39–81 days) to 5 days (range: 2–8 days). However, Xpert detection of Mtb in sputum is more expensive than traditional microscopic examination. In one analysis, it was found that the cost of rapid sputum-based detection is $ 2–4 US dollars, which is close to the cost of conventional sputum smear for microscopy. In order to promote the application of Xpert MTB/RIF, the Foundation for Promoting Innovative Diagnostic Methods (FIND) has initiated negotiations for substantial price reduction. However, with no effectively improved health care system, the promotion of Xpert MTB/RIF cannot be effectively applied for DR-TB control, especially in shortening the time for initial follow-up and initial treatment [90].

4.3 Whole Genome Sequencing (WGS)

Microbial genomics has enabled us to study microbial genetic markers that may affect treatment and prognosis of infections. Because Mtb is transmitted between hosts, whole genome sequencing (WGS) is becoming an effective way to identify microbial evolution in Mtb lineages. Currently, there are two types of sequencers, the first generation sequencer and the second generation sequencer, which has been well known as the next generation sequencer (NGS). The first generation sequencer consumes more time in sequencing, but has high throughput and low cost (about $65 US dollars per bacterial genome). The second generation has lower throughput and higher cost (about $150 US dollars per genome by Illumina® MiSeq) and sequencing of multiple genomes within one day is possible [91].

Compared to Xpert MTB, WGS is capable of more favorable detection of various mutations. In addition, false positive can be avoided in WGS when polymorphism in rifampicin rpoB resistance core region (RRDR) is detected. WGS has not yet been applied as a routine diagnostic technology for TB, partly because Mtb needs to be cultured for several weeks before enough DNA can be extracted. The culture of slow-growing Mtb before DNA extraction is a time-consuming step in WGS. Therefore, it is important to extract DNA directly from frozen isolates rather than re-culture it. There is a reliable and low-cost DNA extraction method in the culture of 1 mL early Mycobacterium growth positive indicator tube (MGIT), which is sufficient for WGS to identify Mycobacterium species and predict antibiotic resistance in clinical specimen. Recently, studies have found a WGS method that does not require pre-culture. Mtb DNA specific biotinylated RNA bait is applied to directly capture the complete Mtb genome in non-sputum culture specimen. And the WGS data can be obtained weeks before DST results are available. DNA sequencing can also be applied to confirm rifampicin resistance detected in Xpert MTB/RIF. However, conventional WGS costs hundreds of US dollars, and only is applied to detect clinical specimens in a few high-income countries.

4.4 Specimen Transportation Media Technology

Sputum specimen processing in clinical laboratories requires an efficient and safe system that cannot be impaired by long-term transportation. Generally speaking, prolonged storage time leads to reduced positive rate. Therefore, specimen transportation media technology plays an important role in the whole procedures for diagnosis of TB. The specimen transportation media system consists of Mtb inactivation and DNA stabilization. Their purpose is to maintain the quality of DNA while obtaining sufficient DNA output. Some known transportation technologies include PrimeStoreTM-Molecular Transport Medium (PS-MTM) and Cetylpyridine Chloride (CPC). PS-MTM inactivates Mtb in specimens and maintains DNA/RNA stability at ambient temperature for further molecular processing and analysis. For Xpert MTB analysis, incubation of sputum with sample reagent (SR) could keep Mtb detection rate stable within 72 h [92].

4.5 Mtb Load Detection

Quantification of Mtb load in TB patients plays an important role in predicting the prognosis. Several detection technologies can be applied to quantify Mycobacterium load, such as BD ProbeTec system and AdvanSure TB/NTM real-time PCR kit. Lee and his colleagues determined the cyclic threshold (Ct) of Mycobacterium load by assessing quantitative AdvanSure TB/NTM real-time PCR kit (LG Life Sciences, Korea) [93]. The Ct value for best positive staining is less than 33.2, with 95.0% sensitivity and 32.0% specificity. These findings suggest that the AdvanSure TB/NTM real-time PCR kit can be applied to quantify the Mycobacterium load. AdvanSure TB/NTM real-time PCR kit is based on IS6110 primers to detect Mycobacterium, and rpoB gene-specific primers and probes are applied to distinguish Mtb from NTM. However, the technology fails to detect the presence of active Mycobacterium organisms in the specimen.

4.6 Serological Diagnosis of Active TB

Serological diagnosis for TB is widely applied in developing countries. In an Indonesian study, Senosaputra and her colleagues found that plasma anti-alpha-crystallin (ACR) level, anti-lipid arabinomannan, anti-trehalose 6,6′-dimycitrate, and anti-TB-glycolipid antigen antibodies in active TB patients are higher than those in latent TB infection (LTBI) and healthy controls. In another study, five lipid antigens show different IgG antibody responses: cord factor (trehalose 6,6′-dimycotic ester) (TDM-T), monoacyl phosphatidylinositol dimannoside (Ac-PIM2), Mycobacterium bovis BCG-isolated Trehalomycetes (TMM-M), Trehalomonas (TMM-M), GPL from Mycobacterium avium complex (MAC) [94]. However, a systematic assessment on the diagnostic accuracy of serological tests revealed that these tests show inaccuracy in the diagnosis of pulmonary and extrapulmonary TB [95]. Serological tests for TB are limited in defining the past history of TB, and are impossible to diagnose active TB. In addition, it has been strongly recommended by WHO that commercially available serological tests should not be applied for clinical diagnosis of pulmonary and extrapulmonary TB.

4.7 Molecular Diagnosis of DR-TB

Drug resistance of Mtb has been increasing. MDR (at least rifampicin and isoniazid resistance) and XDR (increased resistance to fluoroquinolone and kanamycin/amikacin/capreomycin) strains of Mtb have been identified as major threats to the control of TB epidemics. Drug sensitivity test of Mtb to the first-line and second-line anti-tuberculosis drugs is a key component in TB control. To completely understand the drug sensitivity of infected Mtb facilitates formulating chemical treatment regimen to improve efficacy and avoid the abuse of ineffective anti-tuberculosis drugs. Traditional phenotypic DST takes at least 2 weeks, 1 week for preliminary detection of microbial growth and the other week for critical concentration assessment of first-line anti-tuberculosis drugs. Obviously, some new, rapid and accurate DST technologies are urgently needed. In a large multinational trial, BACTEC MGIT960 as a reference standard, MDR/XDR-TB was directly detected based on sputum specimens of patients. The line probe assay (LPA), pyrophosphatic acid sequencing (PSQ), and microscopic drug sensitivity (MODS) technology were compared. The results showed the average time of LPA and PSQ is 1.1 days, while that of MODS and MGIT are 14.3 days and 24.7 days, respectively [95].

There are many options for LPA, such as AID LPA (AID Diagnostika, Germany) [89], Hain LPA (Hain Lifescience, Germany) [96], INNO LPA (Innogenetics, Belgium) [97], GenoType MTBDRplus [25], and GenoType MTBDRsl [98]. INNO LPA and GenoType MTBDRplus have been assessed and validated by a WHO experts team. AID LPA is intended to detect common mutations responsible for resistance to rifampicin, isoniazid, streptomycin, capreomycin, amikacin, ethambutol, and fluoroquinolone. Meanwhile, a comparative study showed that MTBDRplus LPA is more sensitive than Xpert MTB/RIF in detecting rifampicin resistance of Mtb [98]. In summary, different technologies can be applied to explore different drug resistance-related mutations, and the changes in technologies enable us to detect various drug resistance.

The PSQ detection consists of seven PSQ analyses, which are applied to detect mutations in gene or promoter regions.

By these analyses, the causes of drug resistance to the first- and second-line anti-tuberculosis drugs can usually be identified [99]. A study found the correlation between PSQ results and phenotypic DST results, 98.7% for rifampicin, 94.3% for isoniazid, 99.2% for capreomycin, 99.2% for amikacin, 96.4% for kanamycin, and 97.6% for quinolones (levofloxacin, ofloxacin, or moxifloxacin) [100].

GenoType MTBDRsl (MTBDRsl) is the only commercially available molecular assay for detection of resistance to fluoroquinolones (levofloxacin, ofloxacin, and moxifloxacin) and second-line injectable anti-tuberculosis drugs (kanamycin, capreomycin, and amikacin). MTBDRsl has been applied to detect rrs and gyrA gene mutations that are responsible for drug resistance to injectable antibiotics and fluoroquinolones, respectively. In addition, by using MTBDRsl, embB mutations leading to ethambutol resistance are able to be detected. The sensitivity and specificity of MTBDRsl are as follows: fluoroquinolones 87% and 96%, kanamycin 77% and 100%, capreomycin 80% and 98%, amikacin 100% and 100%, ethambutol 57% and 92%, respectively. In a meta-analysis, MTBDRsl showed favorable accuracy in detecting resistance to fluoroquinolones, capreomycin, and amikacin, but it might not be applied to detect drug resistance to ethambutol and kanamycin. However, despite some progress in drug sensitivity test technologies, challenges remain in terms of procedural performance records, long-term financial support, and the number of scientific publications [101].

More rapid and appropriate detection and treatment for TB can effectively reduce the hospitalization rate and occurrence of complications. Meanwhile, unnecessary treatment and false positive cases can be effectively avoided. Advances in molecular diagnosis and detection of active pulmonary TB can improve the population health. Therefore, its development has promising prospects in the future. We still need to consider the requirements of new diagnostic examinations and the ways to assess their diagnostic accuracy, operational feasibility, and ultimate clinical significance [102].

5 Application of Artificial Intelligence in Imaging Precise Diagnosis

TB is a pulmonary infectious disease caused by Mtb. It has been estimated by WHO that deaths due to TB were 1.57 million in 2017 [103]. China has the second largest TB epidemic in the world (following India), with high rates of TB infection, incidence, drug resistance, and mortality. And the risk of simultaneous infection of TB and HIV/AIDS has been increasing. The spread of HIV/AIDS accelerates the prevalence of TB, and TB has been the main cause of death in patients with HIV/AIDS [104]. Therefore, rapid and accurate diagnosis and timely treatment are the key issues for TB control.

Chest X-ray (CXR) and sputum smear for microscopy (SSM) are recommended by WHO as the main ways for screening of TB. CXR is the most widely applied imaging system. In China, CXR has been applied for categorized preliminary screening of TB. In addition to SSM for rapid detection of TB, both technologies are applied for grading diagnosis of TB. But in remote rural areas of China, no experienced and skilled radiologists and laboratory practitioners are available for rapid interpretations of CXR and SSM results.

5.1 Automated Chest Radiography for TB

The advantages of portable digital Chest X-ray (DCXR) to detect TB include high speed, low cost, good sensitivity and specificity. In populations with low prevalence of HIV/AIDS, the sensitivity and specificity of portable CDXR in diagnosis of TB is about 80% and 75%, respectively. And in population with moderate and high prevalence of HIV/AIDS, its sensitivity and specificity to TB is about 90% and 80%, respectively. At present, in some research institutes, researches have been conducted for application of artificial intelligence-based automatic digital system for population screening of pulmonary TB. Such institutions include Delft Imaging Systems in the Netherlands [105–107], AGFA of Belgium, Quer.ai of India, Lunit of Korea, National Library of Medicine from National Institute of Health (NIH) in the U SA, and Shenzhen Chronic Disease Prevention and Control Center and Shenzhen Zhiying Medical Company [104, 108] are the representatives. The software system can automatically score the likelihood of TB on each chest image (Fig. 9.1). Large-scale data test has proven their high detection accuracy.

Efforts have been made jointly by Delft Medical Imaging Corporation of the Netherlands, Radboud University of the Netherlands, and the South African Lung Research Institute in Cape Town. And an intelligent diagnostic software has been developed for its application with DCXR platforms in Africa and Europe [20] [109, 110]. The results of clinical trial showed that the intelligent software outperforms formally trained African clinicians in African hospitals. And it can be applied to diagnose and detect passive and active TB and to screen the prevalence of TB in common population. The intelligent software is capable of automatically analyzing abnormalities in chest images within 1 min and scoring them on a percentage basis. The intelligent software has been tested by several institutions in Africa and Europe, including Zambia, South Africa, the United Kingdom, and Tanzania. In screening of high-risk populations, such as prisoners and homeless population, some cases of TB have been detected. At present, the accuracy of the intelligent detection software for TB in China needs to be improved.

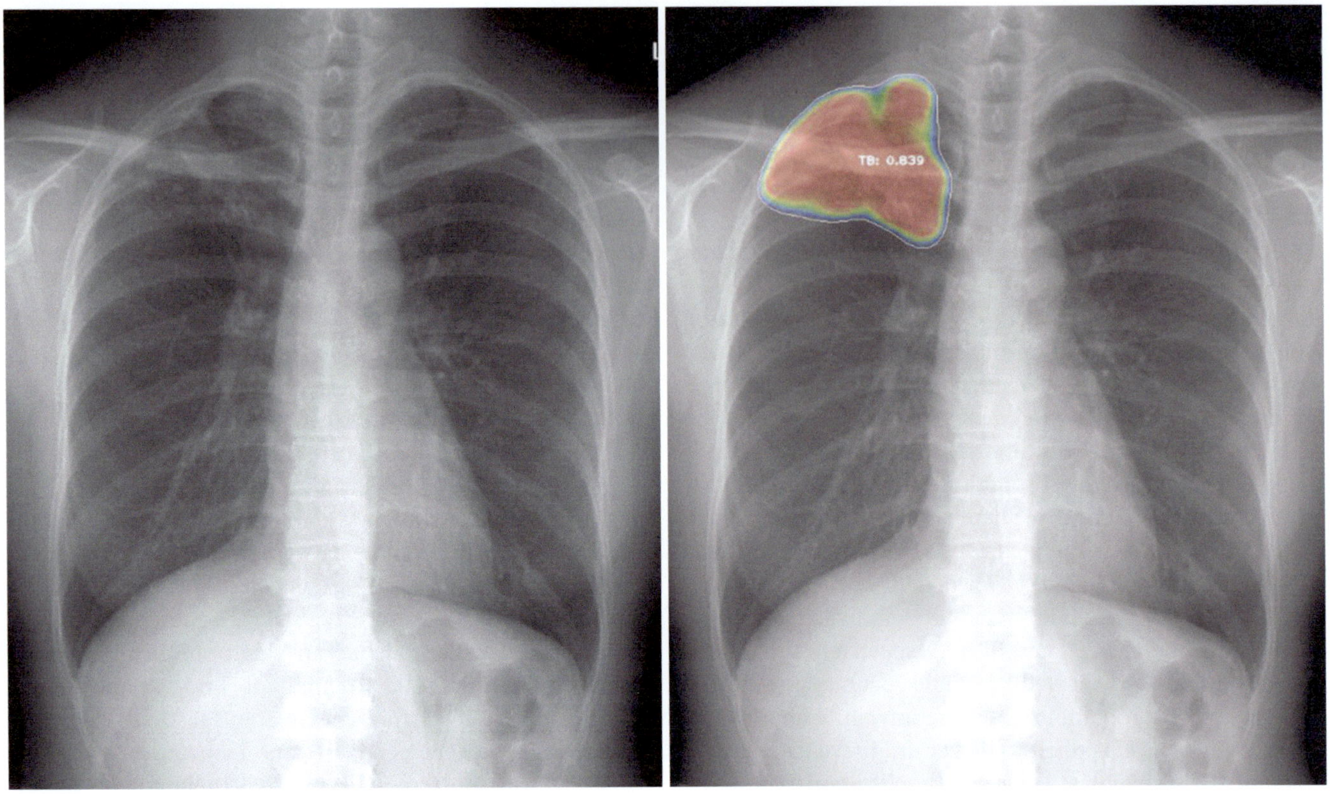

Fig. 9.1 Illustration of original DR image (left) and the detection result (or the heat map) from an AI system (right). The AI-determined TB infected lung area (right) is shown in different color. The red area shows highly infected area on the original image (left) and yellow as moderate infected. The left panel illustrates the simple operation and confidence of TB. In this case, the TB confidence level is 92.1%

Another automated chest system for TB was developed by the National Library of Medicine (NLM) of the National Institutes of Health in the USA [104, 111, 112]. The researchers collaborated with a non-governmental organization in Western Kenya (Academic Model Providing Access to Healthcare, AMPATH) to screen local populations for TB [107]. The portable digital chest system developed by NLM was installed by AMPATH on custom trucks to provide screening in remote rural areas. Intelligent TB screening system runs on low-power computers. Once the digital chest radiographs are obtained, the intelligent TB screening system developed by NLM immediately runs for analysis. The advanced image processing and artificial intelligence learning algorithm are applied in the system for simply display of the test results, which is valuable reference for diagnosis of TB. The research team of NLM has also cooperated with clinical researchers in Shenzhen to explore the diagnostic data from chest radiographs of TB in China and to improve artificial intelligence technology and detection accuracy [104, 113].

Efforts have been made jointly by NLM, Shenzhen Chronic Disease Prevention and Control Center, and Zhiying Healthcare Science and Technology Institution in Shenzhen to develop an intelligent chest radiography TB screening system (NLM/SZ system). The system is a group of modules that can be connected with chest radiograph system. Firstly, the system applies a new automatic lung boundary detection algorithm to detect the lung area automatically, and the detection accuracy reaches up to 92–95%. And the system extracts image features from the detected lung area, and performs a two-class decision on chest radiograph, normal and abnormal chest radiographs. The system also applies multi-resolution image texture and edge curvature as well as artificial intelligence neural network (NN) and deep learning convolutional neural network for classification. The overall accuracy of the neural network classifier can reach 99.3%, and the false positive rate is less than 7%. Therefore, the chest X-ray automatic TB detection system can be applied for mass screening and diagnosis of TB to provide preliminary diagnosis of suspected pulmonary TB, slight abnormalities, or reexamination recommended. NLM/SZ system is also devoted to the development of global health services and diagnostic technology. By using TB data from the Chinese population, the detection algorithms are improved, and low-cost, high-reliability chest X-ray screening system has been developed. At the same time, TB detection technology which is important for HIV/AIDS treatment has been paid close attention [114]. The detection accuracy of AI systems developed by three companies was compared. And the comparison was found that the accuracy of NLM/SZ (AUC) is higher than that of AGFA and Dairyford. The same results have also been obtained by using independent test data.

For TB screening as well to monitor the progress of the effectiveness for treatment, chest radiographs of the same patient for many years are compared, which is very important for the follow-up of TB and the assessment of therapeutic efficacy. There are some subjective judgments during the observation and comparison of chest radiographs by clinicians. Contrast subtraction based on artificial intelligence can correctly align chest X-ray images at different times, and subtract the aligned images to identify the changes [115] (Fig. 9.2). Subtraction technology based on AI registration can markedly identify suspected lesions and help assessment of treatment in the follow-ups of TB.

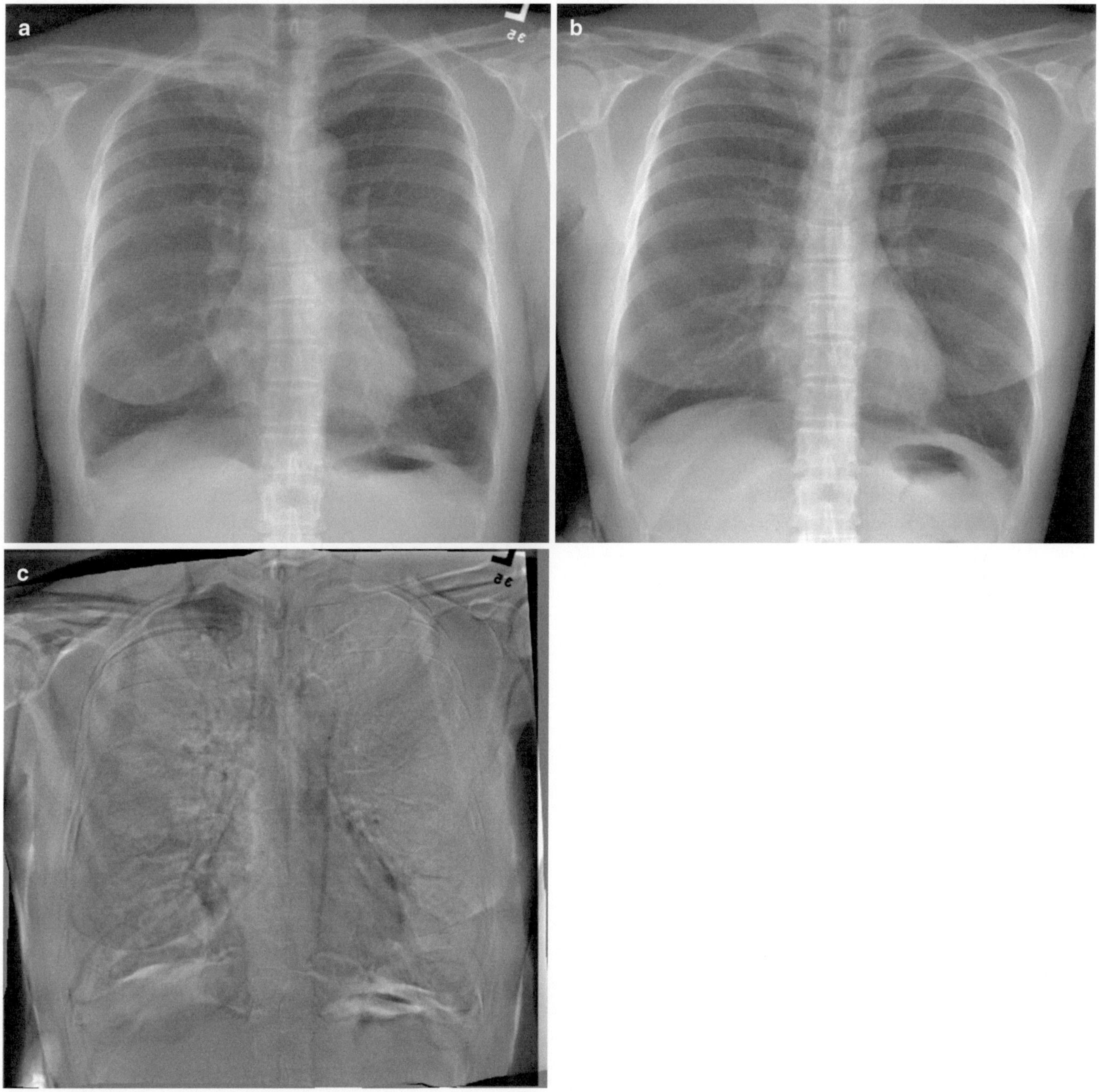

Fig. 9.2 Example of temporal subtraction on two DR images from same patient taken at different time. Upper left is the current DR image, upper left is the prior DR image taken 9 months before the current one. Lower left is the subtracted image between current and prior directly without using temporal subtraction algorithm. Lower right is the resultant image from temporal subtraction algorithm from the current and prior image. AI-based temporal subtraction result (lower right) is able to illustrate the change of abnormality which can not only increase the diagnostic accuracy but also increase the efficacy. (**a**) Current chest radiograph, (**b**) prior chest radiograph of identical patient taken 9 months ago, and (**c**) resultant image from temporal subtraction

5.2 Automated Microscopy for TB

Detection of acid-fast bacilli (AFB) by sputum smear microscopy (SSM) is still the most common diagnostic technology for rapid detection of pulmonary TB infection in clinical practice. A recent statistical analysis has been conducted by WHO in 22 high TB burden countries. It has been estimated that the cost of 42,827 laboratories in sputum smear microscopy is about $137 million US dollars. However, the detection rate of acid-fast bacilli by sputum smear microscopy has been low. In addition to the non-standard sputum specimen, the main reasons are the inadequate hardware and non-standardized detection procedures. The automatic microscopic pulmonary TB detection system can improve the detection rate of acid-fast bacilli and reduce related costs [116, 117].

The automatic microscope system (TBDx) developed jointly by Chinese and American scientists and engineers for efficient detection of acid-fast bacilli has been successfully validated in clinical trials [109, 117–119]. TBDx system applies artificial intelligence detection algorithm to scan high-resolution digital images of fluorescent smears, and automatically score the suspected fluorescein. The intelligent TB detection algorithm includes two main functions: (1) acid-fast bacillus detection and (2) visual field and smear specimen detection. The detection of acid-fast bacilli includes: screening acid-fast bacilli (AFB) by suspicious area segmentation technology, suspicious image area, and other non-acid-fast bacilli suspicious image area. The isolation process distinguishes the category of acid-fast bacilli from non-acid-fast bacilli. The mathematical expressions of false positive objects and true positive suspicious areas in images are calculated by feature extraction algorithm. The suspicious areas and possibilities of acid-fast bacilli are automatically determined by using artificial intelligence classification algorithm for processing and classification. Intelligent detection algorithm identifies the red boundary box around the suspicious image area, indicating that it may be acid-fast bacilli (Fig. 9.3). Based on the acid-fast bacilli grading test, the results of acid-fast bacilli in the visual field and sputum smear specimens are analyzed, and then the positive and negative status of each field and smear as well as the overall acid-fast bacilli density are assessed according to the standards formulated by the International Union for Tuberculosis Prevention and Lung Disease (IUATLD). The sensitivity of the intelligent algorithm can be higher than 90%.

TBDx system integrates high-quality fluorescent microscope, digital camera, automatic carrier, manipulator, smear storage box and artificial intelligence algorithm software to analyze digital images of each visual field. Once the stained sputum smear is placed in the system storage box, the system can automatically load the smear for imaging and analysis. The current system can automatically process one or four sputum smears on a loading platform, or load sputum smears with a manipulator. The loading program can automatically process 50–200 sputum smears. The whole process of a sputum smear takes about 5 min, 10–12 sputum smears in 1 h, and 100 sputum smears in 8 h. The TBDx system can be applied to detect the high density of acid-fast bacteria (e.g., 3+ or 2+) in sputum smears.

In a recent clinical trial at the South African TB Center, two 40-year-old experienced microscopic technicians were assigned to observe smears, with standard culture media as a reference, to evaluate the performance of TBDx. The results showed that the sensitivity of TBDx to positive sputum smear microscopy and culture (SSM+/C+) is 98%, and to negative sputum smear microscopy and culture (SSM−/C+) is 40%. The sensitivity and specificity of TBDx system are 79.8% and 78.9%, respectively. If the TBDx system takes less than one suspicious region of acid-fast bacteria as the normal range, the sensitivity of TBDx decreases to 73.4%, and the specificity increases to 95.7%. The results confirmed that TBDx, as an independent diagnostic system, has been proven to be comparable to experienced microscopic technicians, which provides a quality diagnostic solution for areas with insufficient well-trained microscopic technicians. The results also confirmed that TBDx has the potential to reduce the burden of detectors and the expensive cost of molecular DNA technology by using shunt systems to select strong positive and negative TB specimens. In China, effects have been made jointly by Shenzhen Chronic Disease Control Center and Shenzhen Zhiying Healthcare Science and Technology Company to develop an automatic fluorescence microscopy TB detection system, which has reached the world advanced level in both accuracy and speed.

Researchers have analyzed the combination of TBDx and molecular DNA technology (Xpert®) for the diagnosis of TB [110]. In the clinical trial, 1009 sputum smears were selected from patients with pulmonary TB. The specimens were examined by traditional smear microscopy, TBDx microscopy, and liquid culture medium. The positive specimens assessed by TBDx were processed by Xpert®. The results of this study showed that 90% of the positive TB cases detected by Xpert can be screened positive by TBDx. Meanwhile, TBDx reduces the number of tests required by Xpert® by 73%, which greatly reduces the cost of testing. As pointed out in the study, the application of TBDx automated microscopy has the potential to improve the existing health diagnostic criteria via comparison of Xpert detection and conventional microscopy. The preliminary results of this study have also been achieved in China. For instance, the intelligent detection system developed by Shenzhen Zhiying Healthcare Technology Co., Ltd. integrates AI detection system, contrast subtraction, and acid-fast bacillus detection by AI sputum smears to serve the control of TB in China.

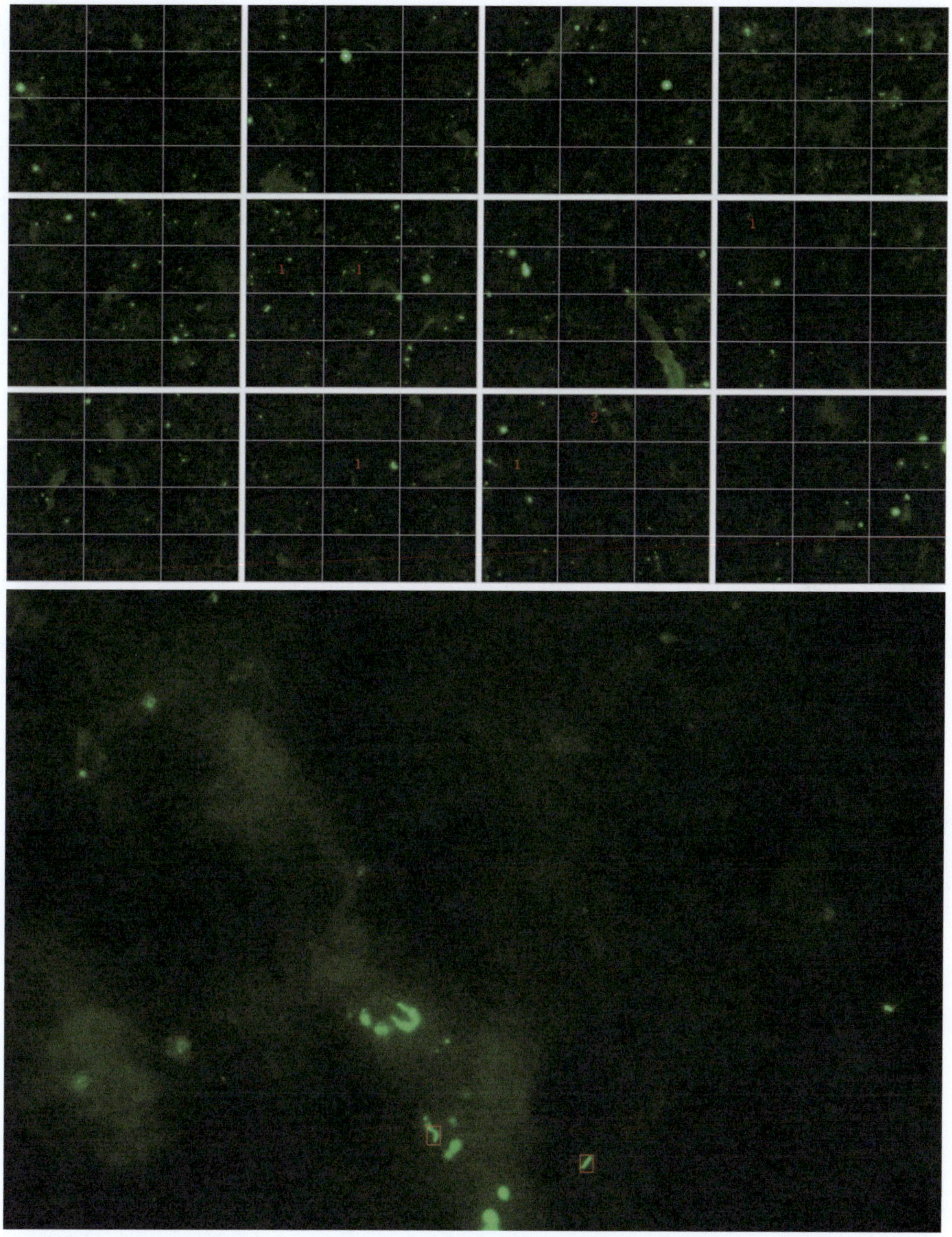

Fig. 9.3 Illustration of AI-based 4-slide automatic fluorescence microcopy TB bacilli detection results including mosaic image from stitching several adjacent field of view (FOV) images in whole slide scanning (top), and an example of FOV (bottom) from the mosaic image. The system can automatically scan 4 sputum slides, perform automatic detection, and generate report. Two operation modes can be selected: (1) automatic scanning of selected 100 FOV (from several thousand FOV) for each slide-based WHO standard and (2) automatic scanning of entire slide in about 8 min to consist of 3000–6000 FOV pending on the size of smear. The overall accuracy can exceed 85%

5.3 Summary

TB is an infectious disease caused by Mtb, which mainly affects lung function and is a major public health problem all over the world. Although the WHO recommended chest X-ray and sputum smear microscopy have been widely applied, their missed diagnosis rates are relatively high. Several large-scale clinical trials have proved that the artificial intelligence and machine learning-based automatic microscopic TB detection system and automatic chest X-ray TB detection system can improve the accuracy of TB screening and diagnosis. In addition, automated microscopic and digital imaging TB screening system can save time for microscopic technicians and radiologists in interpreting sputum smears and images, which greatly improves work efficiency and improves the accuracy of TB diagnosis. It is of great significance for the prevention and treatment of TB. With the development of artificial intelligence technology, the accuracy of TB screening and diagnosis will be further improved. Although significant progress has been made in the application of AI in diagnosis of TB based on chest radiography and sputum smear microscopy recently, a large number of confirmed radiological images and sputum smears with pathological markers are needed to improve AI algorithm. In such a way, an accurate, fast, and convenient AI diagnostic system for clinical application can be developed. In addition, clinical feedbacks and needs from doctors, hospitals, countries, and WHO should be jointly included in the research and development. We look forward to the wide application of accurate AI system in clinical practice to serve patients.

References

1. Zhong D, Zhang YH, Fu YY, et al. Prevalence of TB in migrating population and advances in its control strategy. Mod Prev Med. 2011;4282(20):4277–8.
2. Wu LW. Treatment and management of patients with TB in migrating population in Shanghai and their effects. Shanghai: Fudan University; 2013.
3. Li T, Du X, Shewade HD, et al. What happens to migrant tuberculosis patients who are transferred out using a web-based system in China? PLoS One. 2018;13(11):e206580.
4. Li X, Jiang SW. TB control in migrating population of China and its strategy. Chin J Antituberculosis. 2009;2009(10):561–3.
5. Li T, Zhang H, Shewade HD, et al. Patient and health system delays before registration among migrant patients with tuberculosis who were transferred out in China. BMC Health Serv Res. 2018;18(1):786.
6. Yang YZ. Difficulties of TB control in migrating population and the countermeasures. Guangdong Med. 2010;2010(15):1912–3.
7. Zhou CH, Qin LX, Li BX, et al. Application of diagnostic imaging in TB control system. Chin J Antituberculosis. 2016;2016(11):925–8.
8. Wei JF, Jiang XQ, Zheng XL, et al. Problems of TB control in migrating population of China. China Pract Med. 2007;2007(31):155.
9. Gao CN, Tan SY, Wen WP, et al. Factor analysis on health needs of patients with TB in migrating population. China Health Educ. 2008;2008(6):449–50.
10. Guan HY, Yang YZ, Tan WG, et al. Factors influencing occurrence of drug resistant tuberculosis in migrating population in Shenzhen. Chin J Antituberculosis. 2013;2013(8):557–61.
11. Lin DW, Gong XL. Management of TB in remote mountain areas of China. Chin J Antituberculosis. 2007;29(5):472–3.
12. Guan HY, Yang YZ, Tan WG, et al. Needs analysis on treatment and management of initially treated patients with sputum smear positive TB in migrating population in Shenzhen. Chin J Antituberculosis. 2011;33(7):407–11.
13. Tu DH, Wan LY, Wang LX. Theories and practice of modern TB control. Beijing: Military Medical Science Press; 2013. p. 188.
14. Xie HB, Zhang H, Li X, et al. Analysis on human resources in TB control agencies nationwide. Chin J Antituberculosis. 2011;33(1):12–5.
15. Dorman S. Advances in the diagnosis of tuberculosis: current status and future prospects. Int J Tuberc Lung Dis. 2015;19(5):504–16.
16. Jiang SW. Innovative management of patients with TB for better compliance to treatment. Chin J Antituberculosis. 2017;39(7):673–6.
17. Valencia S, Leon M, Losada I, et al. How do we measure adherence to anti-tuberculosis treatment? Expert Rev Anti-Infect Ther. 2017;15(2):157–65.
18. Tu DH, Wan LY, Wang LX. Modern theories and practice in tuberculosis control. Beijing: Military Medical Science Press; 2013. p. 188.
19. Guan HY, Yang YZ, Tan WG, et al. Survey on demands for treatment and management of initially treated patients with smear positive TB in migrating population of Shenzhen. Chin J Antituberculosis. 2011;33(7):407–11.
20. Hu DY, Wang T, Liu XY, et al. Implementation and factors influencing DOT for patients with smear positive TB in Chongqing. China Healthcare Res. 2006;2006(5):219–21.
21. Zhong T, Liu SY, Zhu MM, et al. Electronic DOT for registered TB patients in Nanshan district of Shenzhen. China Chronic Dis Prev Control. 2016;24(5):332–6.
22. Li RL, Lin HY, Yang YZ, et al. Effects of volunteer implemented DOT on compliance to TB treatment in migrating population. Chin J Antituberculosis. 1999;1999(1):22–5.
23. Zhao J, Duan QH, Zuo T, et al. Factors influencing attitudes and needs towards DOT in 187 patients with TB in Wuhan. Chin J Antituberculosis. 2016;2016(12):1073–7.
24. Yang XR, Huang XP. Effects of family member implemented DOT on compliance to treatment in patients with TB in migrating population. J Nurs Manag. 2013;2013(4):288–9.
25. Li JJ, Zhang JL, Li GG, et al. Effects of family member implemented DOT on compliance to treatment in patients with TB in migrating population. J Med Pest Control. 2013;2013(12):1315–8.
26. Zhou J, Yuan LL, Zhong QH. Health care professionals and family member implemented DOT for patients with TB in migrating population in Foshan. J Clin Pneumol. 2012;2012(5):847–8.
27. Yang XR. Effects of long distance follow ups on compliance to treatment in initially treated patients with TB in migrating population. Mod Clin Nurs. 2012;2012(04):65–7.
28. Gao CN, Xu ZW, Tan QY, et al. Management model for patients with TB in migrating population in Guangzhou. Guangdong Med. 2010;2010(15):1920–2.
29. Wang J, Zhu MM, Lu JJ, et al. Intervention to trans-regional referral management in patients with TB in migrating population. Pract J Card Cereb Pneumol Vasc Dis. 2010;2010(07):891–2.
30. Lin DW, Qin LY, Lin M, et al. Exploration on a predicting system for compliance to treatment in patients with TB. Chin J Antituberculosis. 2016;2016(12):1066–72.
31. Guo XJ, Wang J, Zhong T, et al. Effects of real-time observation and medication reminder mode in eDOT system for TB. Chin J Antituberculosis. 2017;39(7):689–94.
32. Jiang L, Zhong Q, Li JW, et al. Detection, treatment and management of patients with TB in migrating population in Baoan district of Shenzhen. South China Prev Med. 2010;2010(03):47–9.
33. Liu SY, Tan WG, Yang YR, et al. Application of information technology in TB control. J Tuberc Lung Health. 2018;7(1):3–8.
34. Moulding TS. The unrealized potential of the medication monitor. Clin Pharmacol Ther. 1979;25(2):131–6.
35. Moulding T, Onstad GD, Sbarbaro JA. Supervision of outpatient drug therapy with the medication monitor. Ann Intern Med. 1970;73(4):559–64.
36. Peng H, Lu W, Zhu LM, et al. Consistency of electronic drug box based drug dispense and actual intake. Jiangsu Prev Med. 2013;24(1):13–6.
37. Xie YT, Du J, Luo P, et al. Preliminary report on application of APP for management of patients with TB in Tongzhou district of Beijing in 2016. Chin J Antituberculosis. 2017;39(7):708–12.
38. Holzman SB, Zenilman A, Shah M. Advancing patient-centered care in tuberculosis management: a mixed-methods appraisal of video directly observed therapy. Open Forum Infect Dis. 2018;5(4):y46.
39. Lai K, Han YT, Fang HX. Application of video directly observed treatment in management of patients with TB. Chin J Antituberculosis. 2017;2017(7):679–83.
40. Fang HX, Qin YB, Liu CW, et al. Application of internet plus mobile phone video in treatment and management of patients with TB. Chin J Antituberculosis. 2017;2017(7):684–8.
41. Macaraig M, Lobato MN, McGinnis PK, et al. A national survey on the use of electronic directly observed therapy for treatment of tuberculosis. J Public Health Manag Pract. 2018;24:567.
42. Ren H, Yuan ZA, Gu ZR, et al. Development and application of spread trajectory analysis of latent respiratory infectious diseases. Chin J Prev Med. 2013;47(1):63–6.

43. Vazquez-Prokopec GM, Bisanzio D, Stoddard ST, et al. Using GPS technology to quantify human mobility, dynamic contacts and infectious disease dynamics in a resource-poor urban environment. PLoS One. 2013;8(4):e58802.
44. Touray K, Adetifa IM, Jallow A, et al. Spatial analysis of tuberculosis in an urban west African setting: is there evidence of clustering? Tropical Med Int Health. 2010;15(6):664–72.
45. Liu SY, Yang YR, Chen L, et al. Application of information technology in family quarantine of patients with smear positive TB. Chin J Antituberculosis. 2018;40(9):1012–8.
46. Yan BS. Further study on thick smear test for detection of Mycobacterium tuberculosis. Chin J Lab Med.1980;3(3):146–7.
47. Zhang L, Zhou HJ, Feng S. Application of florescent staining in detection of Mycobacterium tuberculosis. Shandong Med. 2014;2014(7):55–7.
48. Peng J, Liu WE, Li HL, et al. Evaluation of our self-designed nanometer silicon membrane sandwich cup system for diagnosing tuberculosis. Clin Respir J. 2016;10(5):647–52.
49. Huang GQ, Cai CZ, He SQ, et al. Study on a new technology for detection of Mycobacterium tuberculosis. Hainan Med. 2016;2016(7):1048–50.
50. Dai ZC. History of anti-tuberculosis in China. Beijing: People's Medical Publishing House; 2013.
51. Liu SY, Tan WG, Yang YR, et al. Application of information technology to promote TB prevention and control. J Tuberc Lung Health. 2018;7(1):3–8.
52. Dainton C, Chu CH. A review of electronic medical record keeping on mobile medical service trips in austere settings. Int J Med Inform. 2017;98:33–40.
53. World Health Organization. Digital heath for the end TB strategy: an agenda for action. Geneva: World Health Organization; 2014.
54. Wade VA, Karnon J, Eliott JA, et al. Home videophones improve direct observation in tuberculosis treatment: a mixed methods evaluation. PLoS One. 2012;7(11):e50155.
55. Jiang SW. Application of innovative management to improve patients' compliance to treatment of TB. Chin J Antituberculosis. 2017;39(7):673–6.
56. Qin YB, Xie YG, Fang HX, et al. Application of text/voice message in management of urban patients with sputum smear positive TB. Chin J Antituberculosis. 2017;39(7):695–701.
57. Shi LJ, Jin JM. Effects of follow ups via telephone or text message on anti-tuberculosis treatment. China Mod Phys. 2013;51(1):119–20, 122.
58. Zhang T, Xi MX. Advances in supervision and management of TB patients. Pract Prev Med. 2017;24(3):382–4, Cover 3.
59. Zhong DL, Huang HA, Liu GF, et al. Effects of internet video based medication supervision on TB control. China Med Eng. 2012;20(4):143–5.
60. Miao YJ, Gao GZ. Research advances in development of mobile health care APP. Nurs Stud. 2018;2018(06):860–2.
61. Cao H, Chen J, Fang J. Effects of internet based health education about TB control in a university. China Sch Health. 2014;35(6):890–2.
62. Wu J, Zhao MW, Ning F, et al. Effects of Wechat public platform based health education about TB control in student volunteers from universities. Chin J Antituberculosis. 2016;38(7):588–91.
63. Liu PP, Lin WB, Zhong NR, et al. Internet Wechat platform based health education about TB control in migrating population. Chin J Antituberculosis. 2017;39(7):713–6.
64. Mirsaeidi M, Farshidpour M, Banks-Tripp D, et al. Video directly observed therapy for treatment of tuberculosis is patient-oriented and cost-effective. Eur Respir J. 2015;46(3):871–4.
65. Xie YT, Du J, Luo P, et al. Preliminary report on application of mobile APP for supervision and management of TB patients in Tongzhou district of Beijing in 2016. Chin J Antituberculosis. 2017;39(7):708–12.
66. Liu SY, Yang YR, Chen L, et al. Application of information technology in family quarantine of patients with sputum smear positive TB. Chin J Antituberculosis. 2018;40(9):1012–8.
67. Bain EE, Shafner L, Walling DP, et al. Use of a novel artificial intelligence platform on mobile devices to assess dosing compliance in a phase 2 clinical trial in subjects with schizophrenia. JMIR Mhealth Uhealth. 2017;5(2):e18.
68. Peng H, Lu W, Zhu LM, et al. Consistency of drug dispensing in electronic medicine box with actual medication in patients with TB in Jiangsu province. Jiangsu Prev Med. 2013;24(1):13–6.
69. Huan ST, Chen R, Liu XQ, et al. Feasibility of drug dispensing record in electronic medicine box for medication supervision in patients with TB. Chin J Antituberculosis. 2012;34(7):419–24.
70. Menzies D, Dion MJ, Francis D, et al. In closely monitored patients, adherence in the first month predicts completion of therapy for latent tuberculosis infection. Int J Tuberc Lung Dis. 2005;9(12):1343–8.
71. Au-Yeung KY, DiCarlo L. Cost comparison of wirelessly vs. directly observed therapy for adherence confirmation in anti-tuberculosis treatment. Int J Tuberc Lung Dis. 2012;16(11):1498–504.
72. Zheng M, Wang P. Presentation of suspected TB cases reported by non-TB control institutions in Zhengzhou during 2010 to 2014. Chin J Antituberculosis. 2016;38(3):228–9.
73. Xu XP. Effects of TB information management system on referral and tracking of TB patients. Public Health Prev Med. 2012;23(6):91–2.
74. Zhang LH, Fang AM, Guo CY. Large-scale data analysis on missed report and missed registry of TB. Public Health Prev Med. 2017;28(4):100–2.
75. An XD. Application of Internet technology in health care service and Internet resources about TB control. Chin J Antituberculosis. 2000;22(3):174–5.
76. Guo XJ, Wang J, Zhong T, et al. Effects of real-time supervision and reminder in electronic DOT management of TB. Chin J Antituberculosis. 2017;39(7):689–94.
77. Lin YH, Zhou L, Wu Y. Student health surveillance information system in Shenzhen. China Sch Health. 2014;35(8):1206–8.
78. Fu XS. Urban social management organization system: introduction of Shenzhen Social Work Committee and its network project. China Inst Reform Manag. 2013;2013(10):8–11.
79. Wang L, Zhang QB, Wu XM, et al. Design and application of TB information system based on GIS. China Digit Med. 2012;7(4):40–3.
80. Fan J, Rao HX, Wu P, et al. Spatial distribution of pulmonary TB during 2012 to 2014 in China. Chin J Epidemiol. 2017;38(7):926–30.
81. Rao HX, Yu J, Guo P, et al. Bartonella Species Detected in the plateau pikas (Ochotona curzoiae) from Qinghai Plateau in China. Biomed Environ Sci. 2015;28(9):674–8.
82. Sun XL, Zhang H, Wang Y, et al. Application and prospects on Internet+ health care service. Health Care Equip. 2017;38(10):132–4.
83. Ghodbane R, Raoult D, Drancourt M. Dramatic reduction of culture time of Mycobacterium tuberculosis. Sci Rep. 2014;4:4236.
84. Drobniewski F, Nikolayevskyy V, Maxeiner H, et al. Rapid diagnostics of tuberculosis and drug resistance in the industrialized world: clinical and public health benefits and barriers to implementation. BMC Med. 2013;11:190.
85. Ou X, Song Y, Zhao B, et al. A multicenter study of cross-priming amplification for tuberculosis diagnosis at peripheral level in China. Tuberculosis (Edinb). 2014;94:428–33.
86. Centers for Disease Control and Prevention (CDC). Update: Nucleic acid amplification tests for tuberculosis. MMWR Morb Mortal Wkly Rep. 2000;49:593–4.
87. Ling DI, Flores LL, Riley LW, et al. Commercial nucleic-acid amplification tests for diagnosis of pulmonary tuberculosis in respiratory specimens: meta-analysis and meta-regression. PLoS One. 2008;3:e1536.

88. WHO guidelines approved by the Guidelines Review Committee. In Xpert MTB/RIF implementation manual: technical and operational 'how-to': practical considerations. Geneva: World Health Organization; 2014.
89. Catanzaro A, Rodwell TC, Catanzaro DG, et al. Performance comparison of three rapid tests for the diagnosis of drug-resistant tuberculosis. PLoS One. 2015;10:e0136861.
90. Bodmer T, Strohle A. Diagnosing pulmonary tuberculosis with the Xpert MTB/RIF test. J Vis Exp. 2012:e3547. https://doi.org/10.3791/3547.
91. Koser CU, Ellington MJ, Peacock SJ. Whole-genome sequencing to control antimicrobial resistance. Trends Genet. 2014;30:401–7.
92. Banada PP, Sivasubramani SK, Blakemore R, et al. Containment of bioaerosol infection risk by the Xpert MTB/RIF assay and its applicability to point-of-care settings. J Clin Microbiol. 2010;48:3551–7.
93. Kim, Y.J., Park, M.Y., Kim, S.Y., et al. [Evaluation of the performances of AdvanSure TB/NTM real time PCR kit for detection of mycobacteria in respiratory specimens]. Korean J Lab Med. 2008;28:34–8.
94. Fujita Y, Doi T, Maekura R, et al. Differences in serological responses to specific glycopeptidolipid-core and common lipid antigens in patients with pulmonary disease due to Mycobacterium tuberculosis and Mycobacterium avium complex. J Med Microbiol. 2006;55:189–99.
95. Steingart KR, Ramsay A, Dowdy DW, et al. Serological tests for the diagnosis of active tuberculosis: relevance for India. Indian J Med Res. 2012;135:695–702.
96. Li Q, Dong HY, Pang Y, et al. Multicenter evaluation of the molecular line probe assay for multidrug resistant Mycobacterium Tuberculosis detection in China. Biomed Environ Sci. 2015;28:464–7.
97. Viveiros M, Leandro C, Rodrigues L, et al. Direct application of the INNO-LiPA Rif.TB line-probe assay for rapid identification of Mycobacterium tuberculosis complex strains and detection of rifampin resistance in 360 smear-positive respiratory specimens from an area of high incidence of multidrug-resistant tuberculosis. J Clin Microbiol. 2005;43:4880–4.
98. Yadav RN, Singh BK, Sharma SK, et al. Comparative evaluation of GenoType MTBDRplus line probe assay with solid culture method in early diagnosis of multidrug resistant tuberculosis (MDR-TB) at a tertiary care centre in India. PLoS One. 2013;8:e72036.
99. Lacoma A, Molina-Moya B, Prat C, et al. Pyrosequencing for rapid detection of Mycobacterium tuberculosis second-line drugs and ethambutol resistance. Diagn Microbiol Infect Dis. 2015;83:263–9.
100. Lin SY, Rodwell TC, Victor TC, et al. Pyrosequencing for rapid detection of extensively drug-resistant Mycobacterium tuberculosis in clinical isolates and clinical specimens. J Clin Microbiol. 2014;52:475–82.
101. Mahendradhata Y, Probandari A, Widjanarko B, et al. Embedding operational research into national disease control programme: lessons from 10 years of experience in Indonesia. Glob Health Action. 2014;7:25412.
102. Lawn SD. Advances in diagnostic assays for tuberculosis. Cold Spring Harb Perspect Med. 2015;5:a017806.
103. WHO. Global tuberculosis control: epidemiology, strategy, financing (WHO report 2018).
104. Jaeger S, Karargyris A, Candemir S, et al. Automatic tuberculosis screening using chest radiographs. IEEE Trans Med Imaging. 2014;33(2):233–45.
105. Maduskar P, Muyoyeta M, Ayles H, et al. Detection of tuberculosis using digital chest radiography: automated reading vs. interpretation by clinical officers. Int J Tuberc Lung Dis. 2013;17(12):1613–20.
106. Hogeweg L, Sanchez C, Maduskar P, et al. Automatic detection of tuberculosis in chest radiographs using a combination of textural, focal, and shape abnormality analysis. IEEE Trans Med Imaging. 2015;34:2429.
107. Muyoyeta M, Maduskar P, Moyo MR, et al. The sensitivity and specificity of using a computer aided diagnosis program for automatically scoring chest X-rays of presumptive TB patients compared with Xpert MTB/RIF in Lusaka Zambia. PLoS One. 2014;9(4):e93757.
108. Folio, L, Sigelman, J, Wang, Y, et al. Automatic identification and classification of tuberculosis findings on chest radiographs for global surveillance programs. Annual Meeting of the American Roentgen Ray Society (ARRS).
109. C. Pangilinan, A. Divekar, G. Coetzee, et al. Application of stepwise binary decision classification for reduction of false positives in tuberculosis detection from smeared slides. Proceedings of the IASTED International Symposia on Imaging and Signal Processing in Healthcare and Technology, 16–18 May 2011, Washington, DC; https://doi.org/10.2316/P.2011.737-035.
110. Ismail NA, Omar SV, Lewis JJ, et al. Performance of a novelalgorithm using automated digital microscopy for diagnosing tuberculosis. Am J Respir Crit Care Med. 2015;191(12):1443–9.
111. Karargyris A, Folio L, Siegelman J, et al. Comparing the performance of man and machine for TB screening in chest radiographs. NIH Intramural Research Festival, Bethesda MD, 6–8 Nov 2013.
112. Lure F, Jaeger S, Antani S, et al. Application of automatic microscopy and digital chest radiography diagnostic system in screening of tuberculosis. Electron J Emerg Inf Dis. 2017;2(1):5–8.
113. Computer-aided TB Screening on Chest X-rays. https://lhncbc.nlm.nih.gov/project/computer-aided-tb-screening-chest-x-rays.
114. Fleming Y. Lure, Stefan Jaeger, Sameer Antani, et al. Automated system for radiologic tuberculosis screening. Chinese Congress of Radiology (CCR) 2017, Shanghai, China, 12–15 Oct 2018.
115. Jaeger S, Candemir S, Antani SK, et al. Two public chest X-ray datasets for computer-aided screening of pulmonary diseases. Quant Imaging Med Surg. 2014;4(6):475–7. https://doi.org/10.3978/j.issn.2223-4292.2014.11.20.
116. Aoki T, Oda N, Yamashita Y, et al. Usefulness of computerized method for lung nodule detection in digital chest radiographs using temporal subtraction images. Acad Radiol. 2011;18(8):1000–5.
117. Kik SV, Denkinger CM, Casenghi M, Vadnais C, Pai M. Tuberculosis diagnostics: which target product profiles should be prioritised? Eur Respir J. 2014;44(2):537–40.
118. James J Lewis, Bernard Fourie, Gerrit Coetzee, Fleming Y. M. Lure, Ajay Divekar, Gavin Churchyard, Susan Dorman. Computer aided detection (CAD) of TB on sputum smear microscope: comparing the performance of a microbiologist's conventional reading with a microbiologist's performance using CAD detection as an aid, in a high HIV prevalent setting. XIX International AIDS Conference (AIDS 2012), 22–27 July 2012, Washington, DC.
119. C. Pangilinan, A. Divekar, G. Coetzee, et al. Application of stepwise classification for detection of tuberculosis on smeared slides under microscope system. Proc. SPIE 8315, Medical Imaging 2012: Computer-Aided Diagnosis, 83153E (February 23, 2012); https://doi.org/10.1117/12.910484; SPIE Medical Imaging Conference, Newport Beach, CA, 4–9 Feb 2012.

Emergency Management of TB Emergency Public Health Events

10

Wei-ye Yu, Xu-jun Guo, and Sheng-yuan Liu

1 Concepts

1.1 Laws, Regulations, and Guidelines

For the surveillance, management, information release, summarization, and evaluation of public health emergencies, the Law of the People's Republic of China on the Prevention and Control of Infectious Diseases, Regulations on Emergency Response to Public Health Emergencies, the National Emergency Plan for Public Health Emergencies, the Measures for the Management of Information Reporting for the Surveillance of Public Health Emergencies and Infectious Diseases, and the Measures for Information Release on Epidemics of Legal Infectious Diseases and Sudden Public Health Events have been issued in China. According to the Regulations on Emergency Response to Public Health Emergencies, provinces, municipalities directly under the Central Government and autonomous regions are responsible to formulate emergency response plans in their respective administrative regions in light of local actual conditions.

For public health emergencies of TB, the relevant laws, regulations, and guidance manual are relatively limited, with no systematic guidance at the national level. Only some laws and regulations are involved, such as the Measures for Management of Tuberculosis Prevention and Control. Since more than 70% of public health emergencies occur in schools in China and more than 80% of school emergencies are epidemic of infectious diseases [1], schools are key places for prevention and control of public health emergencies caused by TB. Other regulations issued in China only standardize the responses to public health emergencies occurring in schools. Such regulations include Technical Procedures for Reporting Sudden Public Health Emergencies of Infectious Diseases in Schools and Kindergartens (trial implementation) in 2006, the Working Standards for TB Prevention and Control in Schools (trial implementation) in 2010, the Work Manual for TB Prevention and Control in Schools, and the Working Standards for TB Prevention and Control in Schools in 2017. Local guidelines for sudden public health events of TB are insufficient. At present, only the Emergency Response Plan for Tuberculosis Public Health Events in Shandong Province can be searched. There are many regional guidelines for TB epidemic and public health emergencies in schools, such as the Management Plan for TB Epidemic in Schools of Shenzhen and the Guideline for Surveillance and Management of TB Epidemic in Schools of Beijing, and the Technical Scheme for Management of TB Epidemic in Schools of Henan Province (Trial Implementation).

Although the local documents have positive effects on the prevention and control of TB public health emergencies, due to the low level of effectiveness, it is difficult to maintain consistency between information and regulations, and their role is relatively limited. In addition, although schools are the key places for TB public health emergencies, other places such as prisons, nursing homes, welfare institutions, and factories are also frequently reported with TB epidemics [2–5]. Therefore, laws and regulations at the national level need to be promulgated urgently to standardize the management and investigation of TB public health emergencies.

The promulgation of rules and regulations for emergency management of TB epidemic in Shenzhen is at the forefront of the country. In addition to the Pre-plan for the Management of Tuberculosis Epidemic in Schools of Shenzhen issued in 2009, the Pre-plan for the Management of Tuberculosis Emergency Public Health Events in Key Places of Shenzhen was recently proposed to include prisons, nursing homes, and welfare homes in the surveillance and pre-planning of TB public health events.

W.-y. Yu (✉)
Department of Tuberculosis, The Shenzhen Center for Chronic Disease Control, Shenzhen, Guangdong, China

X.-j. Guo · S.-y. Liu
Shenzhen Nanshan Center for Chronic Disease Control, Shenzhen, Guangdong, China

W.-y. Yu et al. (eds.), *Tuberculosis Control in Migrating Population*, https://doi.org/10.1007/978-981-32-9763-0_10

1.2 Relevant Concepts

According to the definition of the Emergency Regulations on Public Health Emergencies, public health emergencies refer to outbreaks of major infectious diseases, mass diseases of unknown origin, major food and occupational poisoning, and other events that cause or may cause serious damage to public health. In the National Emergency Plan for Public Health Emergencies, public health emergencies are classified into four levels: particularly significant (Grade I), major (Grade II), larger (Grade III), and general (Grade IV).

Public health emergencies caused by TB are defined in the Emergency Work Scheme for Public Health Emergencies of Tuberculosis in Shandong Province that (1) the occurrence of importing infectious TB, (2) the outbreak of TB in aggregating population, and (3) the loss or leakage of Mtb strains. The occurrence of imported infectious TB is defined as one or more cases of infectious TB from abroad, including: (1) officially informed by foreign health or health quarantine institutions that entry person(s) is (are) patient(s) with infectious pulmonary TB; (2) clinically diagnosed new cases of foreign patients with infectious pulmonary TB; (3) reported information that the entry person(s) is (are) patient(s) with infectious TB. The outbreak of TB in aggregating population is defined as 3 or more associated patients with TB in a short period of time (within 1 month) at collective working places such as schools and construction sites. The loss or leakage of Mtb strains is defined as the loss, leakage, being stolen, or robbed of Mtb strains during transportation and storage. We believe that the scope of TB public health emergencies is insufficiently defined. Although the probability of occurrence is small, it may also include other situations. Because TB is a zoonotic disease and may be transmitted via the gastrointestinal tract, the sudden increase of intestinal TB patients caused by improper animal quarantine and flow of its products into market should also be considered, such as the TB cattle event in the USA. Due to the scarcity of other cases and reports, we focus on the outbreak of TB in aggregating population in this chapter.

As mentioned earlier, school is the focus of public health emergencies caused by TB. So it is necessary to clarify its concept. Public health emergency of TB in schools is clearly defined in the Code for School Tuberculosis Prevention and Control (2017 edition) issued jointly by the National Health and Family Planning Commission and the Ministry of Education. The definition is that when 10 or more epidemiologically associated TB cases or when death occurs from TB in a school in the same semester, the county-level health and family planning administrative department where the school is located is responsible to define whether it is public health emergency based on the results of on-site investigation and public health risk assessment. The administrative department of health and family planning at or above the county level may also directly define the event in accordance with the prescribed working procedures and the actual work of disease prevention and control. Therefore, that 10 or more epidemiologically associated TB cases or occurrence of death from TB in a school in the same semester is the threshold to define the occurrence of public health emergency of TB in schools. However, the occurrence of TB less than 10 cases involves three other concepts: clustering epidemic, epidemic tendency, and sporadic cases.

School tuberculosis epidemic is defined as three or more cases of active TB with epidemiological association in the same school within 1 month in the Technical Standards for Surveillance and Management of Tuberculosis in Schools of Beijing. The epidemic tendency of TB in schools is defined as two or more reported cases of TB in the same school within 1 month. However, there is no unified or accepted conclusion on the concepts of clustering epidemic, epidemic tendency, and sporadic cases. It is generally believed that public health emergencies rank the highest in the surveillance and management of TB, followed by clustering epidemic, epidemic tendency, and sporadic cases.

One of the most important measures in public health emergencies is close contacts screening, and the definition of close contacts remains elusive. In the Technical Standards for School TB Prevention and Control (2017 Edition), the category of close contacts is defined as individuals who have direct contact with TB patient, mainly including teachers and students in the same class, and students in the same dormitory. If one or more new cases of pulmonary TB are detected in the screening of teachers and students in the same class and dormitory, the screening scope of close contacts should be extended to teachers and students in the same teaching building and dormitory floor. Meanwhile, the screening scope can also be appropriately expanded according to the in-site investigation. In addition, family members in close contact with the patient should also be screened. The definition has certain operability in close contact screening in schools, but it fails to define the time, frequency, and mode of close contact. For teachers and students who have direct contact but are in different classes and dormitories, it is difficult to judge whether they should be included in the scope of screening. A retrospective semi-experimental study of TB epidemic management at the University of Rio de Janeiro found that the detection of active TB cases increases from 2% to 2.7% and the detection of latent infection increases from 62% to 69% after changing the operational definition of close contacts from "sharing closed space with index cases for at least 100 h" to "sharing closed space with index cases for at least 4 h per week." The change from 62% to 69% showed significant difference [6]. Therefore, the close contacts need to be carefully defined, which has a significant impact on the detection of active cases and infections.

1.3 Migrating Population and TB Emergency Public Health Events

The migrating population is characterized by low income, poor health awareness, crowded housing, and poor nutritional status. They often fail to present to healthcare institutions after getting sick. Instead, they tend to tolerate or neglect the condition, buy medicine in pharmacies by themselves, or go to illegal healthcare institutions for treatment. The delayed consultation commonly leads to serious and persistent spread of the disease. Therefore, the migrating population is at higher risks of TB infection than local residents [7]. Clustering epidemic of TB and TB public health emergencies occur from time to time in the migrating population, which should be paid more close attention by departments concerning disease prevention and control [8].

2 Emergency Management

2.1 Surveillance and Reporting

According to the Information Reporting in Surveillance of Emergency Public Health Events and Infectious Diseases Epidemics, TB Control Institutions are responsible for surveillance and information reporting of TB epidemics, and are supervised and managed by the health administrative departments at the same level. Their main responsibilities include collecting and verifying the public health event or TB epidemic data after designated working staffs receive reports via the social reporting consultation telephone, establishing epidemiological investigation teams and laboratories for field epidemiological investigation and laboratory testing of biological samples, and establishing information network for maintenance and management of epidemiological data and information analysis. In addition, all healthcare institutions are responsible for reporting public health emergencies within their scope of responsibility. The responsible reporting units and responsible reporting persons who obtain information related to public health emergencies should report to the TB control agencies by telephone or fax within 2 h. After verifying the event by the TB control agency, the event should be reported online directly within 2 h. Meanwhile, the event should also be reported to the health administrative department of the same level by telephone or fax. After the health administrative department receives the information report on public health emergencies, an expert team should be organized for on-site investigation as soon as possible. Public health emergency is confirmed, corresponding measures should be taken according to specific grading of the event. And the event should be reported to the government of the same level within 2 h, and at the same time it should be reported to the health administrative department of the higher level. If the event is defined not to be a public health emergency, the professional TB control institutions should closely follow up the development of the situation and report the changes of the situation at any time.

In Nanshan district of Shenzhen, routine surveillance of TB epidemic is performed according to regulations, and detention places, schools, and enterprises are enlisted as the key places for TB epidemic surveillance and management. Especially for enterprises, Nanshan district is the first in the whole country to enlist enterprises as the key workplace for TB surveillance. For initially presented patients who are suspected with TB, the names and addresses of their working units are collected to establish a database of workplace epidemic surveillance for data screening and comparison. The epidemiological correlation verification is performed if there are overlapping data. And for two or more related cases that constitute epidemic tendency, according to the risk factors of infectious cases, different measures such as on-site investigation, close contacts screening, and health education are performed. For enterprises that have had clustering epidemic or have frequent sporadic cases, work suspension for diagnosis of suspected infectious cases, quarantine after diagnosis, environmental hygiene assessment, DNA homology detection of Mtb strains, cohort follow-up, and healthcare observation can be performed. In addition, the Geographic Information System for Tuberculosis (GIS) jointly developed by Nanshan Chronic Disease Prevention and Control Institute of Shenzhen, and Shenzhen Advanced Technology Research Institute has been applied to establish an API address automatic cleaning, address coding and location platform based on Baidu Map. And via the predicting platform for TB epidemic (based on absolute number and mobile percentage method, webpage version), precise positioning of patient's static address within community has been realized, and community-level monthly outbreak can be predicted.

2.2 Responsible Subject of Management

According to the regulations in the Emergency Response to Public Health Emergencies and the National Emergency Plan for Public Health Emergencies, the State Council and the governments at all levels are responsible for, after public health emergency occurs, establishing national and local emergency response headquarters in accordance with the recommendations of the administrative departments of public health and actual conditions. The emergency response headquarters shall be under their respective heads as commander-in-chief or main leadership. In addition, the State Council and health administrative departments of all levels are responsible for establishing or designating a day-to-day management institutions and expert advisory committees for daily management and technical support of emergency response to public health emergencies.

The administrative departments of public health at or above the county level are responsible for organizing the investigation, control, and medical treatment of emergencies. The healthcare institutions, disease prevention and control institutions, health supervision institutions and entry–exit inspection, and quarantine institutions are professional and technical institutions directly dealing with public health emergencies.

When public health emergencies occur, relevant departments at all levels are responsible for, according to their functions, response to the emergency according to the grading of the event.

The governments at all levels are responsible for mobilizing resources, delimiting control areas, adopting epidemic control measures, migrating population management, implementing traffic health and quarantine, information release, performing mass prevention and mass control, and maintaining social stability. The health administrative departments are responsible for organizing investigation and management, organizing expert committees to assess and grade the event, adopting emergency control measures, supervising and inspecting, information release and communicating, formulating technical standards and norms, health education, and event assessment. The healthcare institutions are responsible for patient treatment and transfer, assisting CDC in investigation and management, preventive measures against nosocomial infection, reporting infectious diseases and poisoning patients, case analysis and summarization, and scientific research and international exchanges. The disease prevention and control institutions are responsible for information reporting of public health emergencies, epidemiological investigation, laboratory test, scientific research and international exchanges, formulation of technical standards and norms, and technical training. The health supervision institutions are responsible for supervising and inspecting the implementation of emergency measures in healthcare institutions and CDC institutions, health supervision and law enforcement inspection, and investigating illegal acts in events. The entry–exit inspection and quarantine institutions are responsible for emergency management at ports, reporting information on public health emergencies at ports and their changes.

2.3 Measures and Procedures in Emergency Management

Before TB public health emergencies occur, adequate preparations should be made. The preparations include establishment of leadership team and working team for epidemic management, establishment of working mechanism for multi-sector cooperation, formulation of public health emergencies management plans, preparation of funds budget and reservation of sufficient amounts, reservation of materials needed in management, and the regular drills for implementation of emergency management plans.

Measures and procedures in investigating and managing public health emergencies of TB, as summarized in various norms, reports, and documents, include case verification, case quarantine and treatment, case investigation, contacts screening, extended investigation, field investigation and environmental hygiene evaluation, disinfection of epidemic spots, health education, psychological support, healthcare observation, strain identification (sputum smear, sputum culture, strain identification, drug sensitivity test, and whole genome sequencing), cohort follow-ups, and prophylactic treatment. The time points of the measures and procedures are shown in Fig. 2. The measures in dealing with TB clustering epidemic, epidemic tendency, and sporadic cases are similar. According to the grading of event and the specific situation of the epidemic site, the measures taken are also different. According to the types and sequence of measures, we summarize as follows (Fig. 10.1).

Detection

TB cases are confirmed via active surveillance, telephone reporting, close contacts screening, and by TB control institutions. And their working place, studying place, and accommodation address are compared with those of other recent confirmed cases of TB to exclude possibility of epidemiological association.

Verification

TB prevention and control institutions are responsible to check the information of clue cases, such as name, gender, age, identity card number, and work unit with the information at the TB reporting card in the special TB reporting system. And the diagnosis of TB is fully verified with the presented healthcare institutions. After the diagnosis and epidemiological association are preliminarily verified, whether it constitutes a public health emergency event should be judged rapidly for initial report.

Field Investigation

Management Notice

The unit with occurrence of TB public health emergency should be informed via Notice of Tuberculosis Emergency Public Health Event Management. And the time and procedures of field management should be timely informed. The scope of close contacts screening is preliminarily determined. And preparations for filed management include suspension and quarantine of TB patients, complete ventilation and sterilization, a place for field investigation and management, the time for inspection, basic information about close contacts, working place, defined or suspected TB patients.

Relevant Personnel and Materials Preparation

A working team for TB public health emergencies (epidemiologist, radiologist, physician, nurses) is established. And vehicles and drivers are coordinated. Materials for inspection, sterilization, protection, and emergency rescuing are prepared. And investigation forms and cameras are prepared for field investigation.

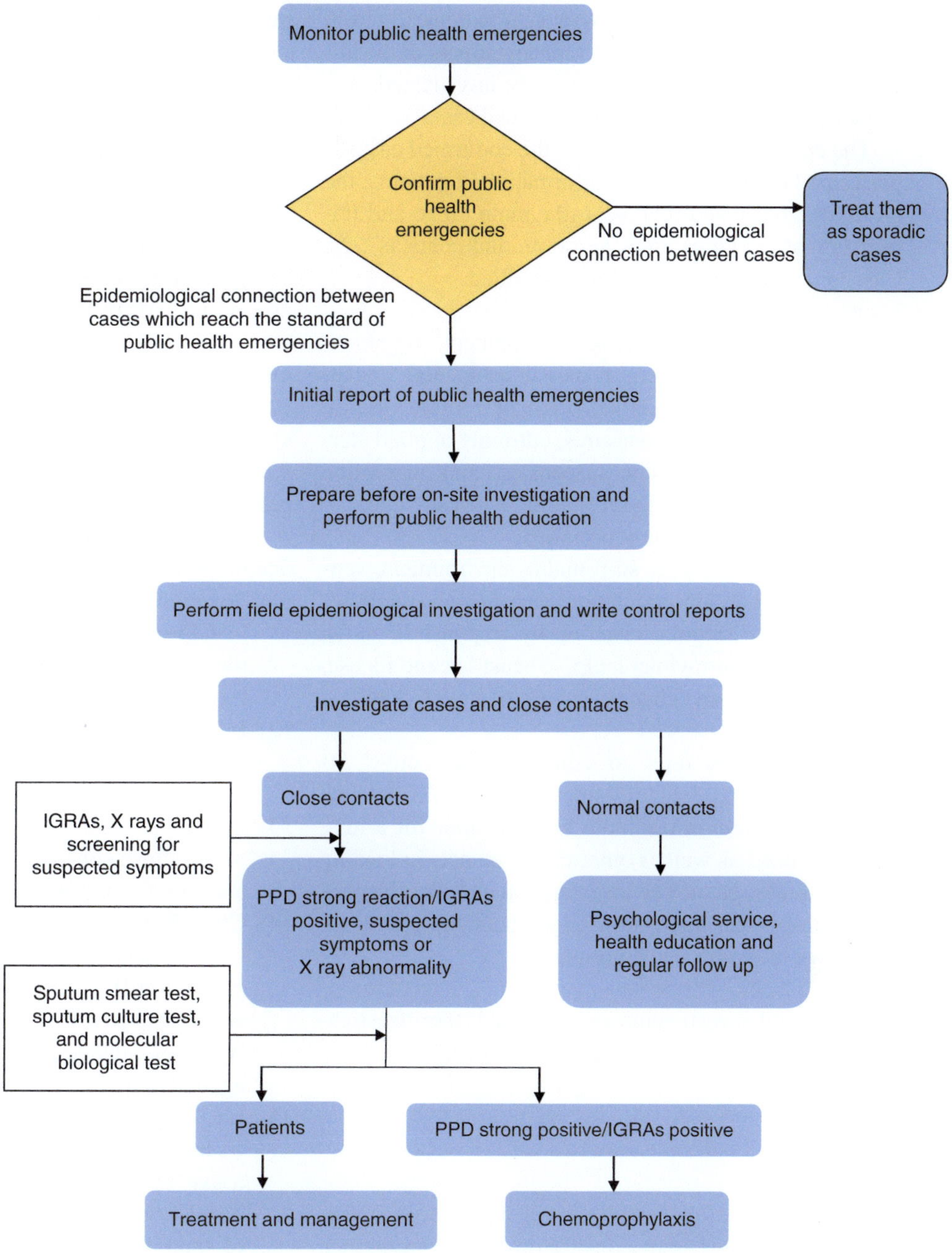

Fig. 10.1 Emergency response when TB breaks out

Field Investigation

Education Before Investigation

The occurrence and responses to TB public health emergencies should be informed to the units with occurrence of TB public health emergencies. Health education about TB control should be performed in the units with occurrence of TB public health emergencies for their active cooperation in the relevant investigations and elimination of panic.

Content of Investigation

The occurrence process, building layout, environmental hygiene, implementation of routine disease prevention and control measures, suspension and quarantine of patients from work/school, and personnel emotions should be investigated in detail to assess the severity of the epidemic. And the time for management and the screening scope of close contacts are determined according to the severity of the epidemic.

The main contents of the investigation include:

(1) Occurrence

The cases should be actively searched. The information about all the patients in the target region, specific population, and healthcare institutions should be collected, and the information should be verified on a case-by-case basis. The detailed case information of confirmed and suspected cases should be collected and sorted chronologically. And the onset, consultation, diagnosis, and treatment of the initial case and subsequent cases should be investigated.

(2) Epidemiological survey of the confirmed cases

The epidemiological survey of the confirmed cases is performed to know the basic information of patients, the onset, diagnosis and treatment, the main range and trajectories of activities after the onset, and contacts. The Case Questionnaire of TB should be filled.

(3) Institution

The address, surrounding environment, organizational structure, number of workers/students, layout, healthcare staffing, implementation of routine disease prevention and control measures, currently applied sterilization, health education, suspension, and quarantine of patients from work/school should be investigated.

(4) The workplace/classroom/dormitory

The number, location, surrounding environment, ventilation (smooth air circulation and regular windows open), hygiene (regular cleaning by responsible staff), air conditioner, ultraviolet lamp, exhaust fan and its use, seat distribution, and changes should be investigated.

(5) Close contacts

Close contacts refer to contacts with active TB patients, especially sputum smear positive TB patients who study or live in the same room or floor for a long period of time, as well as other close contacts judged by the field investigator. The investigation includes the contact of the cases, their knowledge about the epidemic, protective measures and emotions.

After the field investigation is completed, the investigation should be reported by the management team.

Field Control

Health Education

Under the guidance of the health administrative department, the TB control agency is responsible to further strengthen the health education about TB control in the unit with occurrence of TB public health emergency. The health education is intended to eliminate their panic and stabilize their mood for normal work and study.

Health education mainly includes: (1) TB is an infectious disease transmitted through the respiratory tract. (2) Personal protection should be paid close attention, such as exercise to improve the resistance to diseases, wearing face mask, necessity, and importance of patient quarantine, frequent windows open for favorable ventilation. (3) The patients should be encouraged and cared to build up self-confidence and reduce fear. (4) If cough or expectoration occurs, immediate presentation to healthcare institutions for diagnosis of TB is necessary. (5) Patients should be urged to take medicine regularly and receive re-examinations regularly for completion of standardized treatment [9].

Management of Confirmed Cases, Clinically Diagnosed Cases, and Suspected Cases

Confirmed or clinically diagnosed TB cases should receive standardized treatment and management. And the suspected TB cases need to be diagnosed according to the prescribed procedures. All of the confirmed, clinically diagnosed, and suspected cases of TB need to rest and cooperate in the treatment and management. The cases of infectious TB should be suspended and quarantined from work/study for treatment. Only when the patient is cured or the condition is improved, reentry to work/study is permitted with the diagnostic certificate issued by the TB control agency.

Screening and Management of Close Contacts

(1) Screening

Close contacts to patients with active TB should receive screening of TB and the results should be recorded.

(2) Investigation of suspected TB symptoms

All close contacts should receive investigations on suspected TB symptoms.

(3) Tuberculin skin test/Interferon γ release assay

All close contacts should receive tuberculin skin test and interferon γ release assay.

(4) Chest X-ray

Individuals aged under 15 years with PPD strong positive or IFN γ release assay positive, as well as those with suspected symptoms of TB should receive chest X-ray to exclude the possibility of TB. Close contacts aged above 15 years should receive chest X-ray.

(5) Bacteriological test of sputum

Individuals with PPD strong positive, IFN γ release assay positive, suspected symptoms of TB, or chest X-ray abnormalities should receive bacteriological test of sputum. Three sputum specimens are collected, with one for sputum smear test and two for Mtb culture. Those with Mtb culture positive should receive tests for Mtb strain identification, drug sensitivity test, and DNA homology analysis. And those with Mtb culture negative should receive molecular biological examination.

In DNA homology analysis, compared to traditional genotyping such as IS6110-based restriction fragment length polymorphism (IS6110-RFLP), spoligotyping, and mycobacterial interspersed repetitive unit-variable number tandem repeats (MIRU-VNTR), the whole genome sequencing has many advantages, such as high resolution, identification of transmission direction, and detection of super spreader.

Due to these advantages, it has gradually been promoted for application. Walker et al. found that five SNPs from the genome sequencing of Mtb strains isolated from specimens of two cases can be applied as thresholds to identify short-term transmission relationship between the two cases [10]. Their findings provide an important basis for the assessment of public health emergencies.

The new cases of active pulmonary TB detected in close contacts screening, individuals with only PPD strong positive or IFN γ release assay positive, and other close contacts should be managed accordingly.

(1) Individuals with only PPD strong positive or IFN γ release assay positive.

On the basis of informed consent, prophylactic medication is administered.

(2) Other close contacts with no prophylactic medication.

For other close contacts with no prophylactic medication, the unit with occurrence of public health emergencies should strengthen health education and follow-up medical observation. Those presenting with suspected symptoms of TB during follow-ups or medical observations should be reported to TB control agency. The medical observation generally lasts for 2 years. The cohort follow-up refers to the requirement that close contacts with no signs of TB should receive TB-related examinations at TB control agency at 3 months, 6 months, 1 year, and 2 years after the occurrence of public health emergency, as shown in Fig. 3. TB control agencies are responsible for collecting data about medical observation monthly, reporting the number of absence, number of individuals with suspected symptoms of TB, number of presentations in healthcare institutions, number of newly diagnosed TB cases, appropriate screening of the suspected symptoms, and reporting the abnormalities to superior TB control agency.

Environmental Hygiene and Disinfection

The sputum from the confirmed and suspected patients of TB should be sterilized (by mixing 1 volume sputum with 1/5 volume bleaching powder for 2 h). The places that the patients work, study, and live should be disinfected regularly (with fumigation of 0.5–1.0% peracetic acid solution, spray of hydrogen peroxide compound air disinfectant, or ultraviolet radiation).

Extended Screening

If new confirmed cases of TB are detected in close contacts screening, or if there is sufficient air exchange between the epidemic area and other areas detected in the field investigation, or if TB cases are in close contact with personnel in other areas, the investigation and management should also be extended to a wider scope.

Within 2 weeks after the event is managed, the case close report should be finished jointly by the working management team and the participating managing institutions.

The significance of the above-mentioned measures for TB public health emergencies can be summarized as follows: (1) to know well the nature and scale of the epidemic for corresponding management, such as case verification, case investigation, contacts screening, extended screening, strain identification, field investigation and environmental hygiene evaluation, (2) to provide treatment, management, and related healthcare services for the detected cases and contacts, such as case treatment, health education for contacts, psychological support, medical observation, cohort follow-up, and prophylactic treatment, and (3) to prevent further spread of the epidemic, such as case quarantine and disinfection of the related places.

2.4 Information Release

According to the regulations in the Information Release Scheme for Legal Infectious Diseases and Public Health Emergencies of the Ministry of Health, the information of public health emergencies is issued regularly. The Ministry of Health publishes the general information of public health emergencies on the Bulletin of the Ministry of Health and the website of the Ministry of Health monthly and annually. The information of last month is published before the tenth of each month, and the information of last year is published before February 10 each year. If the epidemic reached the criteria of major public health emergency (level II or above), the frequency of information release is increased. If necessary, weekly or daily information release is implemented. Otherwise, the news media is authorized or press conference is held for information release. The main contents of the released information include the general information and case information of public health emergencies. The specific information includes the general situation, distribution, occurrence, and development of public health emergencies and its emergency management, such as the number of public health emergencies, the number of cases and casualties, the nature of the incident, the causes, the place and scope of occurrence, the management and control measures, and the release of compulsory measures. Information on especially major public health emergencies (Grade I) is issued by the Ministry of Health, and information on major public health emergencies (Grade II) and below is issued by the health administrative departments of provinces, autonomous regions, and municipalities directly under the central government.

3 Case Closing and Case Assessment

3.1 Case Closing Report

As the operation manual supplemented to the Working Standards for School TB Prevention and Control (Trial Implementation), the Working Manual for School TB Prevention and Control published in 2012 requires that within 2 weeks after the completion of field investigation and management of TB public health emergencies in schools, the working management team is responsible for a comprehensive summary of the whole event, including the analysis of its causes, and preventive measures against similar events in the future. A detailed and comprehensive investigation report should be written jointly by the health administration department of the same level and the higher level, the school where the event occurred and its administrative department. The main contents of the final investigation report include the basic information about the place where the event occurred, the time of reporting and its verification, the course of the event, the three distributions of the disease, the field investigation and management, the measures adopted for disease prevention and control, the recommendations for following management, the causes of the event, and the conclusions of the investigation. The reference format of the case closing report is also provided [11].

According to the general principles of public health emergencies management, we believe that TB control agency should report the event for three times to the higher health administrative department and the direct superior TB control agency at three different time points for decision making. The specific procedures are described as follows.

TB control agency is responsible for reporting the TB public health emergencies. The staffs in district-level TB control agency in the area where the event occurred are responsible for reporting the TB public health emergencies. The event should be reported to the district-level health administrative department, the directly superior TB control agency, and the unit with the occurrence of TB public health emergency. The report is sent in a paper version with official seal.

Initial Report

After preliminary field investigation and verification, if the event reaches the criteria of public health emergency, the district-level TB control agency is responsible for reporting the event via official paperwork within 2 h. Meanwhile, the field epidemiological survey and management procedures for TB public health emergency should be initiated. In the initial report, the time, place, scope, number of patients, and the course of event should be reported in detail. In addition, the initial report should also include the preliminary investigation results and analysis, the measures already adopted, and the management plan.

Progress Report

After the field investigation is completed, the management team shall, on the basis of the results of the investigation, promptly compile a progress report about the development process, situation assessment, management progress, control measures, and the causes of event.

Case Closing Report

Within 2 weeks after the event is managed, the management team shall organize the participating departments to write a detailed and comprehensive closing reports. The closing report is intended to summarize the occurrence and management of the event, put forward recommendations about the preventive measures against similar events in the future. The specific contents of the closing report should include the reporting of the event, the general situation of the event, the field investigation and management, the causes, consequences, effects, and recommendations of the event [12].

3.2 Event Assessment

After management, the causal analysis of the whole TB public health emergency should be performed. Combined with epidemiological case investigation and close contacts investigation, the relationship between the first case and the following cases in time, space, and distribution should be analyzed in detail. Combined with DNA homology analysis, the source of infection and its transmission chain should be defined. And a conclusion should be made in the closing report.

References

1. Ministry of Health. To strengthen TB prevention and control in schools: Speech by Jiang ZJ, vice Minister of Health at the National Telephone Conference on Strengthening the Management of Primary and Secondary Schools [EB]. http://www.moh.gov.cn/newshtml/16521.htm. 21 Nov 2006.
2. Zhang SR, Ruan W, Li YQ, et al. Experiences of the parents caring for their children during a tuberculosis outbreak in high school: a qualitative study. BMC Public Health. 2014;14(1):1–7.
3. Bergmire-Sweata D, Barnett BJ, Harrisa SL, et al. Tuberculosis outbreak in a Texas prison, 1994. Epidemiol Infect. 1996;117(3):485–92.
4. Dobbins C, Marishta K, Kuehnert P. Tuberculosis outbreak associated with a homeless shelter-Kane County, Illinois, 2007-2011. J Am Med Assoc. 2012;307(23):2480–2.
5. Lai CC, Hsieh YC, Yeh YP, et al. A pulmonary tuberculosis outbreak in a long-term care facility. Epidemiol Infect. 2016;144(7):1455–62.

6. Loredo C, Cailleaux-Cezar M, Efron A, et al. Yield of close contact tracing using two different programmatic approaches from tuberculosis index cases: a retrospective quasi-experimental study. BMC Pulm Med. 2014;7(14):133.
7. Yang C, Lu L, Warren JL, et al. Internal migration and transmission dynamics of tuberculosis in Shanghai, China: an epidemiological, spatial, genomic analysis. Lancet Infect Dis. 2018;18:788.
8. Valin N, Antoun F, Chouaïd C, et al. Outbreak of tuberculosis in a migrants' shelter, Paris, France, 2002. Int J Tuberc Lung Dis. 2005;9(5):528–33.
9. Wang LX, Chen MT. Serial health promotion brochures on TB control planning in China. 2nd ed. Beijing: People's Military Medical Press; 2012. p. 33–4.
10. Walker TM, Ip CL, Harrell RH, et al. Whole-genome sequencing to delineate Mycobacterium tuberculosis outbreaks: a retrospective observational study. Lancet Infect Dis. 2013;13(2):137–46.
11. Wang L, Cheng S, Chen W. Handbook on tuberculosis prevention and control in schools. Beijing: Military Medical Science Publishing House; 2012.03.
12. National Tuberculosis Controllers Association; Centers for Disease Control and Prevention (CDC). Guidelines for the investigation of contacts of persons with infectious tuberculosis. Recommendations from the National Tuberculosis Controllers Association and CDC. MMWR Recomm Rep. 2005;54(RR-15):1–47.